THE ROLE OF NEURAL PLASTICITY IN CHEMICAL INTOLERANCE

ANNALS OF
THE NEW YORK ACADEMY
OF SCIENCES

Volume 933

EDITORIAL STAFF

Executive Editor
BARBARA M. GOLDMAN

Managing Editor
JUSTINE CULLINAN

Associate Editors
STEFAN MALMOLI
MARION GARRY

The New York Academy of Sciences
2 East 63rd Street
New York, New York 10021

THE NEW YORK ACADEMY OF SCIENCES
(Founded in 1817)

BOARD OF GOVERNORS, September 2000 – September 2001

BILL GREEN, *Chairman of the Board*
TORSTEN WIESEL, *Vice Chairman of the Board*
RODNEY W. NICHOLS, *President and CEO* [ex officio]

Honorary Life Governors
WILLIAM T. GOLDEN   JOSHUA LEDERBERG

JOHN T. MORGAN, *Treasurer*

Governors

ELEANOR BAUM	D. ALLAN BROMLEY	KAREN BURKE
LAWRENCE B. BUTTENWIESER	PRAVEEN CHAUDHARI	
JOHN H. GIBBONS	MICHAEL GOLDEN	RONALD L. GRAHAM
ROBERT G. LAHITA	JACQUELINE LEO	WILLIAM J. McDONOUGH
JOHN F. NIBLACK	SANDRA PANEM	RICHARD RAVITCH
RICHARD A. RIFKIND	SARA LEE SCHUPF	JAMES H. SIMONS

HELENE L. KAPLAN, *Counsel* [ex officio]   PETER H. KOHN, *V.P. & Secretary* [ex officio]

ANNALS OF THE NEW YORK ACADEMY OF SCIENCES
Volume 933

THE ROLE OF NEURAL PLASTICITY IN CHEMICAL INTOLERANCE

Edited by Barbara A. Sorg and Iris R. Bell

The New York Academy of Sciences
New York, New York
2001

Copyright © 2001 by the New York Academy of Sciences. All rights reserved. Under the provisions of the United States Copyright Act of 1976, individual readers of the Annals are permitted to make fair use of the material in them for teaching or research. Permission is granted to quote from the Annals provided that the customary acknowledgment is made of the source. Material in the Annals may be republished only by permission of the Academy. Address inquiries to the Permissions Department (editorial@nyas.org) at the New York Academy of Sciences.

Copying fees: For each copy of an article made beyond the free copying permitted under Section 107 or 108 of the 1976 Copyright Act, a fee should be paid through the Copyright Clearance Center, Inc., 222 Rosewood Drive, Danvers, MA 01923 (www.copyright.com).

♾ The paper used in this publication meets the minimum requirements of the American National Standard for Information Sciences—Permanence of Paper for Printed Library Materials, ANSI Z39.48-1984.

Library of Congress Cataloging-in-Publication Data

The role of neural plasticity in chemical intolerance / edited by Barbara A. Sorg and Iris R. Bell.
    p. cm. — (Annals of the New York Academy of Sciences ; v. 933)
    Includes bibliographical references and index.
    ISBN 1-57331-308-4 (cloth : alk. paper) — ISBN 1-57331-309-2 (pbk. : alk. paper)
    1. Multiple chemical sensitivity—Pathophysiology—Congresses. 2. Neuroplasticity—Congresses. 3. Neurotoxicology—Congresses. I. Sorg, Barbara A. II. Bell, Iris. III. Series.

Q11.N5 vol. 933
[RB152.6]
500 s—dc21
[616.8'047]
                                                  2001018333

GYAT / PCP
Printed in the United States of America
ISBN 1-57331-308-4 (cloth)
ISBN 1-57331-309-2 (paper)
ISSN 0077-8923

ANNALS OF THE NEW YORK ACADEMY OF SCIENCES
Volume 933
March 2001

THE ROLE OF NEURAL PLASTICITY IN CHEMICAL INTOLERANCE

Editors and Conference Organizers
BARBARA A. SORG AND IRIS R. BELL

[This volume is the result of a conference entitled *The Role of Neural Plasticity in Chemical Intolerance* held by the New York Academy of Sciences on June 16–19, 2000, at The Rockefeller University in New York, New York.]

CONTENTS

Preface. *By* BARBARA A. SORG AND IRIS R. BELL ix

Part I. Chemical Intolerance in Humans

The Compelling Anomaly of Chemical Intolerance. *By* CLAUDIA S. MILLER .. 1

Controlled Exposures to Volatile Organic Compounds in Sensitive Groups. *By* NANCY FIEDLER AND HOWARD M. KIPEN 24

Sensitization Studies in Chemically Intolerant Individuals: Implications for Individual Difference Research. *By* IRIS R. BELL, CAROL M. BALDWIN, AND GARY E. R. SCHWARTZ 38

The Iowa Follow-up of Chemically Sensitive Persons. *By* DONALD W. BLACK, CHRISTOPHER OKIISHI, AND STEVEN SCHLOSSER 48

Part II. Animal Models for Chemical Intolerance: Role of Central Nervous System Plasticity

Repeated Formaldehyde Effects in an Animal Model for Multiple Chemical Sensitivity. *By* BARBARA A. SORG, MATTHEW L. TSCHIRGI, SAMANTHA SWINDELL, LICHAO CHEN, AND JIDONG FANG 57

Does the Kindling Model of Epilepsy Contribute to Our Understanding of Multiple Chemical Sensitivity? *By* M. E. GILBERT 68

A Genetic Rat Model of Cholinergic Hypersensitivity: Implications for Chemical Intolerance, Chronic Fatigue, and Asthma. *By* DAVID H. OVERSTREET AND VELJKO DJURIC 92

Episodic Exposures to Chemicals: What Relevance to Chemical Intolerance? *By* R. C. MACPHAIL 103

Environmental Risks and Public Health. *By* BERNARD D. GOLDSTEIN 112

Part III. Neural Plasticity in Pathological Pain

Sensitization, Subjective Health Complaints, and Sustained Arousal. *By* HOLGER URSIN AND HEGE R. ERIKSEN 119

Representation of Acute and Persistent Pain in the Human CNS: Potential Implications for Chemical Intolerance. *By* PIERRE RAINVILLE, M. CATHERINE BUSHNELL, AND GARY H. DUNCAN 130

Role of Neurotransmitters in Sensitization of Pain Responses. *By* WILLIAM D. WILLIS, JR. 142

Central Neuroplasticity and Pathological Pain. *By* RONALD MELZACK, TERENCE J. CODERRE, JOEL KATZ, AND ANTHONY L. VACCARINO 157

Spinal Cord Neuroplasticity following Repeated Opioid Exposure and Its Relation to Pathological Pain. *By* JIANREN MAO AND DAVID J. MAYER 175

Part IV. Cytokines, Chronic Fatigue States, and Sickness Behavior

Cytokines and Chronic Fatigue Syndrome. *By* ROBERTO PATARCA 185

Mediators of Inflammation and Their Interaction with Sleep: Relevance for Chronic Fatigue Syndrome and Related Conditions. *By* JANET M. MULLINGTON, DUNJA HINZE-SELCH, AND THOMAS POLLMÄCHER 201

The Role of Cytokines in Physiological Sleep Regulation. *By* JAMES M. KRUEGER, FERENC OBÁL, JR., JIDONG FANG, TAKESHI KUBOTA, AND PING TAISHI 211

Cytokine-Induced Sickness Behavior: Mechanisms and Implications. *By* ROBERT DANTZER 222

Potential Mechanisms in Chemical Intolerance and Related Conditions. *By* DANIEL J. CLAUW 235

Part V. Physiological Stress and the Neuroendocrine Axis

Role of Gaseous Neurotransmitters in the Hypothalamic-Pituitary-Adrenal Axis. *By* CATHERINE RIVIER 254

Plasticity of the Hippocampus: Adaptation to Chronic Stress and Allostatic Load. *By* BRUCE S. MCEWEN 265

Part VI. Neural Conditioning

Acquiring Symptoms in Response to Odors: A Learning Perspective on Multiple Chemical Sensitivity. *By* OMER VAN DEN BERGH, STEPHAN DEVRIESE, WINNIE WINTERS, HENDRIK VEULEMANS, BENOIT NEMERY, PAUL EELEN, AND KAREL P. VAN DE WOESTIJNE 278

Pavlovian Conditioning of Emotional Responses to Olfactory and Contextual Stimuli: A Potential Model for the Development and Expression of Chemical Intolerance. *By* TIM OTTO AND NICHOLAS D. GIARDINO 291

Poster Papers

Central Nervous System Effects from a Peripherally Acting Cholinesterase Inhibiting Agent: Interaction with Stress or Genetics. *By* KEVIN D. BECK, GUANPING ZHU, DAWN BELDOWICZ, FRANCIS X. BRENNAN, JOHN E. OTTENWELLER, ROBERTA L. MOLDOW, AND RICHARD J. SERVATIUS.. 310

Symptom Learning in Response to Odors in a Single Odor Respiratory Learning Paradigm. *By* WINNIE WINTERS, STEPHAN DEVRIESE, PAUL EELEN, HENDRIK VEULEMANS, BENOIT NEMERY, AND OMER VAN DEN BERGH.. 315

Deep Subcortical (Including Limbic) Hypermetabolism in Patients with Chemical Intolerance: Human PET Studies. *By* G. HEUSER AND J. C. WU 319

Elevated Nitric Oxide/Peroxynitrite Mechanism for the Common Etiology of Multiple Chemical Sensitivity, Chronic Fatigue Syndrome, and Post-traumatic Stress Disorder. *By* MARTIN L. PALL AND JAMES D. SATTERLEE 323

INDEX OF CONTRIBUTORS 331

Financial assistance was received from:

Sponsor
- WALLACE RESEARCH FOUNDATION

Major Funder
- DEPARTMENT OF THE ARMY

Supporters
- EASTERN PARALYZED VETERANS ASSOCIATION
- NATIONAL INSTITUTE OF ENVIRONMENTAL HEALTH SCIENCES, NATIONAL INSTITUTES OF HEALTH

The New York Academy of Sciences believes it has a responsibility to provide an open forum for discussion of scientific questions. The positions taken by the participants in the reported conferences are their own and not necessarily those of the Academy. The Academy has no intent to influence legislation by providing such forums.

Preface

> *Wonder is the daughter of ignorance;*
> *and the greater the object of wonder,*
> *the more the wonder grows.*
> —Vico[a]

Chemical intolerance (CI) is a term used to describe a feeling of illness from low levels of environmental chemicals and is sometimes used interchangeably with multiple chemical sensitivity (MCS). Intolerance of chemicals is a hallmark feature of MCS. However, the term refers to a symptom found in a broader range of individuals diagnosed with several other disorders, including MCS, Gulf War syndrome, chronic fatigue syndrome, fibromyalgia, and solvent-exposed workers. CI is an emerging problem in environmental health, and the prevalence of clinically significant CI is estimated to be 5% in the United States. This estimate is based on only a handful of reports, yet the number is staggering from the standpoint of human costs. Individuals with CI can no longer function in the everyday world because of a wide variety of symptoms associated with exposure to common chemicals and foods. These patients are isolated physically and emotionally, the longitudinal course of the illness is unknown, and there is no definitive, widely accepted treatment.

Because of several controversies, no single case definition exists for CI or MCS. The disagreements among researchers and clinicians are many, but all agree that those reporting CI/MCS suffer greatly. There is no doubt that the debate over the authenticity of CI/MCS as distinct disorders will continue.

The goal of this conference was not to address the debate. Many possibilities have been raised regarding the causes of CI and the overlapping disorders mentioned above. Because of the wide variety of symptoms, it has been challenging to find a focal point on which to begin testing specific hypotheses. The best way to continue moving forward in determining the cause(s) for these illnesses was to find that focal point. Several recent studies show that neurological symptoms are the number-one complaint among those reporting CI in different populations. The organizers of the conference believed that research efforts should therefore move toward an understanding of the basic mechanisms underlying the neurobiological changes that are thought to occur in CI.

This conference focused on developing a series of testable hypotheses based upon the postulate that a change in nervous system function, or *neural plasticity*, plays a role in the development and/or maintenance of CI. To formulate these hypotheses, the organizers gathered together top scientists from basic neuroscience subdisciplines who may help explain the debilitating symptoms. The major areas of focus at the conference were (1) CI in humans; (2) animal models for CI and the role of neural plasticity; (3) neural plasticity in pathological pain; (4) cytokines, chronic fatigue states, and sickness behavior; (5) physiological stress and the neuroendocrine axis; and (6) neural conditioning.

---

[a]Vico, Giambattista. 1968. *The New Science of Giambattista Vico*, p. 71, para. 184. Translated by T. G. Bergin and M. H. Fisch. Cornell University Press. Ithaca, New York.

The conference afforded a wonderful opportunity for many fruitful discussions, both during the meeting and between sessions. Intriguing data were presented from all fields. One of the outcomes of the meeting was that basic scientists communicated to clinicians the biological processes involved in fatigue states, chronic pain, brain responses to physiological/psychological stress, and fundamental changes in neural circuitry underlying conditioning. In addition, several of the basic scientists commented that this was an area of study of which they were previously unaware and that it opened up new opportunities for application of their basic biological findings.

Overall, the conference provided a forum for cross-talk between scientists and clinicians and, further, among subdisciplines in the neurosciences. These intriguing, yet debilitating, illnesses may begin to be approached in a logical and feasible manner if clinicians are provided with enough information to make it possible to consider treatment options. Neuroscientists in the various disciplines represented at this conference can provide some of this information, but it is clear we need to expand efforts to offer more complete explanations for these illnesses. The process of the meeting increased the participants' appreciation of (1) the systemwide problems that individuals with CI experience and (2) the need for a comparably systematic and interactive approach to the research questions in this area. Collectively, the overlaps between the seemingly diverse topic areas, such as the observed clinical phenomena, sensitization, sleep/fatigue, pain, conditioning, and stress, may assist in accounting for the phenomenology of CI in total. Future studies will need to consider individual differences, longitudinal outcomes, and repeated measure/within-subject designs. CNS plasticity is a starting point for this work.

The participants in this conference made a significant contribution to the field because, as discussed by one of the presenters, Dr. Mary E. Gilbert, we have "moved the discussion beyond arguments over authenticity [of these illnesses]. Although [this conference] may have done little to resolve the controversy over the veracity of MCS, it has promoted a healthy dialogue regarding potential neurobiological substrates for this and related clinical syndromes."

Our ignorance of the underlying causes of CI and related illnesses should not provide a rationale to dismiss patients' symptoms as illusory. The enigmatic nature of these disorders should instead provoke wonder and the incentive to expand our level of understanding of basic mechanisms of neural plasticity. The conference speakers provided perspectives from their own fields of study. In so doing, they allowed us to broaden our thinking and make it possible to take steps toward integrating existing basic science knowledge with the clinical condition. With this foundation, we can forge new questions about the causes of and treatments for CI and related illnesses.

ACKNOWLEDGMENTS

We wish to thank the conference speakers for their contributions to this volume and for providing fresh perspectives on the puzzling issue of chemical intolerance and related illnesses. We are grateful to the New York Academy of Sciences, especially to Renée Wilkerson-Brown and Rashid Shaikh for exceptional guidance and organization. We are also thankful to Sheila Kane and Stefan Malmoli for organizing the *Annals* volume and to Jenny Baylon for assistance with correspondence. Many thanks as well to the conference audience for promoting lively discussions. We are grateful to Henry Wallace and the Wallace Research Foundation, the Department of the Army, the Eastern Paralyzed Veterans Association, and the National Institute of Environmental Health Sciences–National Institutes of Health for financial support of this conference.

—BARBARA A. SORG
— IRIS R. BELL

The Compelling Anomaly of Chemical Intolerance

CLAUDIA S. MILLER[a]

Environmental and Occupational Medicine, Department of Family and Community Medicine, University of Texas Health Science Center at San Antonio, San Antonio, Texas 78229-3900, USA

> *It may be the all-inclusiveness of potential factors, the difficulty of establishing an animal model, and the lack of measurable endpoints that make acceptance of the hypothesis difficult. It would seem as if almost any combination [of chemicals] that every human being is exposed to might initiate this sequence, and almost any factor may trigger it once established. Therefore, is it the agents or the responder?*
>
> —FREDERICK F. BECKER (LETTER TO THE AUTHOR)
> *University of Texas MD Anderson Cancer Center*

ABSTRACT: In science, anomalies expose the limitations of existing paradigms and drive the search for new ones. In the late 1800s, physicians observed that certain illnesses spread from sick, feverish individuals to those contacting them, paving the way for the germ theory of disease. The germ theory served as a crude, but elegant formulation that explained dozens of seemingly unrelated illnesses affecting literally every organ system. Today, we are witnessing another medical anomaly—a unique pattern of illness involving chemically exposed groups in more than a dozen countries, who subsequently report multisystem symptoms and new-onset chemical, food, and drug intolerances. These intolerances may be the hallmark for a new disease process or paradigm, just as fever is a hallmark for infection. The fact that diverse demographic groups, sharing little in common except some initial chemical exposure event, develop these intolerances is a compelling anomaly pointing to a possible new theory of disease, one that has been referred to as "Toxicant-Induced Loss of Tolerance" ("TILT"). TILT has the potential to explain certain cases of asthma, migraine headaches, and depression, as well as chronic fatigue, fibromyalgia, and "Gulf War syndrome". It appears to evolve in two stages: (1) *initiation*, characterized by a profound breakdown in prior, natural tolerance resulting from either acute or chronic exposure to chemicals (pesticides, solvents, indoor air contaminants, etc.), followed by (2) *triggering* of symptoms by small quantities of previously tolerated chemicals (traffic exhaust, fragrances, gasoline), foods, drugs, and food/drug combinations (alcohol, caffeine). While the underlying dynamic remains an enigma, observations indicating that affected individuals respond to structurally unrelated drugs and experience cravings and withdrawal-like symptoms, paralleling drug addiction, suggest that multiple neurotransmitter pathways may be involved.

[a]Address for correspondence: Environmental and Occupational Medicine, Department of Family and Community Medicine, University of Texas Health Science Center at San Antonio, 7703 Floyd Curl Drive, San Antonio, TX 78229-3900. Voice: 210-567-7760; fax: 210-567-7764.
millercs@uthscsa.edu

Scientific understanding of chemical intolerance remains in its infancy, mired in controversy. The media tends to fuel the controversy by portraying only the most extreme cases, overlaid with a thin veneer of scientific opinion. Patients with this problem are caught up in the acrimonious cross fire between various physician groups. This acrimony is fueled by the different medical paradigms concerning the condition's origins. Litigation and compensation claims lead to adversarial proceedings that draw medical practitioners unwillingly into the conflict. Expert witnesses paint themselves into scientific corners and opinions harden on all sides. Everyone has an opinion, mostly based upon their personal beliefs with no definitive data to support them. However, science is not about belief. It is about "guess and test", that is, formulating hypotheses based upon observation ("guess") and then testing those hypotheses ("test"). All science begins with observation.

The purpose of this paper is to summarize the available, salient observations concerning chemical intolerance. Admittedly, most of these observations are anecdotal. This is normal for new science. The observations presented here constitute the few facts available to us, but there is considerable agreement about them. The next step is formulating a hypothesis that explains these observations, a process that Darwin described as "grouping facts so general laws can be derived from them". Comprehensive fact-gathering is the first critical step. Done well, it will enable us to avoid what Thomas Henry Huxley called "the great tragedy of science—the slaying of a beautiful hypothesis by an ugly fact". In the next section, we will review the "ugly facts" of chemical intolerance, those which any successful hypothesis must be able to explain.

THE UGLY FACTS

Roughly half of those who are chemically intolerant say their illness began following a specific exposure event, referred to as an *initiating* event, for example, a chemical spill, chronic solvent exposure, a pesticide application, indoor air contaminants, combustion products, etc. (FIG. 1).[1] A small subset of individuals exposed in situations like these appear to develop chronic symptoms that persist years, even decades, beyond their original exposure. At first, affected individuals may describe "flu-like" symptoms that just will not go away, or feeling as though they are in a "perpetual fog". Next to develop are multisystem symptoms that seem to wax and wane unpredictably. Subsequently, there may be a dawning awareness of certain new intolerances, for example, for alcoholic beverages or a medication. Over time, these intolerances grow to include a wide variety of common, structurally unrelated chemicals, foods, drugs, caffeine, alcoholic beverages, and skin contactants. This has been termed the "spreading phenomenon". The intolerances may appear suddenly, within weeks following an acute, high-level exposure (e.g., a chemical spill), or, in the case of lower level exposures (e.g., a sick office building), develop insidiously over months or years.

Food intolerances may develop, but go unrecognized at first. Affected individuals may instead report every sort of digestive difficulty, feeling ill after meals, or extreme irritability if a meal is missed or delayed. Symptoms can occur following inhalation, ingestion, mucosal contact, or injection (e.g., drugs) of a substance. Different exposures, for example, fragrances, chemicals outgassing from new fur-

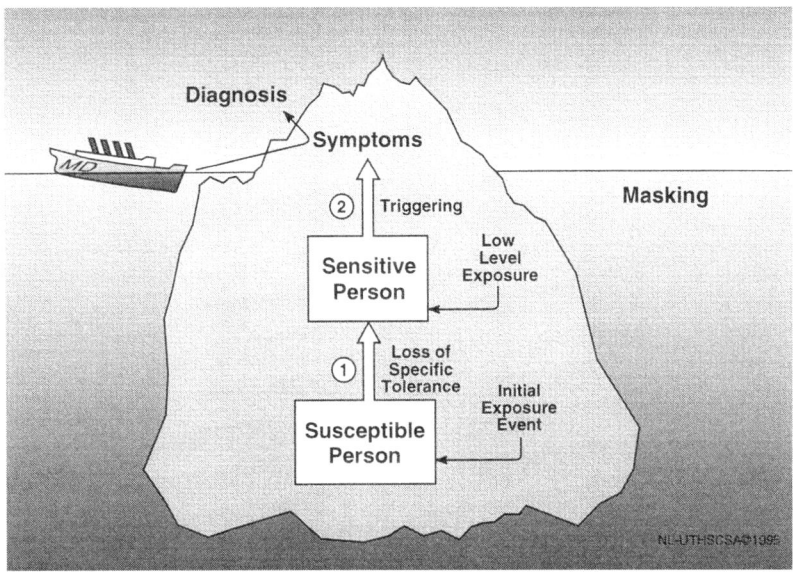

FIGURE 1. Phenomenology of Toxicant-Induced Loss of Tolerance (TILT). Illness appears to develop in two stages: (1) initiation, that is, loss of prior, natural tolerance resulting from an acute or chronic exposure (pesticides, solvents, indoor air contaminants, etc.), followed by (2) triggering of symptoms by small quantities of previously tolerated chemicals (traffic exhaust, fragrances), foods, drugs, and food/drug combinations (alcohol, caffeine). The physician sees only the tip of the iceberg—the patient's symptoms—and formulates a diagnosis based on them (e.g., asthma, depression, chronic fatigue, migraine headaches). Masking hides the relationship between symptoms and triggers. The initial exposure event causing breakdown in tolerance also may go unnoticed (©UTHSCSA 1996).

nishings or carpeting, traffic exhaust, cleaning agents, etc., may trigger different constellations of symptoms that vary from person to person (TABLE 1). There is a certain consistency to these complaints: A *particular* exposure (e.g., diesel exhaust or a fragrance) in a *particular* person is said to elicit a characteristic constellation of symptoms—a *signature response* for that person with that exposure. These responses can occur at below-olfactory-threshold concentrations. Symptoms may flare seconds to hours after a triggering exposure and persist for minutes to days. Patients may report that certain symptoms enable them to identify a specific trigger (e.g., a pesticide), even when no odor is apparent. Hyperresponsiveness to physical stimuli, including bright light, noise, and touch, is commonly reported.[2,3] People who lack a sense of smell (anosmic individuals) may also suffer from chemical intolerances.

Affected individuals generally report that avoiding problem exposures, including foods that bother them, offers relief.[4] In fact, most patients claim that avoidance is the only "treatment" that reliably helps them.[5] Low-level volatile organic chemical (VOC) concentrations in the parts per billion (ppb) or parts per trillion (ppt) range are nearly ubiquitous, making avoidance difficult, as well as socially isolating. Daily exposure to various chemical, food, and drug triggers may hide or "mask" the symp-

TABLE 1. Symptoms commonly reported by chemically intolerant individuals[11]

Neuromuscular
Loss of consciousness
Stumbling/dragging foot
Seizures
Print moving/vibrating on page
Feeling off balance
Tingling in fingers/toes
Double vision
Muscle jerking
Fainting
Numbness in fingers/toes
Clumsiness
Problems focusing eyes
Cold or blue nails/fingers
Uncontrollable sleepiness

Head-related
Head fullness/pressure
Tender face/sinuses
Sinus infections
Tightness in face/scalp
Brain feels swollen
Ringing in ears
Headache
Feeling groggy

Musculoskeletal
Joint pain
Muscle aches
Weak legs
Weak arms
General stiffness
Cramps in toes/legs
Painful trigger points

Gastrointestinal
Abdominal gas
Foul gas
Problems digesting food
Abdominal swelling/bloating
Foul burping
Diarrhea
Abdominal pain/cramping
Constipation

Cardiac
Heart pounding
Rapid heart rate
Irregular heart rate
Chest discomfort

Affective
Feeling tense/nervous
Uncontrollable crying
Feeling irritable/edgy
Depressed feelings
Thoughts of suicide
Nerves feel like vibrating
Sudden rage
Loss of motivation
Trembling hands
Insomnia

Airway
Cough
Bronchitis
Asthma or wheezing
Postnasal drainage
Excessive mucus production
Shortness of breath
Eye burning/irritation
Susceptible to infections
Dry eyes
Enlarged/tender lymph nodes
Hoarseness

Cognitive
Memory difficulties
Problems with spelling
Slowed responses
Problems with arithmetic
Problems with handwriting
Difficult concentration
Difficulty making decisions
Speech difficulty
Feelings of unreality/spacey

Other
Feeling tired/lethargic
Dizziness/lightheadedness

NOTE: Categories were derived via factor analysis of symptoms reported by 112 individuals who said they became ill following exposure to indoor air contaminants ($n = 75$) or cholinesterase-inhibiting pesticides ($n = 37$).

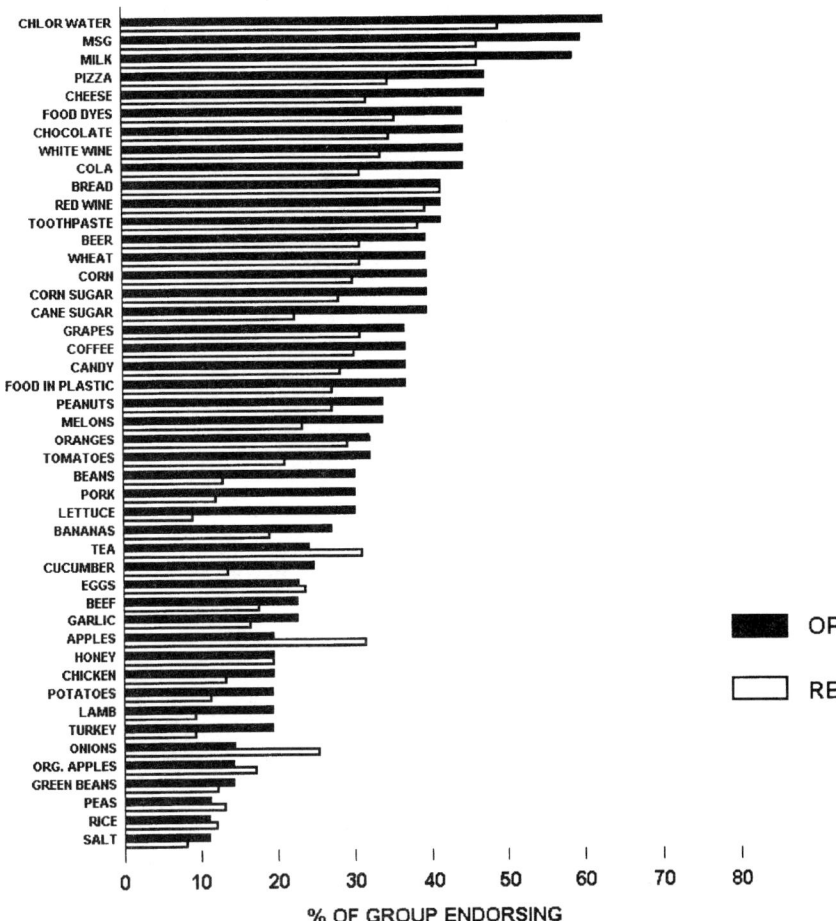

FIGURE 2. Organophosphate-exposed (OP) versus remodeling-exposed (RE): comparison of endorsement rates for all ingestant items.[11]

toms caused by any individual exposure (FIG. 2). For example, a person who uses hair spray and fragrances in the morning, cooks breakfast on a gas stove, and drives through heavy traffic to work in a sick office building may experience near-continuous symptoms.[6,7]

Complicating matters further, repeated exposures (those occurring twice a week or more often) to the *same* trigger, whether indoor air contaminants or caffeine, can cause *habituation*, further obfuscating symptom-exposure relationships. Together, masking and habituation may make it difficult for physicians, and even the patients themselves, to recognize particular triggers. "Withdrawal" symptoms may develop when patients avoid their problem exposures for several days, for example, over a weekend or during a vacation. With reexposure, for example, Monday morning after resuming work, symptoms may return "with a vengeance". Patients sometimes quit their jobs to avoid fragrances, carbonless copy paper, cleaning agents, etc. Others switch employers, occupations, and residences in search of safer surroundings.

About 80% of patients who have participated in clinical studies have been women, with an average age in the fourth decade and educational level of at least two years of college.[8] Among military and industrial populations, primarily males report the problem, likely reflecting underlying gender ratios.[2,3,9] A question remains as to whether females may be disproportionately affected even in these groups. In sick building situations, the condition is more commonly reported by college-educated white females in the middle-age range (30–50 years) and of middle to upper-middle class socioeconomic status.[10] It remains a mystery why more chemically intolerant patients work in office buildings and service industries than in heavy industry where chemical exposures are considered more common, and why more women than men report the problem.[4,11,12] Gender differences may be the result of male/female differences in willingness to report symptoms, something unique about indoor air pollutants present in offices where women tend to be relatively more confined (e.g., as secretaries), or gender-based biological response differences. The paradox that more multiple chemical intolerance cases arise from service industries than heavy industries may be due to "the healthy worker" selection effect, that is, individuals bothered by chemical exposures tend to choose nonchemical jobs; the fact that women, who may be biologically more vulnerable, are less apt to work in heavy industry, mining, construction, etc.; or some unknown, but insidious effect of indoor air chemicals.

A recent, statewide California Department of Health Services study, involving randomized telephone interviews of more than 4000 people, found that both female gender and Hispanic ethnicity were associated with increased self-reporting of chemical intolerance (adjusted odds ratios of 1.63 and 1.82, respectively).[13] As opposed to most clinical studies on chemical intolerance, the California survey did not find employment or education to be associated with chemical sensitivity or doctor-diagnosed MCS; nor was multiple chemical intolerance associated with marital status, geographic location, or income.

People who become chemically intolerant may have had more health problems even before their initial exposure than similarly exposed individuals who do not get sick. For example, aerospace workers who became ill following the introduction of new composite plastic in their workplace averaged 6.2 unexplained physical symptoms *preceding* the change in process versus 2.9 unexplained symptoms in unaffected coworker controls.[9] Fifty-four percent of the chemically intolerant workers had histories of anxiety or depression that preceded their exposure, compared with 4% of controls. Other researchers find that past psychiatric history does not explain the illness.[14] Even if some chemically intolerant individuals do experience depression that predates their initial exposure, the question remains whether their intolerances are caused by depression, whether they are more vulnerable to developing intolerances as a result of preexisting depression (e.g., due to altered brain neurochemistry), or whether their preexposure depression may have resulted from earlier unidentified intolerances.[15]

Most chemically intolerant individuals report multisystem symptoms, with fatigue being the most common (TABLE 2). Symptoms often mimic chronic fatigue syndrome and fibromyalgia, diagnoses many patients eventually acquire.[10,11,16,17] Mood changes (irritability, anxiety, depression) are commonly reported. Gulf War

TABLE 2. Top 20 symptoms (of 119 symptoms) reported by MCS patients attributing their illness to pesticides ($n = 37$) versus remodeling ($n = 75$)[1]

Symptom	Ranking		Mean symptom severity[a]	
	Pesticide	Remodel	Pesticide	Remodel
Tired or lethargic[b]	1	1	2.49	2.44
Fatigue > 6 months[b]	2	3	2.43	2.10
Memory difficulties[b]	3	4	2.32	2.09
Difficulty concentrating[b]	4	2	2.32	2.17
Dizziness, lightheadedness[b]	5	6	2.19	1.85
Depressed feeling[b]	6	8	2.19	1.83
Spacey[b]	7	12	2.19	1.74
Groggy[b]	8	5	2.14	1.96
Loss of motivation[b]	9	7	2.11	1.84
Tense, nervous[b]	10	15	2.11	1.64
Short of breath[b]	11	18	2.11	1.61
Irritable[b]	12	10	2.03	1.79
Problem focusing eyes	13	43	2.03	1.27
Chest pain	14	52	2.00	1.19
Muscle aches[b]	15	11	2.00	1.79
Problems digesting food	16	33	1.97	1.35
Joint pain[b]	17	9	1.95	1.83
Tingling fingers/toes	18	59	1.95	1.12
Headaches[b]	19	14	1.92	1.67
Head fullness or pressure[b]	20	19	1.92	1.60
Difficulty making decisions	21	13	1.89	1.69
Eye irritation	22	16	1.89	1.64
Slowed response	34	17	1.72	1.63
Nausea	36	20	1.65	1.56

NOTE: See reference 1.
[a]Symptoms scored on a 0-to-3 scale: 0 = not a problem; 1 = mild; 2 = moderate; 3 = severe.
[b]Among top 20 symptoms in both pesticide and remodeling patients.

veterans may report sudden rage after particular exposures, a phenomenon referred to as "short fuse syndrome". Fearing they might harm their families, some have handed their guns over to friends for safekeeping. Exposure-related memory and concentration difficulties have led teachers, attorneys, executives, nurses, and other professionals to abandon their cognitively demanding careers.

Different exposure *groups* with different "initiating" exposures describe surprisingly similar symptoms: We compared symptoms reported by 75 chemically intolerant individuals who became ill following building remodeling and 37 who became ill after exposure to a cholinesterase-inhibiting pesticide. Symptoms, ranked in order by severity, were remarkably similar for the two groups, with central nervous system symptoms leading the list. The most common gastrointestinal complaint was "problems digesting food" and the most frequent respiratory complaint was "shortness of breath or being unable to get enough air".[11]

A COMPELLING ANOMALY

In 1989, in a report on multiple chemical intolerance for the New Jersey State Department of Health, Nicholas Ashford and I reviewed the published and "gray" literature in this area and interviewed doctors with divergent views. Our report identified four demographic groups in which "heightened reactivity" to chemicals had been documented:

(1) industrial workers;
(2) occupants of sick buildings, including office workers and school children;
(3) residents of communities with chemically contaminated air or water;
(4) individuals exposed to various chemicals in domestic indoor air, pesticides, drugs, and consumer products.

Although these groups differed greatly in terms of professional and educational attainment, age and sex, and the mix and levels of chemicals involved, we were struck by the fact that individuals in such demographically divergent groups reported similar polysymptomatic complaints triggered by chemical exposures. It suggested to us that perhaps some common thread united these individuals. The similarities between their medical complaints and their exposure histories appeared to be more than coincidental.

Subsequently, with support from the Agency for Toxic Substances and Disease Registry, Howard Mitzel and I conducted an *exposure-driven* study, comparing the outcomes for two well-defined exposure groups: chemically intolerant individuals ($n = 37$) who attributed their illness to a cholinesterase-inhibiting pesticide exposure (an organophosphate or carbamate) and a second group ($n = 75$) who attributed their intolerances to indoor air VOCs associated with new construction or remodeling. We hypothesized the following: if neurotoxic exposures caused multiple chemical intolerance, then the organophosphate group should report more severe symptoms than the VOC group since cholinesterase inhibitors are generally considered more neurotoxic than indoor air VOCs. Indeed, this turned out to be the case. Further, if the condition was caused by chemical exposures, we reasoned that there should be intergroup differences in symptom patterns and severity that reflected the original exposures. Again, the data confirmed significantly greater symptom severity in the pesticide-exposed group than in the VOC group, especially for neuromuscular, affective airway, gastrointestinal, and cardiac symptoms. Cognitive symptoms received the highest mean severity rating for both groups, whereas the largest intergroup difference occurred for cardiac symptoms. Overall, however, *symptom patterns* were near-identical (symptoms in same rank order) for the two groups and they identified similar inhalant and ingestant triggers (TABLE 3, FIG. 2). The fact that the *ordering* of chemical and food intolerances was almost the same for the two groups led us to conclude that, once the illness develops, "similar kinds of substances will trigger symptoms, *irrespective of the chemical nature of the original exposure*" [emphasis added].

Eighty percent of the pesticide and VOC groups were women with an average educational level of almost four years of college. There were no gender-related differences in symptom severity. The vast majority (97%) of participants identified one or more problem foods or other ingestants (e.g., chlorinated tap water, MSG). Sixty percent felt that their diets had been affected "a great deal".

TABLE 3. Inhalant intolerances reported by 80% or more of 112 individuals attributing onset of their illness to organophosphate/carbamate pesticide exposure or indoor air VOCs[11]

Nail polish remover
New carpeting
Detergent aisle in grocery store
Insecticide
Fresh newspaper, newsprint
Felt-tip dry-erase marking pen
Poorly ventilated meeting room
New automobile interior
Fabric store
Hotel room
Perfume
Cigarette smoke
Diesel exhaust
Asphalt or tar
Restroom deodorizer
Particle board
Traffic exhaust
Cigar smoke
Hair spray
Fresh latex paint

Around this same time, Ashford led a nine-country European exploratory study on multiple chemical intolerance, assembling an international research team with expertise in toxicology, occupational medicine, indoor air chemistry, environmental and occupational health, law, and sociology. Just as in the United States, they found that "initiating" exposures involving pesticides were common in Europe. Organic solvent initiating exposures were identified in all nine countries, most involving chronic exposures, that is, repeated solvent use, rather than acute ones. However, there were also potentially informative differences between countries. For example, pesticides were not implicated in Sweden, Finland, or the Netherlands, where cooler temperatures help control insect populations. A so-called "wood preservative syndrome", attributed to pentachlorophenol that had been used to preserve wood for log homes, appeared only in Germany.[18] Although Sick Building Syndrome (SBS) is widely recognized in Scandinavia, it is not commonly associated with multiple chemical intolerance cases in that region. Perhaps this is because Scandinavians are less likely to use pentachlorophenol or pesticides indoors. Scandinavians do, however, associate multiple chemical intolerance with new carpet installation.

In 1993, the chief of staff of the Houston Veterans Administration Hospital asked me to evaluate the first Gulf War veteran referred to their regional center for sick Gulf War veterans. The veteran's principal problem was chemical intolerances. He was experiencing multisystem symptoms with exposures to a host of common chemicals, foods, and medications. After this veteran, I was asked to see the next 58 consecutive Gulf War veterans referred to the center, representing 17 states and a broad cross section of active-duty soldiers and reservists who served in different capacities and locations throughout the Persian Gulf. After reviewing these veterans' exposure histories, it became apparent that no *single* exposure was responsible for their health problems. Other researchers and expert panels have reached the same conclusion.

The different specialists these veterans see assign different labels to their symptoms: a rheumatologist observing diffuse muscle pain diagnoses myalgias; a neurologist hearing head pain and nausea diagnoses migraine headaches; a pulmonologist finding airway reactivity diagnoses asthma; a psychiatrist seeing chronic malaise diagnoses depression; a gastroenterologist noting GI complaints diagnoses irritable bowel syndrome. Nearly all of the veterans seen at the center had symptoms involving several organ systems simultaneously. For these veterans, there was no unifying diagnosis, no known etiology, and no single identifiable disease process. This is not the first time doctors have found themselves baffled by wartime disease. During the Civil War, doctors were faced with a similarly mysterious "syndrome" characterized by fever. Hundreds of thousands of soldiers died. The doctors did what good epidemiologists do today. They classified the cases. Since the hallmark symptom was fever, they classified the cases by fever type—remittent, intermittent, or relapsing. In doing so, they naively lumped together dozens of unrelated illnesses—everything from typhus and typhoid to malaria and tuberculosis.[19] Who would have dreamed it—this germ theory of disease?: this war going on between invisible invaders and the body's immune defenses, with the only outward sign being—literally—the heat of battle.

Is it possible that we are facing the same situation with the Gulf War veterans?: only this time, the hallmark symptom is the newly acquired intolerances these veterans are experiencing—like the mechanic who used to "bathe" in solvents, but now becomes ill after one whiff of gasoline; or the young woman soldier who used to drink any man in her company under the table, but since the war cannot take even one drink without becoming violently ill. The vast majority of sick veterans interviewed reported these same newly acquired intolerances.

During my tenure as environmental medical consultant to the VA referral center, approximately 90% of veterans interviewed described new-onset intolerances to everyday chemical exposures that set off their symptoms: 78% were intolerant of fragrances, tobacco smoke, gasoline vapors, etc.; 78% described food intolerances; 66% reported alcohol intolerance; 25% were intolerant of caffeine; and nearly 40% reported adverse reactions to medications—all since the Gulf War. These intolerances, resulting in flare-ups of symptoms, including fatigue, headaches, GI problems, mood changes, cognitive impairment, and diffuse musculoskeletal pain, are like the fevers experienced by the Civil War soldiers—they are the outward manifestation of the underlying disease process.

What unites the Gulf War veterans and the civilian groups we have studied is their common experience of an initiating chemical exposure followed by newly acquired intolerances and multisystem symptoms. These observations provide compelling scientific evidence for a shared, underlying disease mechanism—one involving a *fundamental breakdown in natural tolerance.* This two-step process—an initiating toxic exposure followed by newly acquired intolerances that subsequently trigger multisystem symptoms—has been referred to with the acronym "TILT", or Toxicant-Induced Loss of Tolerance[b] (FIG. 1).[7,20–23]

This process is the key to understanding these illnesses. It does not appear to matter which exposure caused the breakdown in tolerance—be it pesticides, solvents, smoke from oil fires, or pyridostigmine bromide pills; those substances have long since left these people's bodies. It is the aftermath of these exposures, the new-onset intolerances to low-level chemical exposures, that appear to be perpetuating their symptoms. In some cases, it may be difficult to sort out individual intolerances or "triggers" because of "masking", the confusion of overlapping symptoms that results when individuals are responding to many everyday exposures.

However, the confusion clears when the underlying paradigm is understood. Thus, questions that could not be answered are answered: For example, why is there no generally accepted case definition for multiple chemical intolerance? The diverse symptoms these patients report have thwarted any such case definition attempts, which is to be expected if one is dealing with an entirely new *class of diseases*, paralleling other disease classes such as infectious diseases or immunological diseases.[c] Or, how can structurally unrelated chemicals trigger symptoms, an observation that runs counter to toxicology and allergy as we currently understand them? Once more, if what we are dealing with is a new general disease mechanism, then diverse chemical agents might act as initiators, just as diverse pathogens cause infection and fever.

TILT also explains the following:

- Why affected individuals might remain sick for years after their initial exposure—as a consequence of subsequent triggering by everyday exposures.

- Why some symptoms wax and wane in such a bewildering fashion—as exposures and masking vary over time.

---

[b]The term "Toxicant-Induced Loss of Tolerance" describes a breakdown in prior innate tolerance, like a diabetic's loss of tolerance for sugar. When addictionologists use the term "tolerance", they mean "acquired tolerance", as in an addict following repeated drug use. Here, when we use "tolerance", we mean "natural tolerance". We refer to "habituation", instead of "acquired tolerance", when describing the diminished effect of an agent on a host following repeated administration. Semantics in this realm are difficult, a common problem for new paradigms. Addictionologists use the term "sensitization" to describe an individual's heightened responses following repeated exposure to a drug. Allergists, on the other hand, strenuously object to using "sensitization" in this manner because there is no evidence that heightened responses to most chemicals are immune-mediated. Instead, the allergists invoke the term "intolerance" for non-immunologic adverse responses. With TILT, we prefer the terms "tolerance" and "loss of tolerance" for several reasons: (1) most physicians and laypersons readily grasp the concept; (2) the body's natural ability to tolerate a wide variety of environment exposures is what appears to be lost; and (3) we are at a loss to find another readily recognizable term to convey this concept, short of inventing a new one.

[c]Most proposed case definitions for multiple chemical intolerance (summarized in ref. 10) embody the same principal criteria: chronic, multisystem symptoms triggered by diverse, low-level chemical exposures, with symptoms resolving when exposures are avoided. A recent paper[24] proposes six "consensus criteria" based upon a survey of 89 clinicians and researchers familiar with, but having divergent views of, the illness:[25] (1) a chronic condition (2) with symptoms that recur reproducibly (3) in response to low levels of exposure (4) to multiple unrelated chemicals and (5) improve or resolve when incitants are removed (6) with symptoms that occur in multiple organ systems. The authors urge that multiple chemical intolerance be formally diagnosed *in addition to* any other diagnosable disorders (e.g., migraine, asthma, depression) in all patients in whom the above six criteria are met and for whom "*no single other organic disorder ... can account for all the signs and symptoms associated with chemical exposure.*"

- Why researchers have been unable to isolate a single culprit exposure underlying Gulf War "syndrome"—perhaps a wide variety of exposures culminate in TILT, with individual susceptibility determining who gets sick.

What can be done to diagnose and treat the chemically intolerant? An abundance of anecdotal evidence suggests the chemically intolerant improve when they become aware of what exposures are setting them off and learn to avoid those exposures. To this end, further studies are required using an environmental medical unit (EMU). This EMU is an environmentally controlled inpatient hospital unit where patients can be taken to a "clean" baseline so that their exposure-related symptoms will disappear. The patients can then be exposed to various potential triggers, including caffeine, gasoline, perfume, various foods, medications, and tobacco smoke, one at a time, to determine what is causing their symptoms. Funding for such an EMU is currently being considered.

A validated questionnaire (see APPENDIX) has been described in the medical literature and is currently available for purposes of diagnosis and evaluation of chemically intolerant individuals, as well as aiding researchers in the selection of patients and controls for studies.

To date, researchers have described this phenomenon—groups of individuals developing multisystem symptoms and new-onset intolerances following an initial chemical exposure event—in more than a dozen industrialized countries, including the United States, Canada, Australia, New Zealand, and nine European nations.[10,26] These groups include the following: radiology workers from New Zealand and elsewhere exposed to X-ray developer solution containing glutaraldehyde and other solvents;[27] federal employees in the EPA headquarters building in Washington, D.C., exposed to volatile organic chemicals outgassing from new carpet and construction materials;[28,29] German home owners exposed to pentachlorophenol wood preservative used in log homes;[30] sheep dippers in Great Britain exposed to organophosphate pesticides;[10,31,32] hospital workers in Nova Scotia exposed to building air contaminants;[10] and casino card dealers in Lake Tahoe, Nevada, exposed to solvents and pesticides,[33] among others.

As Kuhn notes, science begins with a list of observations like those we have just summarized.[34] Patterns then emerge. Next, scientists develop a model that forms their observations into a "coherent whole" for purposes of study. Mounting evidence supports TILT as a model for multiple chemical intolerance:

- The fact that the similar multisystem symptoms and new-onset intolerances have appeared in different demographic groups in more than a dozen countries following well-defined exposures to pesticides, solvents, indoor air contaminants, etc.
- The fact that these new-onset intolerances are not limited to chemical inhalants, but also involve foods, caffeine, alcohol, medications, and skin contactants.
- Striking parallels between this phenomenon and addiction (discussed further below), suggesting shared neural mechanisms.[7]
- The identification of an anatomical substrate—the nervous system—whose malfunction may explain these problems.
- Recent animal models replicating features of TILT.[35–37]

ADDICTION AND ABDICTION

Randolph was first to observe the striking similarities between chemical intolerance and drug addiction. Both conditions, he noted, are characterized by stimulatory and withdrawal symptoms, cravings, and cross-addiction/intolerances to structurally diverse substances. One theory is that *both* addiction and chemical intolerance (or "abdiction") might involve loss of tolerance, whether due to repeated drug use or chemical exposures, resulting in amplification of stimulatory and withdrawal symptoms.[7,22] Addicts become addicted, in part, in order to avoid unpleasant withdrawal symptoms. In contrast, chemically intolerant individuals, once they identify specific triggers, tend to avoid them, but *for the same reason addicts remain addicted—in order to avoid unpleasant withdrawal symptoms.* Initially, many chemically intolerant individuals consume caffeine, unaware that it may bother them. In fact, they may experience an initial brief lift, but overlook caffeine withdrawal symptoms occurring days later. Could it be that these apparent polar opposites—addiction and abdiction—are in fact mirror-image strategies for avoiding withdrawal symptoms resulting from TILT?[21,22]

While it seems almost inconceivable that here, in the twenty-first century, we would only now be stumbling upon a new theory of disease, it is worth remembering that other two-step theories of disease now widely accepted, that is, carcinogenesis and the immune theory of disease, were just as controversial in the past century.

CHALLENGES

Various economic interests have hindered research in this area. Some companies hire physicians and researchers as expert witnesses or sponsor their own scientific meetings in an effort to protect vested financial interests. It is the tobacco wars all over again, this time involving not one industry, but a host of industries, including carpet and rug manufacturers, fragrance makers, pesticide producers, building owners' associations, etc.

There is little economic incentive to look further into the condition. Researchers, who respond lemming-like to funding opportunities, find scant opportunities in this realm. Medical research support comes from government sources (e.g., NIH) and pharmaceutical manufacturers, neither of which has shown much interest in this problem. Drug companies and government agencies can hardly be expected to invest in an illness whose very existence remains in doubt. Pharmaceutical companies are often owned by chemical corporations whose products patients may have blamed for causing their illness. Even if this were not the case, one could hardly expect pharmaceutical manufacturers to support research to help people who have trouble tolerating drugs.

Despite significant controversy and funding concerns, multiple chemical intolerance may be one of the most challenging and important puzzles that a researcher could tackle, for several reasons. First, it suggests a new theory of disease, one that has the potential to explain a wide variety of common illnesses whose prevalence has been increasing in recent decades (FIG. 3). Second, multiple chemical intolerance may be a very prevalent problem, perhaps the most common chemically induced illness in the United States. The California Department of Health Services' chemical intolerance prevalence study, a randomized sample of more than 4000 people, found that 6.3% reported having a physician's diagnosis of multiple chemical sensitivity or environmental illness.[13] Some researchers feel this is an underestimate because people may be oblivious to system-exposure relationships due to the masking phenomenon.

Researchers at this meeting will be proposing specific mechanisms for multiple intolerances. Their hypotheses must embrace all of the salient observations for this condition, not just a subset of them. A recent newspaper notice announced, "Industrial Boulevard is empty because it is a road to nowhere. Work is under way to extend it." If the hypotheses proposed here fail to fit *all* of the salient observations concerning this condition, we will be on the road to nowhere too.

At present, stress and its role in this and other illnesses is a favored funding area. There is no question that these patients' symptoms look exactly like those we associated with stress—headaches, fatigue, irritability, depression, and memory and concentration difficulties. There is an understandable tendency to attribute the illness to stress, particularly when existing paradigms do not explain what we are seeing. We must not forget, however, that tens of thousands of chemically intolerant individuals, many holding advanced degrees, are telling us, as loudly and clearly as they can, that *chemical exposures directly and reproducibly* cause their anxiety, headaches, fatigue, irritability, depression, short-term memory difficulties, etc. Thus, we are in a chicken-and-egg situation here. If I have one major bias, it is against the current tendency to zero in on psychological explanations for this illness, when what we need to do is to back up and test the pivotal question first—that is, "is there a subset of people who respond aversely to extraordinary low levels of common chemicals, foods, and drugs?"

Many well-intentioned and well-credentialed researchers stand ready to study the role of stress in this condition. They apply for grants. Peer review committees and government panels meet to decide which studies will be funded, but most lack adequate understanding of the problem. Which studies do you think they will fund? There are approximately 37,000 psychiatrists and 241,000 psychologists in the United States.[38,39] Any suggestion that chemical exposures might cause psychological symptoms can expect a less than enthusiastic reception.

Several government-sponsored consensus workshops have recommended that, as a first step, the EMU studies be conducted to determine whether these people are responding to low-level exposures. For research purposes, challenges would be done in a double-blinded, placebo-controlled manner. The advantage of this approach is that it would not matter whether the patients were experiencing bronchoconstriction that could be objectively measured with a spirometer or if they experienced mood changes that they rated subjectively on a scale. The findings would be equally valid.

The EMU is the only clear pathway for cracking the key conundrum, that is, whether the condition is toxigenic, psychogenic, or both, or different things in different people? This is the question that doctors and policy makers most urgently need answered. Until it is answered, the patients will remain in limbo. There is an ancient Chinese saying—"When you don't know where you're going, any road will take you there." The problem is that it may take decades to get there, especially when research funds are constrained by the very paradigmatic controversy they are needed to settle.

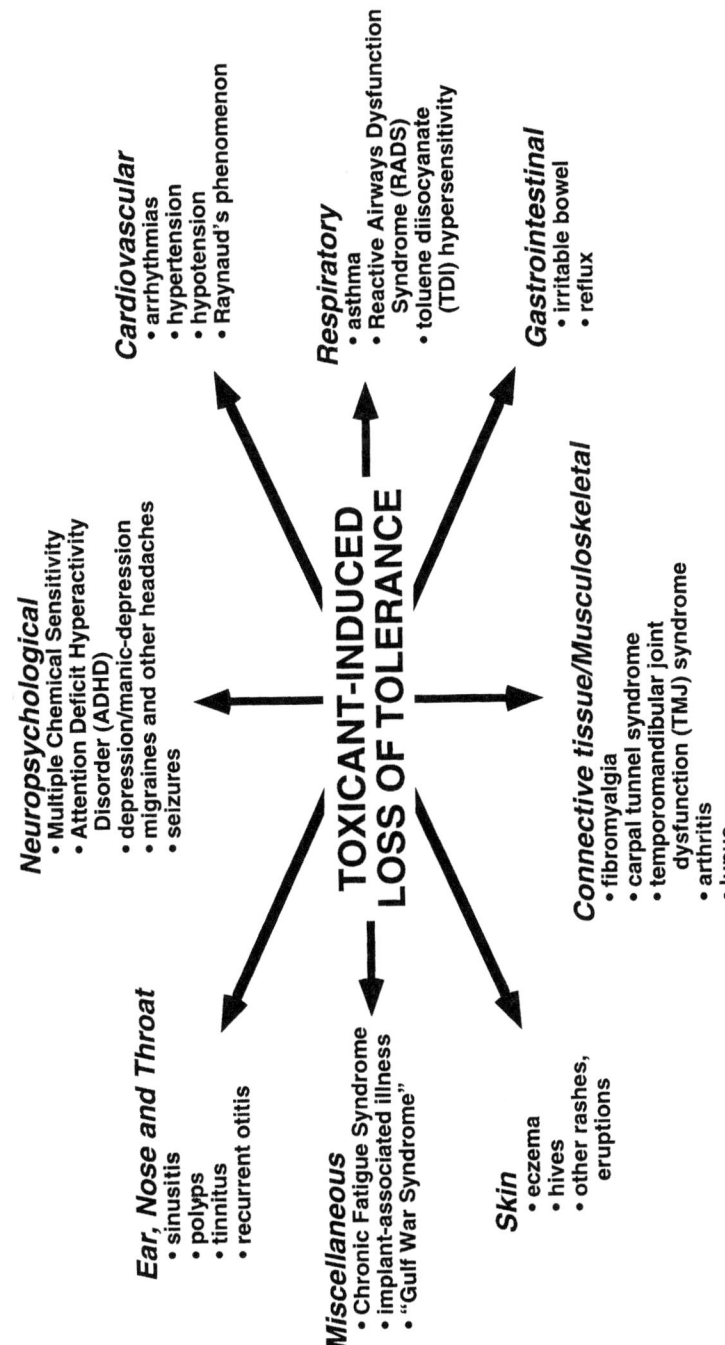

FIGURE 3. Conditions that may have their origins in TILT.

There is nothing wrong with thoughtfully contemplating potential mechanisms that might underlie this illness. However, at the same time, we need to move forward by performing the "crucial experiment"—in this case, human challenge studies in an environmentally controlled hospital unit. Kuhn[34] defined crucial experiments as those able to discriminate sharply between competing paradigms. The EMU experiment has the potential to do just that and will help set medicine and public health on the proper path.

Any theory that is proposed for chemical intolerance:

- Must make sense ("... the first duty of a hypothesis is to be intelligible"—Huxley).
- May be neither simple nor practical ("Make things as simple as possible, but no simpler"—Einstein).
- May require new tools to prove (the microscope allowed us to see germs; an EMU may be necessary to "see" this problem).
- May be unpopular (Copernicus showing that the Earth was not the center of the universe).
- Must be aesthetic, that is, fit existing data and allow prediction; any successful theory must be able to explain all of the salient observations, not just some of them.
- May initially seem strange and implausible (e.g., Einstein's curved space; "What is plausible depends upon the biological knowledge of the time"—Hill).
- May transform neighboring sciences.

Chemical intolerance is no ordinary scientific anomaly. It is a "crisis-provoking" one.[34] As such, it has the potential to transform the fields of environmental health, medicine, psychiatry, psychology, addiction, and toxicology.

The inertia inherent in established paradigms is enormous. Even when the crucial experiment is complete, there are those who will remain skeptical. This is to be expected. Scientific revolutions proceed glacially, but inevitably. The natural history of new paradigms is known: "A new scientific truth does not triumph by convincing its opponents and making them see the light, but rather because its opponents eventually die, and a new generation grows up that is familiar with it" (Max Planck, *Scientific Autobiography*).

BIOSKETCH

Claudia S. Miller, M.D., M.S., is an Associate Professor in Environmental and Occupational Medicine in the Department of Family Practice of the University of Texas Health Science Center at San Antonio. She is board-certified in Allergy/Immunology and Internal Medicine, and has a master's degree in Public Health/Environmental Health. Her research interests include the health effects of low-level chemical exposures, pesticides, indoor air pollution, and Gulf War veterans' illnesses. She has held appointments to several federal advisory committees, including the National Advisory Committee on Occupational Safety and Health, the National Toxicology Program Board of Scientific Counselors, and the Department of Veterans Affairs Persian Gulf Expert Scientific Advisory Committee. She is coauthor of the WHO-award-winning *New Jersey Report on Chemical Sensitivity* and a professionally acclaimed book, *Chemical Exposures: Low Levels and High Stakes*.[10]

REFERENCES

1. MILLER, C. 1994. White paper: chemical sensitivity—history and phenomenology. Toxicol. Ind. Health **10**(4/5): 253–276.
2. MILLER, C. & T. PRIHODA. 1999. The Environmental Exposure and Sensitivity Inventory (EESI): a standardized approach for measuring chemical intolerances for research and clinical applications. Toxicol. Ind. Health **15**: 370–385.
3. MILLER, C. & T. PRIHODA. 1999. A controlled comparison of symptoms and chemical intolerances reported by Gulf War veterans, implant recipients, and persons with multiple chemical sensitivity. Toxicol. Ind. Health **15**: 386–397.
4. LAX, M. & P. HENNEBERGER. 1995. Patients with multiple chemical sensitivities in an occupational health clinic: presentation and follow-up. Arch. Environ. Health **50**(6): 425–431.
5. JOHNSON, A. 1996. MCS Information Exchange. Brunswick, ME.
6. MILLER, C. 1996. Chemical sensitivity: symptom, syndrome, or mechanism for disease? Toxicology **11**: 69–86.
7. MILLER, C. 1997. Toxicant-induced loss of tolerance: an emerging theory of disease? Environ. Health Perspect. **105**(suppl. 2): 445–453.
8. FIEDLER, N. & H. KIPEN. 1997. Chemical sensitivity: the scientific literature. Environ. Health Perspect. **105**(suppl. 2): 409–415.
9. SIMON, G., W. KATON & P. SPARKS. 1990. Allergic to life: psychological factors in environmental illness. Am. J. Psychiatry **147**: 901–906.
10. ASHFORD, N. & C. MILLER. 1998. Chemical Exposures: Low Levels and High Stakes. Wiley. New York.
11. MILLER, C. & H. MITZEL. 1995. Chemical sensitivity attributed to pesticide exposure versus remodeling. Arch. Environ. Health **50**(2): 119–129.
12. BLACK, D., A. RATHE & R. GOLDSTEIN. 1990. Environmental illness: a controlled study of 26 subjects with "20th Century Disease". J. Am. Med. Assoc. **264**: 3166–3170.
13. KRUETZER, R., R. NEUTRA & N. LASHUAY. 1999. Prevalence of people reporting sensitivities to chemicals in a population-based survey. Am. J. Epidemiol. **150**(1): 1–12.
14. FIEDLER, N., C. MACCIA & H. KIPEN. 1992. Evaluation of chemically sensitive patients. J. Occup. Med. **34**: 529–538.
15. DAVIDOFF, A. & L. FOGARTY. 1994. Psychogenic origins of multiple chemical sensitivity syndrome: a critical review of the research literature. Arch. Environ. Health **49**(5): 316–325.
16. CHESTER, A. & P. LEVINE. 1994. Concurrent sick building syndrome and chronic fatigue syndrome: epidemic neuromyasthenia revisited. Clin. Infect. Dis. **18**(suppl. 1): S43–S48.
17. BUCHWALD, D. & D. GARRITY. 1994. Comparison of patients with chronic fatigue syndrome, fibromyalgia, and multiple chemical sensitivities. Arch. Intern. Med. **154**: 2049–2053.
18. SCHIMMELPFENNIG, W. 1994. Zur problematik der begutachtung umweltbedinger toxischer gesundheitsschäden. Bundesgesundheitsblatt **37**: 377.
19. SARTIN, J. 1993. Infectious diseases during the Civil War: the triumph of the "Third Army". Clin. Infect. Dis. **16**: 580–584.
20. GOLOMB, B.A. 1999. Pyridostigmine bromide: review of the scientific literature as it pertains to Gulf War illnesses. Volume 2. RAND. Santa Monica, CA.
21. NEWLIN, D. 1997. A behavior-genetic approach to multiple chemical sensitivity. Environ. Health Perspect. **105**(suppl. 2): 505–508.

22. MILLER, C. 1999. Are we on the threshold of a new theory of disease? Toxicant-induced loss of tolerance and its relationship to addiction and abdiction. Toxicol. Ind. Health **15:** 284–294.
23. MILLER, C., N. ASHFORD, R. DOTY *et al.* 1997. Empirical approaches for the investigation of toxicant-induced loss of tolerance. Environ. Health Perspect. **105**(suppl. 2): 515–519.
24. BARTHA, L., W. BAUMZWEIGER, D. BUSCHER *et al.* 1999. Multiple chemical sensitivity: a 1999 consensus. Arch. Environ. Health **54**(3): 147–149.
25. NETHERCOTT, J., L. DAVIDOFF, B. CURBOW *et al.* 1993. Multiple chemical sensitivities syndrome: toward a working case definition. Arch. Environ. Health **48:** 19–26.
26. ASHFORD, N. 1995. Letter to the editor. Am. J. Ind. Med. **28:** 611–612.
27. GENTON, M. 1998. Shedding light on darkroom disease: progress and challenges in understanding radiology workers' occupational illness. Can. J. Med. Radiat. Technol. **2**(2): 60–66.
28. HIRZY, J. & R. MORRISON. 1989. Carpet/4-phenylcyclohexene toxicity: the EPA headquarters case. Presented at the Annual Meeting of the Society for Risk Analysis, San Francisco.
29. EPA (ENVIRONMENTAL PROTECTION AGENCY). 1989. Report to Congress on Indoor Air Quality. Volume II: Assessment and Control of Indoor Air Pollution.
30. ASHFORD, N., B. HEINZOW, K. LÜTJEN *et al.* 1995. Chemical Sensitivity in Selected European Countries: An Exploratory Study. A Report to the European Commission. Ergonomia. Athens, Greece.
31. MONK, J. 1996. Farmers fight chemical war. Chem. Ind. **February:** 108.
32. STEPHENS, R., A. SPURGEON, I. CALVERT *et al.* 1995. Neuropsychological effect of long-term exposure to organophosphates in sheep dip. Lancet **345:** 1135–1139.
33. CONE, J. & T. SULT. 1992. Acquired intolerance to solvents following pesticide/solvent exposure in a building: a new group of workers at risk for multiple chemical sensitivity. Toxicol. Ind. Health **8**(4): 29–39.
34. KUHN, T. 1970. The Structure of Scientific Revolutions. University of Chicago Press. Chicago.
35. OVERSTREET, D., C. MILLER, D. JANOWSKY *et al.* 1996. Potential animal model of multiple chemical sensitivity with cholinergic supersensitivity. Toxicology **111:** 119–134.
36. SORG, B. 1996. Proposed animal model for multiple chemical sensitivity in studies with formalin. Toxicology **111:** 135–145.
37. ROGERS, W., C. MILLER & L. BUNEGIN. 1999. A rat model of neurobehavioral sensitization to toluene. Environ. Health Perspect. **152:** 356–369.
38. ROBACK, G., L. RANDOLPH, B. SEIDMAN *et al.* 1994. Physician Characteristics and Distribution in the United States. American Medical Association. Chicago.
39. STATISTICAL ABSTRACTS OF THE UNITED STATES. 1994. Bernan Press. Lanham, MD.

Appendix

THE QEESI©

The Quick Environmental Exposure and Sensitivity Inventory (QEESI©) was developed as a screening questionnaire for multiple chemical intolerances (MCI) (see FIG. A1). The instrument has four scales: symptom severity, chemical intolerances, other intolerances, and life impact. Each scale contains 10 items, scored from 0 = "not a problem" to 10 = "severe or disabling problem". A 10-item masking index gauges ongoing exposures that may affect individuals' awareness of their intolerances as well as the intensity of their responses to environmental exposures. Potential uses for the QEESI© include the following:

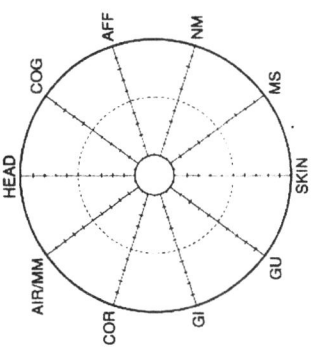

FIGURE A1. The QEESI© questionnaire.

SYMPTOMS

The following questions ask about symptoms you may have experienced commonly. Rate the severity of your symptoms on a 0-10 scale. Do not leave any items blank.

0 = not at all a problem
5 = moderate symptoms
10 = disabling symptoms

For each item, circle one number only:

1	Problems with your muscles or joints, such as pain, aching, cramping, stiffness or weakness?	MS 0 1 2 3 4 5 6 7 8 9 10
2	Problems with burning or irritation of your eyes, or problems with your airway or breathing, such as feeling short of breath, coughing, or having a lot of mucus, post-nasal drainage, or respiratory infections?	AIR/MM 0 1 2 3 4 5 6 7 8 9 10
3	Problems with your heart or chest, such as a fast or irregular heart rate, skipped beats, your heart pounding, or chest discomfort?	COR 0 1 2 3 4 5 6 7 8 9 10
4	Problems with your stomach or digestive tract, such as abdominal pain or cramping, abdominal swelling or bloating, nausea, diarrhea, or constipation?	GI 0 1 2 3 4 5 6 7 8 9 10
5	Problems with your ability to think, such as difficulty concentrating or remembering things, feeling spacey, or having trouble making decisions?	COG 0 1 2 3 4 5 6 7 8 9 10
6.	Problems with your mood, such as feeling tense or nervous, irritable, depressed, having spells of crying or rage, or loss of motivation to do things that used to interest you?	AFF 0 1 2 3 4 5 6 7 8 9 10
7.	Problems with balance or coordination, with numbness or tingling in your extremities, or with focusing your eyes?	NM 0 1 2 3 4 5 6 7 8 9 10
8.	Problems with your head, such as headaches or a feeling of pressure or fullness in your face or head?	HEAD 0 1 2 3 4 5 6 7 8 9 10
9.	Problems with your skin, such as a rash, hives or dry skin?	SKIN 0 1 2 3 4 5 6 7 8 9 10
10.	Problems with your urinary tract or genitals, such as pelvic pain or frequent or urgent urination? (For women: or discomfort or other problems with your menstrual period?)	GU 0 1 2 3 4 5 6 7 8 9 10

3

Total Symptom Score (0-100): ☐

MASKING INDEX

The following items refer to ongoing exposures you may be having. Circle "0" if the answer is NO, or if you don't know whether you have the exposure. Circle "1" if the answer is YES, you do have the exposure. Do not leave any items blank.

Circle "0" or "1" only:

1.	Do you smoke or dip tobacco once a week or more often?	NO=0 YES=1
2.	Do you drink any alcoholic beverages, beer, or wine once a week or more often?	NO=0 YES=1
3.	Do you consume any caffeinated beverages once a week or more often?	NO=0 YES=1
4.	Do you routinely (once a week or more) use perfume, hairspray, or other scented personal care products?	NO=0 YES=1
5.	Has either your home or your workplace been sprayed for insects or fumigated in the past year?	NO=0 YES=1
6.	In your current job or hobby, are you routinely (once a week or more) exposed to any chemicals, smoke or fumes?	NO=0 YES=1
7.	Other than yourself, does anyone routinely smoke inside your home?	NO=0 YES=1
8.	Is either a gas or propane stove used for cooking in your home?	NO=0 YES=1
9.	Is a scented fabric softener (liquid or dryer sheet) routinely used in laundering your clothes or bedding?	NO=0 YES=1
10.	Do you routinely (once a week or more) take any of the following: steroid pills, such as prednisone; pain medications requiring a prescription; medications for depression, anxiety, or mood disorders; medications for sleep; or recreational or street drugs?	NO=0 YES=1

Masking Index (0-10):
(Total number of YES answers) ☐

4

IMPACT OF SENSITIVITIES

If you are sensitive to certain chemicals or foods, on a scale of 0-10 rate the degree to which your sensitivities have affected various aspects of your life. If you are not sensitive or if your sensitivities do not affect these aspects of your life, answer "0." Do not leave any items blank.

0 = not at all
5 = moderately
10 = severely

How much have your sensitivities affected:

1. Your diet	0 1 2 3 4 5 6 7 8 9 10
2. Your ability to work or go to school	0 1 2 3 4 5 6 7 8 9 10
3. How you furnish your home	0 1 2 3 4 5 6 7 8 9 10
4. Your choice of clothing	0 1 2 3 4 5 6 7 8 9 10
5. Your ability to travel to other cities or drive a car	0 1 2 3 4 5 6 7 8 9 10
6. Your choice of personal care products, such as deodorants or makeup	0 1 2 3 4 5 6 7 8 9 10
7. Your ability to be around others and enjoy social activities, for example, going to meetings, church, restaurants, etc.	0 1 2 3 4 5 6 7 8 9 10
8. Your choice of hobbies or recreation	0 1 2 3 4 5 6 7 8 9 10
9. Your relationship with your spouse or family	0 1 2 3 4 5 6 7 8 9 10
10. Your ability to clean your home, iron, mow the lawn, or perform other routine chores	0 1 2 3 4 5 6 7 8 9 10

Total Life Impact Score (0-100): ☐

For additional copies of the **QEESI**, call 210-567-7760. For more information about this questionnaire, refer to Chemical Exposures: Low Levels and High Stakes (2nd Edition) by Nicholas A. Ashford and Claudia S. Miller, John Wiley & Sons, Inc., 1998. To order, call toll-free 1-800-225-5945.

5

FIGURE A1. The QEESI© questionnaire — *continued.*

(1) Research—to characterize and compare study populations and to select subjects and controls.
(2) Clinical evaluations—to obtain a profile of patients' self-reported symptoms and intolerances. The QEESI© can be administered at intervals to follow symptoms over time or to document responses to treatment or exposure avoidance.
(3) Workplace or community investigations—to identify and assist those who may be more chemically susceptible or who report new intolerances. Affected individuals should have the option of discussing results with investigators or their personal physicians.

Individuals whose symptoms began or intensified following a particular exposure event can fill out the QEESI© using two different ink colors, one showing how they were before the event and the second how they have been since the event. On the cover of the QEESI© is a "Symptom Star" (FIG. A2), which provides a graphical representation of patients' responses on the symptom severity scale.

For additional copies of the QEESI©, contact Claudia S. Miller at the address given on page 1 of this article. For further information, see *Chemical Exposures: Low Levels and High Stakes* by Ashford and Miller [1998, Wiley (1-800-225-5945)].

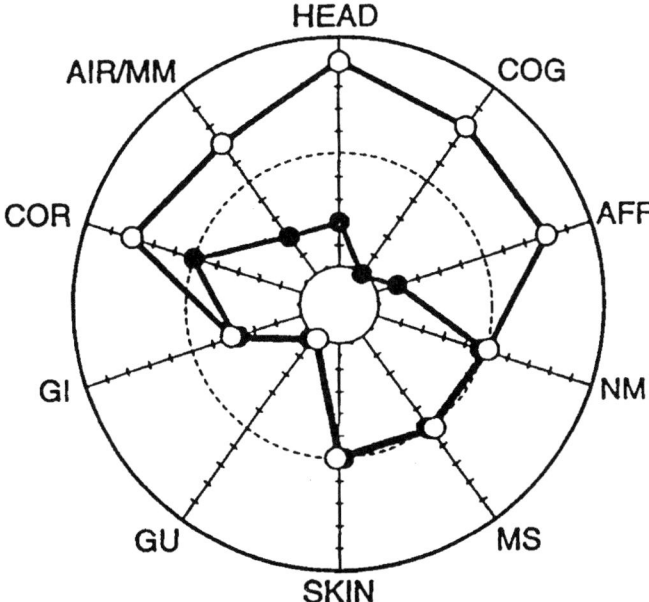

FIGURE A2. QEESI© Symptom Star illustrating symptom severity in an individual before and after an exposure event (e.g., pesticide application, indoor air contaminants, chemical spill). Terms: HEAD = head-related symptoms; COG = cognitive symptoms; AFF = affective symptoms; NM = neuromuscular symptoms; MS = musculoskeletal symptoms; SKIN = skin-related symptoms; GU = genitourinary symptoms; GI = gastrointestinal symptoms; COR = heart/chest-related symptoms; AIR/MM = airway or mucous membrane symptoms; (●) before exposure event; (○) after exposure event.

TABLE A1. Criteria for low, medium, and high scale scores

Scale/Index	Score		
	Low	Medium	High
Symptom severity	0–19	20–39	40–100
Chemical intolerance	0–19	20–39	40–100
Other intolerance	0–11	12–24	25–100
Life impact	0–11	12–23	24–100
Masking index	0–3	4–5	6–10

TABLE A2. Distribution of subjects by group using "high" cutoff points for symptom severity (≥ 40) and chemical intolerances (≥ 40), with masking low or not low (<4 or ≥ 4)

	Risk criteria[a]			Percentage of each group meeting risk criteria				
Degree to which MCI is suggested[b]	Symptom severity score	Chemical intolerance score	Masking score	Controls ($n = 76$)	MCS: no event ($n = 90$)	MCS: event ($n = 96$)	Implant ($n = 87$)	Gulf War veterans ($n = 72$)
Very suggestive	≥ 40	≥ 40	≥ 4	7	16	23	39	45
Very suggestive	≥ 40	≥ 40	<4	0	65	66	36	4
Somewhat suggestive	≥ 40	<40	≥ 4	3	1	2	16	26
Not suggestive	≥ 40	<40	<4	0	0	2	3	6
Problematic	<40	≥ 40	≥ 4	7	3	1	1	0
Problematic	<40	≥ 40	<4	3	13	4	2	0
Not suggestive	<40	<40	≥ 4	68	1	0	2	18
Not suggestive	<40	<40	<4	12	1	2	1	1
				100	100	100	100	100

[a]Subjects must meet all three criteria, that is, symptom severity, chemical intolerance, and masking scores, as indicated in each row of this table.

[b]Terms: "very suggestive" = high symptom and chemical intolerance scores; "somewhat suggestive" = high symptom score, but possibly masked chemical intolerance; "not suggestive" = either (1) high symptom score, but low chemical intolerance score with low masking, or (2) low symptom and chemical intolerance scores; "problematic" = low symptom score, but high chemical intolerance score. Persons in this category with low masking (<4) may be sensitive individuals who have been avoiding chemical exposures for an extended period (months or years).

INTERPRETING THE QEESI©

In a study of 421 individuals, including four exposure groups and a control group, the QEESI© provided sensitivity of 92% and specificity of 95% in differentiating between persons with MCI and the general population.[1,2]

Cronbach's alpha reliability coefficients for the QEESI©'s four scales—symptom severity, chemical intolerances, other intolerances, and life impact—were high (0.76–0.97) for each of the groups, as well as over all subjects, indicating that the questions on the QEESI© form scales showing good internal consistency. Pearson correlations for each of the four scales with validity items of interest, that is, life quality, health status, energy level, body pain, ability to work, and employment status, were all significant and in the expected direction, thus supporting good construct validity.

Information on the development of this instrument, its interpretation, and results for several populations have been published.[1,2] Proposed ranges for the QEESI©'s scales and guidelines for their interpretation appear in TABLES A1 and A2.

REFERENCES

1. MILLER, C. & T. PRIHODA. 1999. The Environmental Exposure and Sensitivity Inventory (EESI): a standardized approach for measuring chemical intolerances for research and clinical applications. Toxicol. Ind. Health **15:** 370–385.
2. MILLER, C. & T. PRIHODA. 1999. A controlled comparison of symptoms and chemical intolerances reported by Gulf War veterans, implant recipients, and persons with multiple chemical sensitivity. Toxicol. Ind. Health **15:** 386–397.

Controlled Exposures to Volatile Organic Compounds in Sensitive Groups

NANCY FIEDLER[a] AND HOWARD M. KIPEN[b]

UMDNJ–Robert Wood Johnson Medical School, Environmental and Occupational Health Sciences Institute, Piscataway, New Jersey 08854, USA

> ABSTRACT: Sensitivities to chemicals are characterized by symptoms in multiple organ systems in response to low-level chemical exposures. This paper reviews studies of controlled exposures to odorants and to mixtures of volatile organic compounds. Sensitive subgroups include subjects who met Cullen's 1987 criteria for multiple chemical sensitivity (MCS), Gulf War veterans with chronic fatigue syndrome and chemical sensitivity (CFS/CS), and subjects with specific self-reported sensitivities to methyl terbutyl ether (MTBE) in gasoline (MTBE-sensitive). All studies include comparison of age- and sex-matched healthy controls. Studies of olfaction did not support unusual sensitivity, defined as lower odor thresholds, among MCS subjects; however, a dose-response pattern of symptoms was observed in response to suprathreshold concentrations of phenyl ethyl alcohol. In blinded, controlled exposures to clean air, gasoline, gasoline/11% MTBE, and gasoline/15% MTBE, a threshold effect was observed with MTBE-sensitive subjects reporting significantly increased symptoms to gasoline/15% MTBE exposure. Autonomic arousal (heart and respiration rate; end-tidal CO_2) in response to odor of chemical mixtures may mediate symptoms for subjects with generalized chemical sensitivities, but not for those whose sensitivities are confined to specific chemicals. For example, Gulf War veterans with CFS/CS experienced reduced end-tidal CO_2 when exposed to diesel fumes, while exposure to MTBE did not produce any psychophysiologic changes in MTBE-sensitive subjects. Controlled olfactory and exposure studies reveal that significant responses can be observed in chemically sensitive subjects even when de-adaptation has not occurred. However, these studies suggest that symptoms are not necessarily accompanied by changes in physiologic arousal. Subject characteristics play a critical role in outcomes.

Multiple chemical sensitivity (MCS) is a perplexing clinical phenomenon in which individuals report numerous physical and psychological symptoms that they associate with low-level chemical exposures.[1–4] Because the symptoms occur in multiple organ systems and are inconsistent with known organic and/or exposure-related illness, MCS has not been recognized as a distinct illness.[5] In 1987, Cullen proposed

---

[a]Address for correspondence: UMDNJ–Robert Wood Johnson Medical School, Environmental and Occupational Health Sciences Institute, 170 Frelinghuysen Road, Room 210, Piscataway, NJ 08854. Voice: 732-445-0123, ext. 625; fax: 732-445-0130.
nfiedler@eohsi.rutgers.edu
[b]Voice: 732-445-0123, ext. 629; fax: 732-445-3644.
kipen@eohsi.rutgers.edu

criteria for the purpose of defining commonalities, at least conceptually, in this patient population. Cullen's criteria emphasized that no other organic illness or laboratory test could explain the symptoms reported and that the onset of MCS began with an identifiable chemical exposure. To date, however, this proposition of chemical causation has never been tested. Other investigators[3] include MCS on a continuum with well-understood medical illnesses such as autoimmune disorders, all of which are attributed to chronic, low-level chemical exposures. The purpose of this paper is to review what we have learned from clinical investigations of MCS as defined by Cullen[6] and from controlled exposure studies of self-reported sensitive subgroups.

BACKGROUND AND CROSS-SECTIONAL COMPARISONS

Several investigators have evaluated the psychiatric, neuropsychological, and immunological status of MCS subjects relative to positive (chronic fatigue syndrome, chronic back pain) and negative control groups.[7-9] In our laboratory as well as others,[8-10] the psychiatric disorders of highest prevalence among MCS subjects are depression and anxiety disorders measured either with psychometric instruments such as the Beck Depression Inventory[11] or with structured psychiatric interviews such as the Diagnostic Interview Survey.[12] In contrast, MCS subjects do not show an increased prevalence of substance abuse/dependence, bipolar disorder, or psychosis.[10,13] This greater prevalence of anxiety and depression exceeds that found in healthy controls and in chronic pain patients,[8] but not that found for other syndromes with medically unexplained symptoms such as CFS.[7] In contrast, however, MCS subjects do not show consistent cognitive impairment or changes in immunologic function relative to healthy controls.[7,8] Earlier reports of compromised verbal and visual memory[14] have not been replicated either in our laboratory or by other investigators.[7,8] Thus, the most consistent finding is an excess of psychiatric comorbidity among MCS subjects. From this evidence, we have developed research strategies, discussed in more detail below, that incorporate rather than exclude psychiatric comorbidity and associated risk factors.

SUBJECT DESCRIPTION

Our studies of chemical sensitivity have evaluated three different sensitive subgroups. Subjects classified as MCS met the Cullen[6] criteria and were compared to age- and gender-matched healthy controls. Gulf War veterans were those who had fatiguing illness with 83% (10/12) who met the 1994 criteria for chronic fatigue syndrome (CFS)[15] and reported sensitivities on the Chemical Odor Intolerance Index[16] to chemicals such as paint, pesticides, and car exhaust at a level comparable to that observed among those diagnosed with MCS (see FIG. 1), yet most did not report lifestyle changes[8] and did not meet the Cullen[6] criteria for MCS (2/12; 17%). Thus, veterans were classified as CFS with chemical sensitivity (CFS/CS) and were compared to age- and gender-matched healthy Gulf War veterans. Finally, individuals report-

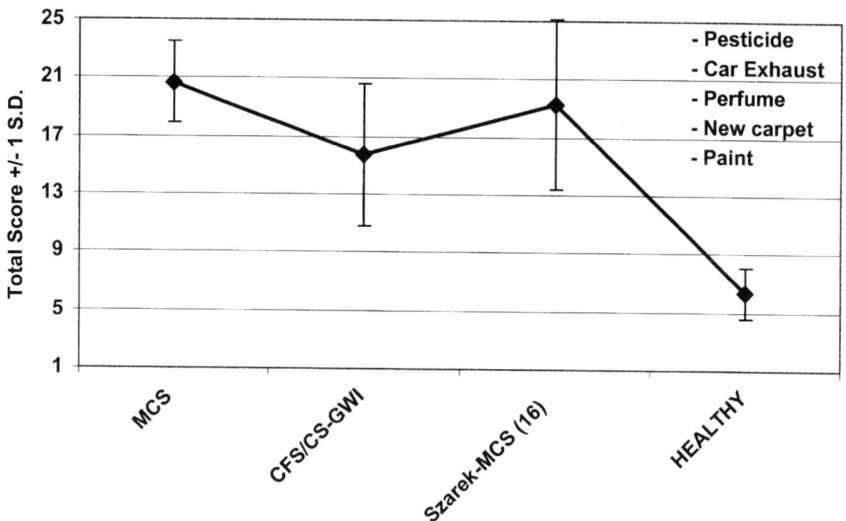

FIGURE 1. Chemical odor intolerance index.

ing sensitivity to methyl tertiary butyl ether (MTBE), an additive used to oxygenate gasoline, were recruited based on responses to a questionnaire on MTBE-related symptoms as defined by Moolenaar[17] (e.g., headache, cough).[18] These individuals did not report that they were unusually sensitive to chemicals such as paint or pesticides and therefore did not meet criteria for MCS or CS. To clearly distinguish them from other self-reported sensitive groups, they will be referred to in the present paper as MTBE-sensitive subjects. In contrast, we[18] labeled these subjects as self-reported sensitives. MTBE-sensitive subjects were also compared to age- and gender-matched healthy controls.

All subjects completed a physical examination that included a history and physical and standard laboratory tests. Subjects with the following conditions were excluded from the studies: neurologic disease or history of brain injury, occupational exposure to neurotoxicants, stroke or cardiovascular disease, serious pulmonary disease (e.g., asthma), liver or kidney disease, serious gastrointestinal disorders, nasal polyps, nasal surgery, sinus disease, major psychiatric disorders to include psychoses, bipolar disorder, alcoholism, or drug abuse. Smokers and pregnant or lactating women were also excluded, as were individuals on beta and alpha blockers, anxiolytics, antidepressants, and steroids. TABLE 1 gives the demographic characteristics for each of the subject groups described above. Subjects from the sensitive groups did not differ in age; however, MTBE-sensitive subjects were significantly more educated than the MCS subjects and CFS/CS veterans. Gender was significantly different between groups with MCS dominated by females and CFS/CS dominated by males sampled from a veteran population. Prior to participation, all subjects signed an informed consent in accordance with Robert Wood Johnson Medical School Institutional Review Board requirements.

TABLE 1. Demographics

	MCS (n = 38)	MTBE-sensitive (n = 12)	CFS/CS-GWI (n = 12)	F	p
Age (mean/SD)	46.0 (7.3)	42.3 (11.9)	40.2 (8.1)	2.59	NS
Years educ. (mean/SD)	15.5 (2.6)	17.1 (4.6)	14.1 (2.1)	4.10	0.02
Gender (females/males)	22/8	6/6	4/11		0.006[a]

[a]Fisher's exact test.

CONTROLLED EXPOSURE METHODOLOGY

Our controlled environment facility is a 7.3-ft (height) by 13.5-ft (width) by 9-ft (depth) stainless steel room in which air flow, temperature, and humidity are controlled (see reference 18 for a complete description of the facility and exposure methods). Our approach to controlled exposure studies has been to select exposure mixtures and concentrations relevant to our subjects. Thus, unlike most previous controlled exposure studies,[19] our focus has not been on the main effect of a given chemical, but on the interactive effect of individual sensitivities and chemical mixtures at low concentrations. This entails surveying subjects to determine the chemicals or mixtures to which they report symptoms. In the MTBE study, for example, the selection of exposure mixtures was driven by the specific gasoline mixture that was associated with symptoms in epidemiologic studies.[17,20] In addition, our studies modeled concentrations of mixtures based on environmental sampling where exposures were likely to occur. For example, we had previous data to estimate the concentrations to which motorists are exposed during refueling of automobiles.[21] Similarly, our sample of Gulf War veterans reported diesel fumes to be one of several substances that elicited symptoms during their service in the Persian Gulf and presently. For this subject group, however, the selection of diesel fumes was only one of several chemical mixtures that was reported to cause symptoms.[22,23] Among the possible choices for an exposure study, we selected diesel fumes because of its relevance to the military and because veterans reported ongoing exposure and illness exacerbation in civilian life. Such an exposure study would then allow us to test current responses of veterans reporting ongoing illness that includes chemical odor intolerance. Again, the concentration of 5 ppm for diesel vapors was chosen based on estimates of concentrations found where diesel-powered vehicles are under repair and represents the upper limit of environmental exposures.[24] Thus, for both MTBE and diesel, exposure concentrations were well below occupational exposure limits in an effort to model the effect of low-level environmental exposures.[18]

Selection of dependent measures was determined by symptom complaints of the target sensitive group. For example, reported symptoms (e.g., headache, dizziness) overlap those induced by stress reactions to exposure. Therefore, psychophysiologic measures such as heart rate, blood pressure, end-tidal CO_2, and muscle tension were measured at baseline before exposure and throughout the controlled exposure to monitor sympathetic and parasympathetic responses to exposure. Questionnaires to monitor symptoms and odor ratings were completed before, during, and after expo-

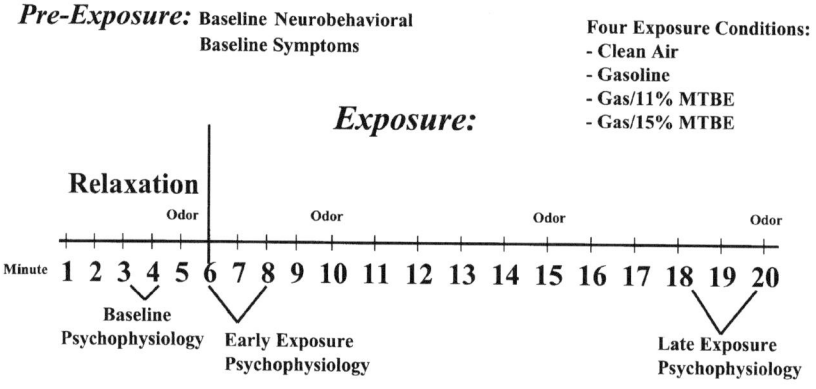

FIGURE 2. MTBE protocol timeline. See reference 18.

sure to assess target and nontarget symptoms. For example, symptoms associated in the epidemiologic literature with MTBE were monitored along with symptoms associated with anxiety, depression, respiratory distress, and solvent exposure.[25] Cognitive complaints of poor concentration and memory invariably accompany exposure and were assessed with a neurobehavioral performance measure of vigilance that simulates a driving task.[26] FIGURE 2 illustrates the procedures for a typical exposure session. Thus, we emphasized measurement of subjective and objective responses to exposure and took into account potential baseline differences between subject groups and within individuals on different exposure days. These baseline differences are particularly critical in this work since subject groups are not homogeneous despite the careful application of case definitions.[7,27,28]

ANXIETY, DEPRESSION, AND MCS

The discussion regarding the relationship between psychiatric disorders and MCS often focuses on whether the psychopathology observed is primary or secondary to MCS. However, a more important question may be whether this comorbidity reflects a biological and/or psychological substrate that affects susceptibility (Bell, this conference). For example, several investigators argue that a hyperventilation response among some MCS subjects may play a role in the symptoms of MCS,[10,29–31] while Bell (this conference) has argued that both MCS and some forms of psychopathology may share factors that increase the risk for neural sensitization.

For example, in addition to the higher prevalence of psychiatric disorders, we find increased scores on measures of traits such as negative affect and anxiety sensitivity. Negative affect is the tendency to experience negative, distressing emotions and may

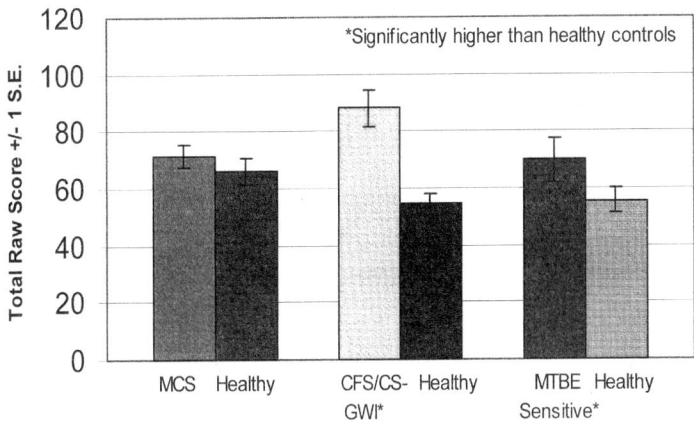

FIGURE 3. Trait neuroticism: NEO Personality Inventory.[33]

encompass symptoms of both anxiety and depression,[32,33] while anxiety sensitivity or fear of anxiety is based on the belief that the symptoms have harmful consequences.[34,35] In community samples of MCS subjects, Gulf War veterans with CFS/CS, and MTBE-sensitive subjects, we found negative affect, assessed with the Neuroticism subscale of the Neuroticism, Extraversion, Openness Scale (NEO),[33] to be elevated relative to healthy controls (see FIG. 3). In addition, in one study of MCS subjects, we also evaluated and found significantly elevated levels of anxiety sensitivity (MCS mean = 18.9; controls mean = 10.2; $p = 0.002$). The latter has been found predictive of the tendency to experience panic attacks that often include hyperventilation.[36] Finally, among Gulf War veterans with CFS/CS and similar to Black et al.,[10] we found significantly elevated rates of current anxiety disorders to include panic and PTSD.[37]

These cross-sectional findings suggest that, regardless of the sensitive subgroup, controlled exposure studies should evaluate anxiety and/or neuroticism as independent variables that contribute to the exposure response. Thus, in our controlled exposure studies, we have included symptom responses to exposure and psychophysiologic measures of sympathetic and parasympathetic arousal as indicators of anxiety responses to exposure.

SYMPTOMS IN RESPONSE TO INHALATION EXPOSURES: RESPONDERS OR RESPONSE BIAS?

For each of the subject groups we have tested, the hallmark for identifying and selecting sensitive subgroups is self-report of symptoms in response to exposure. Often, the goal of controlled exposure studies is to validate the responses that subjects report to occur in the general environment. A significant factor, at least with volatile organic compounds, is the effect that odor alone may have on symptom reporting.[38] For example, clinical reports led some investigators to hypothesize that MCS subjects have an enhanced ability to detect and identify odors,[39] presumably causing symptoms to occur at levels of exposure undetected by many people. However, to date, this hypothesis has not been validated[39,40] when olfactory thresholds of MCS were compared to healthy controls, nor were MCS subjects any better at identifying odors on the multiple-choice University of Pennsylvania Smell Identification Test.[40]

Regardless of the concentration at which odors are detected, increased symptom reporting may occur simply because the subject knows, from odor cues, that exposure is occurring. However, several different mechanisms may be hypothesized to explain these responses to odor. For example, if the subject believes the exposure will be harmful, symptom reports will be influenced either consciously or unconsciously by knowledge of exposure through odor cues. On the other hand, Bolla-Wilson[41] and Van den Bergh[42] suggested that symptom reports could arise as a result of a conditioned physiologic response to the odor such that previous associations of illness with exposure have now been conditioned to that and similar odors. Alternatively, symptoms may be secondary to an anxiety state such as panic that, similar to a conditioned response, initially occurred during previous episodes of exposure. Regardless of the mechanism, symptoms triggered by odor may not reflect a direct physiologic dose response to a chemical exposure. Thus, investigators have discussed several methods for masking or blocking the odor of exposure to then determine the direct effect of chemical exposure.[43]

Data collected from our study of subjects reporting sensitivity to MTBE as well as responses to suprathreshold levels of PEA in MCS subjects from the community both suggest that odor alone either as a cue for exposure or as a conditioned stimulus producing physiologic responses does not account entirely for the symptoms reported. Our MTBE-sensitive subjects reported a sensitivity, defined as increased symptoms, specifically in response to gasoline with 15% MTBE.[18] Since MTBE has a distinctive odor and the purpose of our study was to determine health effects not due to odor, masking of the odor was considered. Initially, we conducted an odor discrimination study to determine whether MTBE-sensitive subjects and age- and sex-matched controls could reliably detect the difference between (i) gasoline with MTBE (15% MTBE v/v) versus gasoline and (ii) gasoline with MTBE (15% MTBE v/v) and re-odorant versus gasoline. The re-odorant was a mixture designed to change the odor of gasoline with MTBE such that the odor of MTBE was no longer recognizable. Six MTBE-sensitive subjects and 8 controls completed two sessions in which they completed a forced choice procedure to determine if 28 bottle pairs contained the same or different mixtures. We[44] found that neither group was able to reliably distinguish gasoline/MTBE with or without the re-odorant from gasoline alone. While the MTBE-sensitive subjects were not accurate in distinguishing gasoline mixtures with and without MTBE, they reported that bottle pairs were different significantly more than did controls regardless of the content of the bottle pairs. While their response bias was to believe they were smelling different odors, the lack of reliability in distinguishing MTBE from gasoline did not support the necessity for odor masking in a repeated measures design.

One possible limitation of the odor discrimination study was that subjects were only allowed a single sniff of each bottle in each pair. It has been suggested that multiple sniffs may be necessary to accurately identify the components of a mixture.[45] Our odor discrimination task did not require subjects to identify components, but simply to discriminate. Therefore, we regarded the experiment as valid for making

TABLE 2. Subjects' awareness of exposure (percent accuracy): MTBE exposure study

Exposure condition	MTBE-sensitive (%)	Controls (%)
Clean air	75	47
Gasoline	25	16
Gas/11% MTBE	42	53
Gas/15% MTBE	25	21

NOTE: From reference 18.

the decision about the controlled exposure masking. This decision was further validated by the fact that subjects were unable, with 15 minutes of exposure time and thus multiple sniffs, to identify accurately the gasoline exposure conditions.[18] However, they were accurate beyond a chance level in detecting that exposure to a gasoline mixture rather than clean air occurred. Regardless of accuracy, MTBE-sensitive subjects were also no more likely to identify an exposure as containing MTBE than were controls (see TABLE 2). Thus, during the controlled exposures, MTBE-sensitive subjects did not exhibit a response bias toward reporting MTBE exposure.

In fact, we found that, relative to controls, the MTBE-sensitive subjects reported significantly more symptoms in the gasoline/15% MTBE condition than in the clean air or gasoline/11% MTBE conditions.[18] Based on the inability of subjects to discriminate gasoline exposure conditions, we did not attribute the increased symptoms of the MTBE-sensitive subjects to knowledge or beliefs about exposure to MTBE. Moreover, if the odor of MTBE was the determinant of symptoms, then we would have expected significantly increased symptoms in the gasoline with 11% MTBE exposure conditions; however, those were not observed.

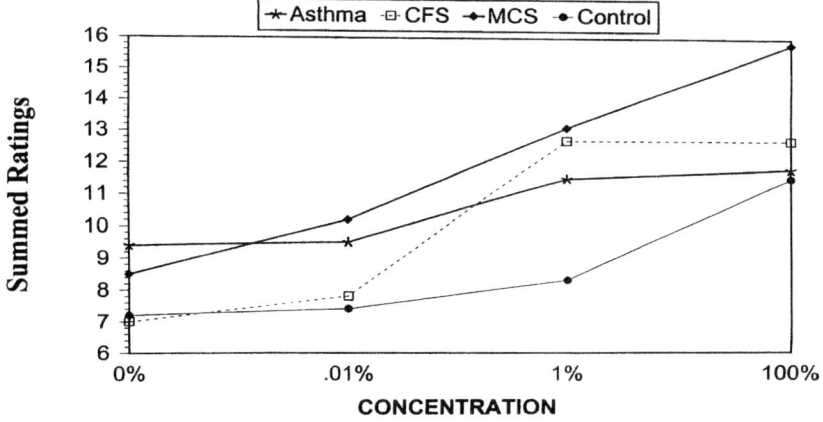

FIGURE 4. Mean trigeminal symptoms to PEA—burning, stinging/pricking, temperature: 1 = low to 9 = high. See reference 40.

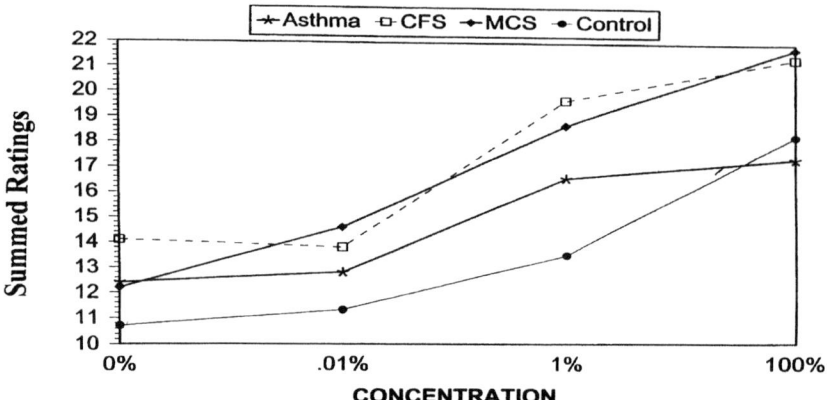

FIGURE 5. Mean aesthetic responses to PEA—intensity: 1 = very weak to 9 = very strong; pleasantness: 1 = pleasant to 9 = very unpleasant; safety: 1 = very safe to 9 = very unsafe. Source: reference 40.

Our studies evaluating aesthetic and trigeminal responses to phenyl ethyl alcohol (PEA) and pyridine (PYR) also do not support that the effects observed reflect purely a negative response to odor. In separate trials for PEA and PYR, subjects were asked to sniff, in random order, bottles that contained three levels of suprathreshold concentrations plus one with 0% of PEA and PYR, but they were not told what concentration was in each bottle.[40] As can be seen in FIGURES 4 and 5, MCS subjects' responses to PEA showed a linear increase in trigeminal symptoms and in negative aesthetic ratings as the suprathreshold concentration increased. However, this pattern was not evident for PYR (not shown). This is particularly remarkable since PYR is an unpleasant, irritating odor, while PEA is generally regarded as pleasant. If responses were purely based on the response bias to report symptoms in response to odor, one would not necessarily expect responses to increase with PEA only. In this experiment, however, we did not ask whether subjects thought the concentration was increased. Therefore, we cannot clearly rule out the effect of subjects' awareness of the concentration on their ratings. However, if subjects knew the concentration, one would have expected the same results for PYR and these also were not found.

On the other hand, MCS subjects' response to PEA could still be explained as a conditioned response since PEA is a constituent of perfume and perfume is reported to elicit symptoms in most MCS subjects.[46] PYR may be encountered less frequently and may not have the same associations as those substances known to elicit symptoms. In fact, a conditioned response may also show the same proportional response pattern as that seen for PEA. Thus, conditioning cannot be ruled out based on these data.

ANXIETY, ODOR, AND CONTROLLED CHEMICAL EXPOSURE

Previously cited studies in our laboratory suggest that exposure to odors, even noxious odors, does not reliably produce increased symptoms among sensitive subgroups.[18,40] Knowledge of exposure also did not reliably increase symptoms. This selectivity of response does not support a generalized response bias towards symptom reporting with odor exposure. However, this selective odor response could still be explained by a classically conditioned anxiety response based on symptoms associated with specific odors. Thus, a parallel question we have investigated is the role of anxiety when subjects report symptoms in response to exposures.

Several investigations,[30] including our own study of anxiety sensitivity, suggest that symptoms, reported by MCS patients, resemble many of those reported by patients with anxiety disorders.[7,10,47] Many chemical exposures that elicit responses are accompanied by distinctive odors.[38] Thus, anticipatory anxiety in response to the odor of the exposure could trigger symptoms characteristic of MCS. Anxiety can be measured both subjectively with symptom reports and with associated psychophysiologic measures of sympathetic and parasympathetic arousal such as heart and respiration rate, respiratory sinus arrhythmia, end-tidal CO_2, and finger temperature. Thus, in our controlled exposure to MTBE and to diesel vapors, psychophysiologic measures were taken at baseline and throughout the onset and duration of exposure as indicators of reaction to odor and to body burden of chemical exposure. For example, in the controlled exposure study of MTBE-sensitive subjects, we took psychophysiologic measures during each baseline period before exposure and during each 15-minute exposure to the following conditions: clean air, gasoline, gasoline/11% MTBE, gasoline/15% MTBE.[18] During the first 5 minutes of the exposure periods for gasoline, gasoline/11% MTBE, and gasoline/15% MTBE, when the odor of the exposure was initially perceived, MTBE-sensitive subjects and controls did not differ on any indicators of psychophysiologic arousal including end-tidal CO_2, which is associated with hyperventilation. Thus, the odor of the gasoline mixtures, to which subjects reported sensitivity, did not result in either sympathetic (e.g., hyperventilation) or parasympathetic arousal (e.g., heart rate variability). Moreover, no significant psychophysiologic differences in response were noted after 15 minutes of exposure had occurred when a body burden of MTBE was documented.[18]

On the other hand, preliminary results of an unblind, controlled exposure to diesel vapors indicate that Gulf War veterans diagnosed with CFS/CS show significantly reduced end-tidal CO_2 during the first 5-minute period of a 45-minute exposure to 5 ppm of diesel vapors (see FIG. 6). These veterans reported that diesel vapors were among those substances that made them ill during their service in the Persian Gulf. Thus, similar to our MTBE exposure study, the diesel exposure selected was one expected to be relevant for the subjects. In both studies, subjects knew that the chemical exposure occurred. Although the MTBE-sensitive subjects were unable to identify accurately which of the three exposure conditions was occurring, they were significantly more accurate in distinguishing clean air from any exposure.[18] Similarly, Gulf War veterans had only one exposure session and knew they were exposed to diesel vapors. Thus, knowledge of a chemical exposure has not produced a consistent psychophysiologic response.

Upon closer examination, however, differences in the subject groups offer a plausible explanation for these divergent results. While the Gulf War veterans met diagnostic criteria for CFS, 16% also met DSM-IV criteria for a current anxiety disorder (i.e., panic disorder and/or PTSD) based on a Diagnostic Interview Survey.[12] The anxiety facet of the Neuroticism scale (CFS/CS mean = 17.5, SD = 5.3; MTBE-sensitive mean = 13.5, SD = 4.7; $t = 1.95$; $p = 0.06$) was higher for the Gulf war vet-

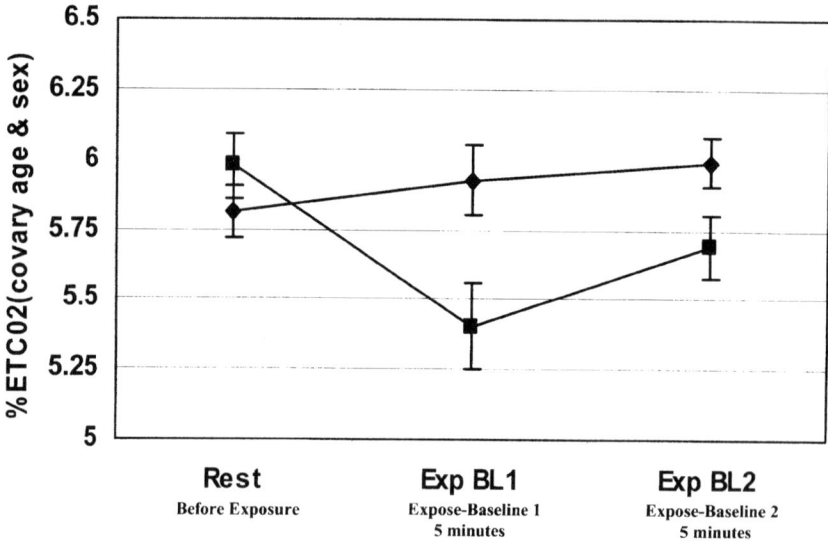

FIGURE 6. Percent end-tidal CO_2: (♦) healthy; (■) CFS/CS-GWI. See reference 22.

erans than for the MTBE-sensitive subjects. Moreover, veterans with CFS/CS reported a generalized chemical sensitivity, while the MTBE-sensitive subjects did not report themselves to be unusually sensitive to chemicals such as paints or pesticides. These comparisons further support previous observations regarding the potential relationship between hyperventilation, anxiety, and the responses of chemically sensitive subjects. It would be interesting to compare subjects who have chemical sensitivity without a comorbid anxiety disorder to determine whether the psychophysiologic response observed is a function of anxiety disorder rather than chemical sensitivity.

FUTURE DIRECTIONS

Neither cross-sectional descriptive studies nor chemical challenge studies can address whether negative affect or anxiety sensitivity preceded the development of chemical sensitivities. They do, however, reveal a pattern of results suggesting these may be enduring traits at least among a subset of those who develop sensitivity to chemicals. Therefore, to investigate prospectively the effect of negative affect in subjects who have not developed chemical sensitivity, we are conducting a study in which women who are high in negative affect and who also report odor intolerance, but not MCS, will be significantly more symptomatic than those low in negative affect when exposed to a mixture of volatile organic compounds found in poorly ventilated buildings.[48,49] This study is directly relevant to MCS since it evaluates only women, for whom MCS is more prevalent, and it evaluates the traits hypothesized to precede MCS rather than MCS itself. Moreover, building-related illness shares many of the same symptoms and features of MCS, and exposure to poor indoor air has been linked to the onset of MCS in at least some subjects.[3]

Our studies of both MCS and MTBE-sensitive subjects suggest that noxious odors do not consistently produce a symptomatic response that differs from controls; that is, MCS subjects responded differently from controls only to suprathreshold levels of a rose-scented chemical (PEA), but not to a noxious odorant (PYR). In addition, MTBE-sensitive subjects responded symptomatically to gasoline with 15% MTBE, but not to gasoline alone or to gasoline with 11% MTBE. Moreover, despite previous hypotheses, it does not appear that chemically sensitive subjects can identify or detect odors more accurately than healthy controls. Thus, sensitive subjects do not exhibit a universal symptomatic response to chemical odors. However, subjects are accurate in distinguishing clean air from chemical mixtures. Thus, masking the clean air conditions recommended by Dick *et al.*[50] will further clarify effects of exposure. This strategy has been successfully employed in several exposure studies of methyl ethyl ketone and acetone.[50] Essentially, a pulse of a lower concentration is given for 5 minutes periodically during the clean air exposure. Odor cues will thus be present and breath samples can be used to validate body burdens for both exposure and clean air conditions.

A significant subset of Gulf War veterans who reported sensitivity to multiple chemicals hyperventilated in response to diesel vapors. This finding is consistent with other studies of MCS subjects in whom hyperventilation has been documented under several different exposures, including CO_2,[31] lactate infusion,[30] and multiple chemicals.[29] In contrast, the MTBE-sensitive subjects did not hyperventilate in response to exposure. Comparison of the subject groups between these studies reveals that our Gulf War veterans were comparable to MCS subjects in their level of chemical odor intolerance, while the MTBE-sensitive subjects were intentionally selected because they did not regard themselves as unusually sensitive to chemicals. Thus, the MTBE-sensitive subjects did not exhibit the same generalized chemical sensitivity nor the same hyperventilation response to odor.

The role of the hyperventilation response in the symptoms reported by MCS subjects during chemical exposures, however, remains to be resolved. In our study of Gulf War veterans, for example, the hyperventilation response resolved after 10 minutes of exposure and, therefore, does not readily account for symptoms that persisted throughout the 45-minute exposure period. None of the previous studies documenting hyperventilation among MCS subjects were designed to follow the course of symptoms during a continuous exposure. Further studies will be needed to address how hyperventilation contributes to the exposure-related symptoms reported by MCS patients.

In conclusion, our results to date suggest that subjects who report specific sensitivities may not respond in the same manner as those with more generalized chemical sensitivities. Ideally, subjects who have chemical sensitivity with and without anxiety should be compared to separate the contributions of these subject characteristics to symptoms and physiologic endpoints. Finally, blinded or masked exposure studies would augment our understanding of the effects of chemical exposure from those attributable to the odor of exposure. Since masking of chemical mixtures has proven problematic, masking of the clean air exposure may be a preferable option for exploring the effects of odor apart from the effects of exposure.[50]

REFERENCES

1. GRAVELING, R.A., A. PILKINGTON, J.P.K. GEORGE et al. 1999. A review of multiple chemical sensitivity. Occup. Environ. Med. **56:** 73–85.
2. SPARKS, P.J., W. DANIELL, D.W. BLACK et al. 1994. Multiple chemical sensitivity syndrome: a clinical perspective. II. Evaluation, diagnostic testing, treatment, and social considerations. J. Occup. Med. **36:** 731–737.
3. ASHFORD, N.A. & C.S. MILLER. 1998. Chemical Exposures: Low Levels and High Stakes. Wiley. New York.
4. KREUTZER, R., R.R. NEUTRA & N. LASHUARY. 1999. The prevalence of people reporting sensitivities to chemicals in a population-based survey. Am. J. Epidemiol. **150:** 1–12.
5. AMERICAN COLLEGE OF PHYSICIANS. 1989. American College of Physicians position statement: clinical ecology. Ann. Intern. Med. **111:** 168–178.
6. CULLEN, M.R. 1987. Workers with Multiple Chemical Sensitivities, pp. 655–662. Hanley & Belfus. Philadelphia.
7. FIEDLER, N., H. KIPEN, J. DELUCA et al. 1996. A controlled comparison of multiple chemical sensitivity and chronic fatigue syndrome. Psychosom. Med. **58:** 38–49.
8. SIMON, G.E., W. DANIELL, H. STOCKBRIDGE et al. 1993. Immunologic, psychological, and neuropsychological factors in multiple chemical sensitivity: a controlled study. Ann. Intern. Med. **119:** 97–103.
9. BLACK, D.W., A. RATHE & R. GOLDSTEIN. 1990. Environmental illness—a controlled study of twenty-six subjects with 20th century diseases. JAMA **264:** 3166–3170.
10. BLACK, D.W., B.N. DOEBBELING, M.D. VOELKER et al. 1990. Multiple chemical sensitivity syndrome. Arch. Intern. Med. **160:** 1169–1176.
11. BECK, A.T. 1978. Beck Depression Inventory. The Psychological Corporation. Harcourt Brace Jovanovich. San Antonio, TX.
12. ROBINS, L.N. & J.E. HELZER. 1985. Diagnostic Interview Schedule (DIS) Version III-A. Washington University School of Medicine. St. Louis, MO.
13. FIEDLER, N. & H.M. KIPEN, Eds. 1997. Experimental approaches to chemical sensitivity. Environ. Health Perspect. **105:** 409–547.
14. FIEDLER, N., C. MACCIA & H. KIPEN. 1992. Evaluation of chemically sensitive patients. J. Occup. Med. **34:** 529–538.
15. FUKUDA, K., S.E. STRAUS, I. HICKIE et al. 1994. The chronic fatigue syndrome: a comprehensive approach to its definition and study. Am. College Physicians **121:** 953–959.
16. SZAREK, M.J., I.R. BELL & G.W. SCHWARTZ. 1997. Validation of a brief screening measure of environmental chemical sensitivity: the chemical odor intolerance index. J. Environ. Psychol. **17:** 345–351.
17. MOOLENAAR, R.L., B.J. HEFFLIN, D.L. ASHLEY et al. 1994. Methyl tertiary butyl ether in human blood after exposure to oxygenated fuel in Fairbanks, Alaska. Arch. Environ. Health **49:** 402–409.
18. FIEDLER, N., K. KELLY-MCNEIL, S. MOHR et al. 2000. Controlled human exposure to methyl tertiary butyl ether in gasoline: symptoms, psychophysiologic and neurobehavioral responses of self-reported sensitives. Environ. Health Perspect. **108:** 753–763.
19. DICK, R.B. 1995. Neurobehavioral assessment of occupationally relevant solvents and chemicals in humans. In Handbook of Neurotoxicology, pp. 217–322. Dekker. New York.
20. HEALTH EFFECTS INSTITUTE. 1996. The Potential Health Effects of Oxygenates Added to Gasoline: A Review of the Current Literature, pp. 1–158. Topsfield, MA.
21. LIOY, P.J., C.P. WEISEL, W-K. JO et al. 1994. Microenvironmental and personal measurements of methyl tertiary butyl ether (MTBE) associated with automobile use activities. J. Exposure Anal. Environ. Epidemiol. **4:** 427–447.
22. FIEDLER, N., G. LANGE, L. TIERSKY et al. 2000. Stressors, personality traits, and coping of Gulf War veterans with chronic fatigue. J. Psychosom. Res. **48:** 525–535.
23. WOLFE, J., S.P. PROCTOR, J.D. DAVIS et al. 1998. Health symptoms reported by Persian Gulf War veterans two years after return. Am. J. Ind. Med. **33:** 104–113.
24. RUDELL, B., M.C. LEDIN, U. HAMMARSTROM et al. 1996. Effects on symptoms and lung function in humans experimentally exposed to diesel exhaust. Occup. Environ. Med. **53:** 658–662.

25. DALTON, P., C.J. WYSOCKI, M.J. BRODY et al. 1997. Perceived odor, irritation, and health symptoms following short-term exposure to acetone. Am. J. Ind. Med. **31:** 558–569.
26. MILLS, K.C., K.M. PARKMAN & S.E. SPRUILL. 1996. A pc-based software test for measuring alcohol and drug effects in human subjects. Alcohol. Clin. Exp. Res. **20:** 1582–1591.
27. SPARKS, P.J., W. DANIELL, D.W. BLACK et al. 1994. Multiple chemical sensitivity syndrome: a clinical perspective. I. Case definition: theories of pathogenesis and research needs. J. Occup. Med. **36:** 718–730.
28. POLLET, C., B.J. NATELSON, G. LANGE et al. 1998. Medical evaluation of Persian Gulf veterans with fatigue and/or chemical sensitivity. J. Med. **29:** 101.
29. LEZNOFF, A. 1997. Provocative challenges in patients with multiple chemical sensitivity. J. Allergy Clin. Immunol. **99:** 438–442.
30. BINKLEY, K.E. & S. KUTCHER. 1997. Panic response to sodium lactate infusion in patients with multiple chemical sensitivity syndrome. J. Allergy Clin. Immunol. **99:** 570–574.
31. POONAI, N., M. ANTONY, K.E. BINKLEY et al. 2000. Carbon dioxide inhalation challenges in idiopathic environmental intolerance. J. Allergy Clin. Immunol. **105:** 358–363.
32. WATSON, D. & J.W. PENNEBAKER. 1989. Health complaints, stress, and distress: exploring the central role of negative affectivity. Psychol. Rev. **96:** 234–254.
33. COSTA, P.T. & R.R. MCCRAE. 1985. The NEO Personality Inventory. Psychological Assessment Resources, Inc. Odessa, FL.
34. REISS, S.P.R.A., D.M. GURSKY & R.J. MCNALLY. 1986. Anxiety sensitivity, anxiety frequency, and the prediction of fearfulness. Behav. Res. Ther. **24:** 1–8.
35. TAYLOR, S., W.J. KOCH & R.J. MCNALLY. 1992. How does anxiety sensitivity vary across the anxiety disorders? J. Anxiety Disord. **6:** 249–259.
36. HOLLOWAY, W. & R.J. MCNALLY. 1987. Effects of anxiety sensitivity on the response to hyperventilation. J. Abnorm. Psychol. **96:** 330–334.
37. LANGE, G., L. TIERSKY, J. DELUCA et al. 1999. Psychiatric diagnoses in Gulf War veterans with fatiguing illness. Psychiatry Res. **89:** 39–48.
38. SHUSTERMAN, D. 1992. Critical review: the health significance of environmental odor pollution. Arch. Environ. Health **47:** 76–87.
39. DOTY, R.L., D.A. DEEMS, R.E. FRYE et al. 1988. Olfactory sensitivity, nasal resistance, and autonomic function in patients with multiple chemical sensitivities. Arch. Otolaryngol. Head Neck Surg. **114:** 1422–1427.
40. CACCAPPOLO, E., H. KIPEN, K. KELLY-MCNEIL et al. 2000. Odor perception: multiple chemical sensitivities, chronic fatigue, and asthma. J. Occup. Environ. Med. **42:** 629–638.
41. BOLLA-WILSON, K., R.J. WILSON & M.L. BLEECKER. 1988. Conditioning of physical symptoms after neurotoxic exposure. J. Occup. Med. **30:** 684–686.
42. VAN DEN BERGH, O., K. STEGEN, I. VAN DIEST et al. 1999. Acquisition and extinction of somatic symptoms in response to odors: a Pavlovian paradigm relevant to multiple chemical sensitivity. Occup. Environ. Med. **56:** 295–301.
43. STAUDENMAYER, H. & J.C. SELNER. 1990. Neuropsychophysiology during relaxation in generalized, universal "allergic" reactivity to the environment: a comparison study. J. Psychosom. Res. **34:** 259–270.
44. OPIEKUN, R.E., K. KELLY-MCNEIL, S. KNASKO et al. 2000. A controlled short-term exposure study to investigate the odor differences among three different formulations of gasoline. Chem. Senses **25:** 395–400.
45. LAING, D.G. 1983. Natural sniffing gives optimum odor perception for humans. Perception **12:** 99–117.
46. KIPEN, H.M., W. HALLMAN, K. KELLY-MCNEIL et al. 1995. Measuring chemical sensitivity prevalence: a questionnaire for population studies. Am. J. Public Health **85:** 574–577.
47. STEWART, D.E. & J. RASKIN. 1985. Psychiatric assessment of patients with "20th century disease" ("total allergy syndrome"). Can. Med. Assoc. J. **133:** 1001–1006.
48. WOODS, J.E. 1989. Cost avoidance and productivity in owning and operating buildings. Occup. Med. State Art Rev. **4:** 753–770.
49. KREISS, K. 1990. The sick building syndrome: where is the epidemiologic basis? Am. J. Public Health **80:** 1172–1173.
50. DICK, R.B., J.V. SETZER, B.J. TAYLOR et al. 1989. Neurobehavioural effects of short duration exposures to acetone and methyl ethyl ketone. Br. J. Ind. Med. **46:** 111–121.

Sensitization Studies in Chemically Intolerant Individuals: Implications for Individual Difference Research

IRIS R. BELL,[a,b,c,d,f,h] CAROL M. BALDWIN,[d,g,h] AND GARY E. R. SCHWARTZ[c,d,e]

[b]*Program in Integrative Medicine, Department of Medicine;* [c]*Department of Psychiatry;* [d]*Department of Psychology;* [e]*Department of Neurology;* [f]*Department of Family and Community Medicine; and* [g]*Respiratory Sciences Center/Department of Medicine, University of Arizona, Tucson, Arizona, USA*

[h]*Department of Psychiatry, Southern Arizona Veterans Affairs Health Care System, Tucson, Arizona, USA*

ABSTRACT: Chemical intolerance (CI) is an individual difference trait in which persons report feeling ill in multiple physiological systems from low levels of a wide range of chemically unrelated environmental substances. This paper discusses the neural sensitization model for progressive host amplification of polysymptomatic responses elicited by chemical exposures following an initiating event. The sensitization model accommodates hypotheses for initiating and eliciting CI in human populations that involve both environmental chemicals and physical or psychological stressors. Recent studies in this laboratory have demonstrated sensitization in individuals with CI over repeated sessions for dependent variables such as electroencephalographic (EEG) activity and diastolic blood pressure. Psychological distress variables alone do not explain these findings. Individuals with CI and/or vulnerability to sensitization share specific characteristics, for example, female gender, certain genetic background (offspring of alcohol-preferring parents), and personal preference for high sugar/carbohydrate intake. Overall, the data suggest that the 15–30% of the general population who report heightened CI are highly sensitizable. Sensitizability may serve an adaptive, sentinel function in threatening environments with poor signal-to-noise ratios. However, as sensitization gradually shifts operating set points of physiological systems out of the normal range in response to allostatic load, this process may contribute to the development of chronic, polysymptomatic health conditions such as multiple chemical sensitivity and/or fibromyalgia. Individual response specificity and stereotypy rather than toxicant properties may determine which types of central, autonomic, and/or peripheral nervous system dysfunctions manifest at subclinical and clinical levels.

INTRODUCTION

Chemical intolerance (CI) is the subjective experience of negative hedonics and polysymptomatic illness from low levels of environmental chemicals.[1] CI is the core symptom of multiple chemical sensitivity (MCS), but it is also a prominent feature

[a]Address for correspondence: Iris R. Bell, M.D., Ph.D., Program in Integrative Medicine, University of Arizona Health Sciences Center, P.O. Box 245153, Tucson, AZ 85724-5153. Voice: 520-626-3512; fax: 520-626-3518.
IBELL@U.ARIZONA.EDU

in subsets of several other controversial conditions, for example, fibromyalgia, chronic fatigue syndrome, Persian Gulf syndrome, and occupational solvent-induced encephalopathy.[2] In different individuals, the manifestations may range from subclinical to clinical in their intensity and impact on quality of life.[1–4] However, a common aspect of CI-related conditions is that the concomitant symptoms emerge in unique patterns for each individual and typically involve the systemic, organism level of organization (e.g., fatigue, cognitive problems, headache, palpitations, gastrointestinal distress, and joint pains) more than a single bodily subsystem.[3–6] The symptom pictures that chemically unrelated agents elicit are often stereotypic for the individual rather than specific to the toxicants' properties.[2,5]

As a result, investigations of individual differences in persons affected with CI offer greater potential for understanding the nature of the problem than do those of chemical toxicity per se. Psychiatric labels for clinical conditions involving CI (e.g., somatoform disorder) offer little toward understanding the possible mechanisms by which symptoms occur.[1,2] The most applicable concepts derive from the following: (i) basic research in the neurosciences on host response sensitization (amplification over time) to repeated, intermittent exposures to substances and/or environmental stressors;[7,8] (ii) McEwen and Stellar's[9,10] model for the effects of repeated environmental stressors on shifting operating set points for multiple subsystems out of the normal range, that is, allostatic load leading to chronic disease; and (iii) Lacey's[11,12] human psychophysiology research on individual response specificity and stereotypic patterning across multiple different stimuli or stressors.

For purposes of this discussion, the term "stressor" refers to an environmental factor of any category (chemical, physical, or psychological) that the individual experiences as significant and thus places demands for adaptation upon the organism as a whole.[7] Sensitization is the progressive amplification of host responses to repeated, intermittent exposures to an initiating stimulus or stressor.[8] Allostasis is "the regulation of the internal milieu through dynamic change in a number of hormonal and physical variables in which there is anything but steady state."[9] The compensatory and anticipatory nervous system and neuroendocrine changes that produce short-term coping for the individual lead to "allostatic load" and long-term costs from development of chronic disease. Sensitization is one pathway into allostatic load. The manifestations of chronic disease for persons with CI reflect individual differences in genetic and gender potential for dysfunction in different physiological subsystems interacting with the current environment.[1]

NEURAL SENSITIZATION IN CHEMICAL INTOLERANCE: THE SENSITIZABLE INDIVIDUAL

Sensitization is a mechanism for host response amplification over time. Initially, novel stimuli with salience or threat for the organism can set sensitization into motion. Repeated, intermittent exposures to the same or to cross-sensitizing stimuli can subsequently elicit the enhanced responses. Drugs, environmental toxicants, exogenous physical or psychological stressors, and endogenous mediators can all initiate the process.[1,7,8] Basic researchers have documented sensitization of behavioral, neurochemical, hormonal, autonomic, and immune system functions.[7] Molecular mechanisms of sensitization may involve persistent changes in cell function, but not necessarily structure.[13,14] In human studies, investigators have demonstrated sensitization from repeated exposures to ingested alcohol[15] and stimulant drugs.[16]

Review of the animal literature reveals certain individual differences that predict a greater susceptibility to sensitization.[2,4] These include female gender, genetic line (substance-preferring parents), spontaneous preference for sucrose, hyperreactivity to novel environments, and lateral asymmetry in response to a test dose of the initiating agent. In parallel, the data consistently show that persons with CI, in both clinical and nonclinical samples, are primarily women (70–80%).[1–5] The replicated presence of the gender finding prompted our laboratory to evaluate populations with CI for parallels to the other individual differences listed above.

The findings indicate that persons with CI score higher than controls on questionnaires regarding carbohydrate craving[17] and endorse family, especially paternal, histories of drug and/or alcohol problems.[2,4,18,19] Interestingly, sober alcoholics also exhibit an extreme preference for highly concentrated sucrose solutions.[20] Sons of male alcoholics demonstrate sensitization and/or failure to habituate autonomic nervous system responses such as finger pulse amplitude or skin conductance over repeated sessions of alcohol ingestion.[15] Notably, sons of alcoholics also show cardiovascular patterns of hyperreactivity to cognitive stressors that predict susceptibility to hypertension and cardiac disease later in life.[21] In another overlap, our studies have shown that persons with CI report increased parental histories of heart disease[22] and that elderly with CI sensitize heart rate and diastolic blood pressure in the laboratory over time.[23]

Thus, the data suggest that persons with CI may be more sensitizable in multiple subsystems. The manifestations of the sensitizability vary, driven by individual differences in genetic- and gender-related vulnerability of various target organs and by the prevailing environmental context. Within the different branches of the nervous system, for example, central nervous system (CNS) sensitization can lead to cravings for certain exogenous substances such as foods;[24] autonomic nervous system (ANS) sensitization can lead to progressive increases in heart rate, blood pressure, visceral contractions, sweating response, or pupillary response;[15,25] and peripheral nervous system (PNS) sensitization can lead to progressive increases in muscle tension with resultant chronic pain.[26–28] It is also unlikely that the sensitization occurs in only one branch of the nervous system at a time. Basic research, for example, shows that the development of a condition such as chronic pain requires involvement and interaction of central and peripheral nervous systems for sensitization to take hold.[28] At a clinical level, the predicted results are polysymptomatic conditions affecting multiple behaviors and various organ subsystems of affected individuals. The manifestations at any given time, however, vary in terms of the capacity for response in the affected subsystems of a given organism.[29,30]

INTERACTIONS OF INDIVIDUAL DIFFERENCES IN GENDER AND GENETICS

Sensitization

How might gender and genetics interact to modulate the manifestations of sensitizability? What differences, for instance, might being a daughter versus a son of an alcoholic make? The potential interaction of the gender and genetic differences in CI offers a way to make sense of many seemingly diverse empirical findings reported in the CI population—that is, much research on sons of alcoholics indicates that these males have an increased risk for developing alcoholism. In contrast, the epidemiological evidence is that adopted-away daughters of alcoholics exhibit somatoform disorders, not alcoholism, at increased rates.[31] Many different researchers have observed increased somatic symptomatology in CI-related disorders, for example, MCS, fibromyalgia, chronic fatigue syndrome, and Persian Gulf syndrome.[32-35]

Consequently, it is possible that the subset of women with CI who have family histories of substance abuse have inherited an enhanced capacity for sensitization, but one that leads in part to craving certain foods rather than alcohol per se.[3,4,6] Previous research in several different laboratories indicates that MCS patients and persons with CI have higher scores on rating scales not only for somatization,[36,37] but also increased reports of specific food cravings and specific food intolerances.[3-6] CI probands themselves report extremely poor tolerance for small amounts of alcohol and prescription and recreational drugs.[3-6] Those persons with CI also score higher than controls for sensitivity to a wide range of external and internal stimuli, including the Anxiety Sensitivity Inventory, the Barsky Somatic Symptom Amplification Scale, and the Noise Sensitivity Scale.[38]

Thus, daughters of alcoholics may inherit a capacity for sensitization, but manifest the CNS sensitization differently from their brothers, that is, develop cravings for sweets or other foods rather than for alcohol and develop behavioral hypersensitivity to many different exogenous and endogenous stimuli. Furthermore, the women who sensitize will exhibit more adverse somatic reactions to various exogenous substances because of greater capacity to sensitize autonomic and peripheral nervous system physiological functions than their male counterparts.

Allostatic Load

When the organism makes chronic, dynamic adjustments to cope with the impact of acute stressors, the price of this adaptability is allostatic load.[9,10] In time, allostatic load can lead to chronic diseases.[10] We have replicated the finding of increased life stress ratings for persons with CI as compared with those of normal controls, starting in childhood.[6,17,38] Women with CI also report prior histories of sexual, emotional, and/or physical abuse at higher rates than do normals.[17] Therefore, the data suggest that a subset of persons with CI experience environmental stressors over many years. These stressors could provide an initiating stimulus for sensitization that subsequent cross-sensitizing stressors such as low-level chemicals later in life could then elicit.[32] In animals, higher estrogen:progesterone ratios facilitate neural sensitization,[39] while higher testosterone levels inhibit neural sensitization.[40]

As a result, sensitized women would be pushing their operating set points for ANS and PNS function out of the normal ranges more readily than would sensitized men in response to exogenous stimuli of all types. In anticipation of larger and larger (sensitized) responses to environmental stressors, the organism as a whole would experience greater and greater chronic disturbances of normal functions. In short, allostatic load from adapting to amplified stressor reactivity should lead to chronic health disorders sooner in more sensitizable than in less sensitizable individuals. FIGURE 1 summarizes the potential flow of events.

Sensitizing stimuli → Allostatic load → Multisystem dysfunctions → Clinical conditions

FIGURE 1. Sensitization induces allostatic disturbances and gradual evolution of clinical conditions.

Data from our laboratory show diastolic blood pressure sensitization in both middle-aged women[17] and elderly persons with CI.[23] It is striking that the average age of onset of clinically significant difficulties in MCS patients is usually in the thirties to forties.[5,6] Middle age may be a point in the life span when the allostatic load begins to impair adaptability to environmental stressors. It follows that a testable hypothesis is that CI in prospective studies will be a risk factor for earlier onset of frank hypertension and associated cardiovascular diseases.

It may also be that CI confers greater persistent impact on physiology than do negative life experiences from exogenous psychosocial stressors alone. For example, women with CI (but no sexual abuse histories) and women with sexual abuse histories (but no CI) both show EEG alpha sensitization to low-level chemical exposures in the laboratory. However, the CI group has higher levels of EEG alpha at all time points throughout the three-session study as compared with both the abused women and the normal controls.[41] In other words, the CI women never get their EEG patterns back to a normal baseline, even in the absence of an eliciting chemical exposure. Allostatic load may have changed the set point for their CNS function.

Ingesting alcohol, drugs, and even foods might become aversive because of the greater vulnerability for sensitization of somatic symptomatology in women compared with men. Physical and psychological stress could also add to the dysfunction by furthering the ANS and PNS sensitization in the women more intensively than in the men. TABLE 1 summarizes a small number of possible examples of manifestations that nervous system sensitization could facilitate. These dysfunctions fall along a continuum; at some arbitrary cutoffs, physicians define the severity as sufficient to merit a clinical label.

We recently tested elements of the model above by comparing fibromyalgia (FM) patients with and without CI versus normal controls. Consistent with the hypotheses

TABLE 1. Examples of possible subclinical and clinical manifestations of nervous system sensitization in highly sensitizable individuals

	Central nervous system	Autonomic nervous system	Peripheral nervous system
Subclinical	Alcohol craving Drug craving Food craving	Blood pressure and heart rate hyperreactivity to stressors	Painful neck or back muscle spasms
	Anxiety	Abdominal pain Nasal congestion & discharge	
Clinical	Alcoholism Drug addiction Bulimia or obesity Panic disorder	Hypertension Cardiac arrhythmias Irritable bowel Vasomotor rhinitis	Torticollis Chronic back pain

above, FM with CI had the highest scores on the Carbohydrate Addicts Test, the SCL-90-R Somatization and Obsessiveness Subscales, the Limbic Symptom Checklist Sensory and Behavior Subscales, and the Harm Avoidance dimension of the Tridimensional Personality Questionnaire.[42] The FM with CI also showed progressive increases in EEG beta-1 activity (12–14 Hz, a frequency typically associated with behavioral activation or arousal) over three sessions of sucrose ingestion, not seen in the FM-only and normal groups.[43]

CHEMICAL INTOLERANCE PHENOMENOLOGY AND INDIVIDUAL RESPONSE STEREOTYPY

As previously reviewed in detail, CI is a symptom reported to varying degrees in persons with clinical conditions as well as in approximately 15–30% of the general population.[1,2] CI can be merely annoying or completely disabling in its impact on quality of life. Moreover, as described above, the environmental sensitivities of persons with CI frequently extend far beyond chemicals to multiple other factors. These include common foods, prescription and recreational drugs, noise, light, and certain tastes.[4,5] Models for explaining CI-related illnesses must consider these observations as well.

For example, at least 25% of patients with MCS have no clinical psychiatric disorders.[32] Women with depression and CI have higher resting levels of EEG alpha activity (8–12 Hz, typically associated with relaxed wakefulness) than do those with depression only or normals.[44] The women with both depression and CI also sensitize (progressively increase) alpha activity at rest and during chemical exposures over repeated laboratory sessions, whereas comparison groups with depression only or normals habituate under the same conditions. Therefore, psychiatric illness per se cannot be a sufficient explanation for CI or MCS. Psychiatric illness is not necessary for CI to be present, and the addition of CI to psychiatric disturbance leads to CNS physiology that differs significantly from the physiology of persons with the psychiatric disturbance alone.

Notably, again consistent with a CNS sensitization model for CI, sons and daughters of alcoholics do exhibit a similar increase in EEG alpha activity compared with offspring of nonalcoholics.[45,46] Although there is a great deal of psychiatric comorbidity in alcoholism and somatization disorder, it is not necessary to have any such comorbidity to have the core condition. *By analogy, we propose that CI is more related by genetics and biological susceptibility to alcoholism (or, at least, to the sensitization-relevant characteristics of alcoholism) than to any affective disorder per se.*

In addition, we have repeatedly found increased rates of physician-diagnosed breast and ovarian cysts in women with CI.[6,38] Other investigators have already associated limbic nervous system sensitization to hypothalamic dysfunction and consequent alterations in reproductive hormone milieu at the local tissues.[47] In other words, sensitization could contribute meaningfully to breast and ovarian cyst formation in women with CI by changing hormone status. It behooves researchers who propose other possible mechanisms for CI to address the whole clinical picture and the available data in the context of their models.

Importantly, each finding represents data on group averages and summary statistics. It is possible to find persons with CI who do not have a given trait, behavior, symptom, personal diagnosis, or family history. Thus, any given observation becomes a clue, but only a permissive rather than essential aspect of the problem. The implication of this point is that the total population of persons with CI is highly heterogeneous. CI is manifest as the outcome of some final common pathway to which multiple upstream, interactive variables contribute. Potential mechanisms for CI are likely complex and multivariate in nature. It may be necessary to utilize sophisticated methodological approaches such as latent variable modeling to capture the entire process in group studies.[48]

However, the systemic patterning of symptoms that persons with CI show is not specific to particular chemicals, foods, stressors, or other factors. Such patterns instead may reflect the individual response specificity and stereotypy that Lacey *et al*.[11,12] postulated and demonstrated in the field of psychophysiology almost 50 years ago. Individual response stereotypy involves the concept that individuals react to exogenous stressors in characteristic ways, with maximal response in specific physiological subsystems and not others.[49] Even though some stimuli or activities can in general elicit arousal, while others evoke relaxation, the subsystems showing the largest response may vary in accord with the individual's potential for responding in specific physiological subsystems more than with the stimulus properties per se.

For example, classic psychophysiology studies demonstrated that it was the same physiological variable in a given normal individual that responded the most to any of four different stressors (cold pressor, mental arithmetic, letter association, hyperventilation).[12] In patient studies, Moos and Engel[50] found that hypertensives exhibited greater blood pressure responses, whereas arthritics showed greater electromyographic signal increases to the same stressors. Furthermore, when multiple physiological subsystems were recorded simultaneously, researchers showed particular patterns of responses within the various subsystems of a given individual across all types of stimuli (e.g., mental arithmetic, proverb interpretation, cold pressor, exercise, loud noise).[51] Such observations suggest that the unique symptom patterns of different individuals with CI may reflect varying degrees of sensitization in various subsystems and functions.

CONCLUSIONS

The operative factor determining the manifestations of CI-related conditions is the individual, not the toxicant or the stressor. A potentially productive focus for research should be the patterns of nervous system dysfunction (CNS, ANS, PNS) that emerge in the course of sensitization to exogenous stimuli. In persons prone to CI, allostatic load may extract a heavy toll in the gradual development of disorders in various subsystems where multiple set points have moved out of the normal range of function because of sensitization to multiple exogenous and endogenous stimuli. Existing data also indicate a need to extend the construct of individual response specificity and stereotypy to research on CI in order to begin sorting out the heterogeneous presentations of affected persons.

CI offers a possible missing conceptual link between the basic and clinical neuroscience of sensitization, the allostatic load model of chronic disease development, and individual difference psychophysiology. Sensitization per se may provide the individual and/or social groupings (e.g., family or coworkers) to which she/he belongs with an early warning system for danger or threat from the environment in the short term. However, the long-term cost to the individual for this sentinel capability may be chronic physiological dysfunctions and clinical disorders. It is feasible and reasonable to proceed with rigorous tests of the hypotheses that derive from this model.

ACKNOWLEDGMENTS

This work was supported in part by grants from the National Dairy Council, the Environmental Health Foundation, the Wallace Genetic Foundation, the American Fibromyalgia Syndrome Association, the U.S. Department of Veterans Affairs, and the National Institutes of Health (Grant No. K24AT00057-01 to I. R. Bell).

REFERENCES

1. BELL, I.R., C.M. BALDWIN & G.E.R. SCHWARTZ. 1998. Illness from low levels of environmental chemicals: relevance to chronic fatigue syndrome and fibromyalgia. Am. J. Med. Suppl. **105**(3A): 74S–82S.
2. BELL, I.R., C.M. BALDWIN, M. FERNANDEZ & G.E. SCHWARTZ. 1999. Neural sensitization model for multiple chemical sensitivity: overview of theory and empirical evidence. Toxicol. Ind. Health **15**: 295–304.
3. MILLER, C.S. 1996. Chemical sensitivity: symptom, syndrome, or mechanism for disease? Toxicology **111**: 69–86.
4. BELL, I.R., E. HARDIN, C.M. BALDWIN & G.E. SCHWARTZ. 1995. Increased limbic system symptomatology and sensitizability of young adults with chemical and noise sensitivities. Environ. Res. **70**: 84–97.
5. ASHFORD, N.A. & C.S. MILLER. 1998. Chemical Exposures: Low Levels and High Stakes. Second edition. Van Nostrand–Reinhold. Princeton, NJ.
6. BELL, I.R., J.M. PETERSON & G.E. SCHWARTZ. 1995. Medical histories and psychological profiles of middle-aged women with and without self-reported illness from environmental chemicals. J. Clin. Psychiatry **56**: 151–160.
7. ANTELMAN, S.M. 1994. Time-dependent sensitization in animals: a possible model of multiple chemical sensitivity in humans. Toxicol. Ind. Health **10**: 335–342.
8. SORG, B.A., J.R. WILLIS, R.E. SEE *et al.* 1998. Repeated low-level formaldehyde exposure produces cross-sensitization to cocaine: possible relevance to chemical sensitivity in humans. Neuropsychopharmacology **18**: 385–394.
9. MCEWEN, B.S. & E. STELLAR. 1993. Stress and the individual: mechanisms leading to disease. Arch. Intern. Med. **153**: 2093–2101.
10. SCHULKIN, J., B.S. MCEWEN & P.W. GOLD. 1994. Allostasis, amygdala, and anticipatory angst. Neurosci, Biobehav. Rev. **18**: 385–396.
11. LACEY, J.I., D.E. BATEMAN & R. VAN LEHN. 1953. Autonomic response specificity: an experimental study. Psychosom. Med. **15**: 8–21.
12. LACEY, J.I. 1959. Psychophysiological approaches to the evaluation of psychotherapeutic process and outcome. *In* Research in Psychotherapy, pp. 173–192. American Psychological Association. Washington, D.C.
13. POST, R.M. 1992. Transduction of psychosocial stress into the neurobiology of recurrent affective disorder. Am. J. Psychiatry **149**: 999–1010.
14. KALIVAS, P.W. & J. STEWART. 1991. Dopamine transmission in the initiation and expression of drug- and stress-induced sensitization of motor activity. Brain Res. Rev. **16**: 223–244.
15. NEWLIN, D.B. & J.B. THOMSON. 1991. Chronic tolerance and sensitization to alcohol in sons of alcoholics. Alcohol. Clin. Exp. Res. **15**: 399–405.

16. STRAKOWSKI, S.M., K.W. SAX, M.J. SETTERS & P.E. KECK. 1996. Enhanced response to repeated *d*-amphetamine challenge: evidence for behavioral sensitization in humans. Biol. Psychiatry **40:** 872–880.
17. BELL, I.R., C.M. BALDWIN, L.G. RUSSEK *et al.* 1998. Early life stress, negative paternal relationships, and current chemical odor intolerance in middle-aged women: support for a neural sensitization model. J. Women's Health **7:** 1135–1147.
18. BELL, I.R., C.M. BALDWIN, M. FERNANDEZ & G.E.R. SCHWARTZ. 2000. Paternal alcoholism in multiple chemical sensitivity: a genetic link with the biology of neural sensitization? J. Nerv. Ment. Dis. In press.
19. BLACK, D.W., C. OKIISHI, J. GABEL & S. SCHLOSSER. 1999. Psychiatric illness in the first-degree relatives of persons reporting multiple chemical sensitivities. Toxicol. Ind. Health **15:** 410–414.
20. KAMPOV-POLEVOY, A., J.C. GARBUTT & D. JANOWSKY. 1997. Evidence for preference for a high-concentration sucrose solution in alcoholic men. Am. J. Psychiatry **154:** 269–270.
21. HARDEN, P.W. & R.O. PIHL. 1995. Cognitive function, cardiovascular reactivity, and behavior in boys at high risk for alcoholism. J. Abnorm. Psychol. **104:** 94–103.
22. BALDWIN, C.M. & I.R. BELL. 1998. Increased cardiopulmonary disease risk in a community-based sample with chemical odor intolerance: implications for women's health and health care utilization. Arch. Environ. Health **53:** 347–353.
23. BELL, I.R., G.E. SCHWARTZ, R.R. BOOTZIN & J.K. WYATT. 1997. Time-dependent sensitization of heart rate and blood pressure over multiple laboratory sessions in elderly individuals with chemical odor intolerance. Arch. Environ. Health **52:** 6–17.
24. ROBINSON, T.E. & K.C. BERRIDGE. 1993. The neural basis of drug craving: an incentive-sensitization theory of addiction. Brain Res. Rev. **18:** 247–291.
25. YOSHIDA, K., A. MORIMOTOR, T. MAKISUMI & N. MURAKAMI. 1993. Cardiovascular, thermal, and behavioral sensitization to methamphetamine in freely moving rats. J. Pharmacol. Exp. Ther. **267:** 1538–1543.
26. URSIN, H.., I.M. ENDRESEN, E.M. HALAND & N. MJELLEM. 1993. Sensitization: a neurobiological theory for muscle pain. *In* Progress in Fibromyalgia and Myofascial Pain, pp. 413–427. Elsevier. Amsterdam/New York.
27. URSIN, H. 1997. Sensitization, somatization, and subjective health complaints. Int. J. Behav. Med. **4:** 105–116.
28. CODERRE, T.J., J. KATZ, A.L. VACCARINO & R. MELZACK. 1993. Contribution of central neuroplasticity to pathological pain: review of clinical and experimental evidence. Pain **52:** 259–285.
29. WENGER, M.A., D.R. COLEMAN, T.D. CULLEN & B.T. ENGEL. 1961. Autonomic response specificity. Psychosom. Med. **23:** 185–193.
30. STERNBACH, R.A. 1966. Principles of Psychophysiology. Academic Press. New York.
31. BOHMAN, M., C.R. CLONINGER, A.L. VON KNORRING & S. SIGVARDSSON. 1984. An adoption study of somatoform disorders. III. Cross-fostering analysis and genetic relationship to alcoholism and criminality. Arch. Gen. Psychiatry **41(9):** 872–878.
32. FIEDLER, N., H.M. KIPEN, J. DELUCA *et al.* 1996. A controlled comparison of multiple chemical sensitivities and chronic fatigue syndrome. Psychosom. Med. **58:** 38–49.
33. HUDSON, J.I., D.L. GOLDENBERG, H.G. POPE *et al.* 1992. Comorbidity of fibromyalgia with medical and psychiatric disorders. Am. J. Med. **92:** 363–367.
34. JOHNSON, S.K., J. DELUCA & B.H. NATELSON. 1996. Assessing somatization disorder in the chronic fatigue syndrome. Psychosom. Med. **58:** 50–57.
35. BELL, I.R., L. WARG-DAMIANI, C.M. BALDWIN *et al.* 1998. Self-reported chemical sensitivity and wartime chemical exposures in Gulf War veterans with and without decreased global health ratings. Mil. Med. **163:** 725–732.
36. BLACK, D.W., A. RATHE & R.B. GOLDSTEIN. 1990. Environmental illness: a controlled study of 26 subjects with "20th century disease". JAMA **264:** 3166–3170.
37. SIMON, G.E., W.J. KATON & P.J. SPARKS. 1990. Allergic to life: psychological factors in environmental illness. Am. J. Psychiatry **147:** 901–906.
38. BELL, I.D., C.S. MILLER, G.E. SCHWARTZ *et al.* 1996. Neuropsychiatric and somatic characteristics of young adults with and without self-reported chemical odor intolerance and chemical sensitivity. Arch. Environ. Health **51:** 9–21.

39. PERIS, J., N. DECAMBRE, M.L. COLEMAN-HARDEE & J.W. SIMKINS. 1991. Estradiol enhances behavioral sensitization to cocaine and amphetamine-stimulated striatal [^{3}H] dopamine release. Brain Res. **566:** 255–264.
40. ROBINSON, T.E., J.B. BECKER & S.K. PRESTY. 1982. Long-term facilitation of amphetamine-induced rotational behavior and striatal dopamine release produced by a single exposure to amphetamine: sex differences. Brain Res. **253:** 231–241.
41. FERNANDEZ, M., I.R. BELL & G.E.R. SCHWARTZ. 1999. Sensitization during chemical exposure in women with and without chemical sensitivity of unknown etiology. Toxicol. Ind. Health **15:** 305–312.
42. BELL, I.D., C.M. BALDWIN, E. STOLTZ et al. 2000. Concomitant environmental chemical intolerance modifies the neurobehavioral presentation of women with fibromyalgia. Submitted.
43. BELL, I.R., C.M. BALDWIN, E. STOLTZ et al. 2000. EEG beta 1 oscillation and sucrose sensitization in fibromyalgia with chemical intolerance. Int. J. Neurosci. In press.
44. BELL, I.R., G.E. SCHWARTZ, E.E. HARDIN et al. 1998. Differential resting qEEG alpha patterns in women with environmental chemical intolerance, depressives, and normals. Biol. Psychiatry **43:** 376–388.
45. EHLERS, C., E. PHILLIPS & B.L. PARRY. 1996. Electrophysiological findings during the menstrual cycle in women with and without late luteal phase dysphoric disorder: relationship to risk for alcoholism? Biol. Psychiatry **39:** 720–732.
46. EHLERS, C.L. & M.A. SCHUCKIT. 1991. Evaluation of EEG alpha activity in sons of alcoholics. Neuropsychopharmacology **4:** 199–205.
47. HERZOG, A.G., M.M. SEIBEL, D. SCHOMER et al. 1984. Temporal lobe epilepsy: an extrahypothalamic pathogenesis for polycystic ovarian syndrome? Neurology **34:** 1389–1393.
48. NORMAN, G.R. & D.L. STREINER. 2000. Principal components and factor analysis, path analysis, and structural equation modeling. *In* Biostatistics: The Bare Essentials, pp. 163–200. Decker, Inc. Hamilton, Canada.
49. ANDREASII, J.L. 1995. Psychophysiology: Human Behavior and Physiological Response. Third edition. Erlbaum. Hillsdale, NJ.
50. MOOS, R.H. & B.T. ENGEL. 1962. Psychophysiological reactions in hypertensive and arthritic patients. J. Psychosom. Res. **6:** 227–241.
51. ENGEL, B.T. 1960. Stimulus-response and individual response specificity. Arch. Gen. Psychiatry **2:** 305–313.

The Iowa Follow-up of Chemically Sensitive Persons

DONALD W. BLACK,[a,b] CHRISTOPHER OKIISHI,[c] AND STEVEN SCHLOSSER[b]

[b]*Department of Psychiatry, University of Iowa College of Medicine, Iowa City, Iowa, USA*
[c]*University of Iowa Health Care, Iowa City, Iowa, USA*

ABSTRACT: Clinical symptoms and self-reported health status in persons reporting multiple chemical sensitivities (MCS) are presented from a 9-year follow-up study. Eighteen (69%) subjects from a sample of 26 persons originally interviewed in 1988 were followed up in 1997 and given structured interviews and self-report questionnaires. In terms of psychiatric diagnosis, 15 (83%) met DSM-IV criteria for a lifetime mood disorder, 10 (56%) for a lifetime anxiety disorder, and 10 (56%) for a lifetime somatoform disorder. Seven (39%) of subjects met criteria for a personality disorder using the Personality Diagnostic Questionnaire-IV. Self-report data from the Illness Behavior Questionnaire and Symptom Checklist-90-Revised show little change from 1988. The 10 most frequent complaints attributed to MCS were headache, memory loss, forgetfulness, sore throat, joint aches, trouble thinking, shortness of breath, back pain, muscle aches, and nausea. Global assessment showed that 2 (11%) had "remitted", 8 (45%) were "much" or "very much" improved, 6 (33%) were "improved", and 2 (11%) were "unchanged/worse". Mean scores on the SF-36 health survey showed that, compared to U.S. population means, subjects reported worse physical functioning, more bodily pain, worse general health, worse social functioning, and more emotional-role impairment; self-reported mental health was better than the U.S. population mean. All subjects maintained a belief that they had MCS; 16 (89%) acknowledged that the diagnosis was controversial. It is concluded that the subjects remain strongly committed to their diagnosis of MCS. Most have improved since their original interview, but many remain symptomatic and continue to report ongoing lifestyle changes.

The multiple chemical sensitivity syndrome (MCS) is a condition that has been attributed to extreme sensitivity to low concentrations of chemicals tolerated by most people. The diagnosis, often referred to as "environmental illness", remains controversial and is not generally recognized by mainstream medicine.[1–3] Recently, the World Health Organization[4] held a conference to consider MCS. Although conceding that the validity of MCS had not been established, conferees urged that research continue. They proposed the neutral term, "idiopathic environmental intolerance", because many persons diagnosed with MCS are thought to develop symptoms in response to environmental agents other than chemicals.

---

[a]Address for correspondence: Psychiatry Research–MEB, University of Iowa College of Medicine, Iowa City, IA 52242-1000.

Persons diagnosed with MCS are generally polysymptomatic and report sensitivities to multiple unrelated substances.[5] Environmental physicians, a group of practitioners who claim special expertise in diagnosing and treating MCS, believe that the disorder is widespread and is responsible for substantial suffering and disability in the general population. Cross-sectional studies[6–8] indicate that persons diagnosed with MCS have impaired social and occupational adjustment and suffer other indices of disability, including a greater likelihood of being considered medically disabled, receiving disability and unemployment compensation, having a higher frequency of physician visits and emergency department visits, and having more inpatient hospital days. In a recent study of quality of life and MCS, Black et al.[9] used the Medical Outcome Studies Short Form-36[10] and found that subjects meeting criteria for MCS had lower scores on each of the 10 subscales than did comparison subjects, including physical functioning, bodily pain, vitality, social function, and emotional and mental health scales. Other researchers have suggested that MCS is life-threatening and that subjects with MCS are at great risk for early death; these allegations have never been substantiated.

Despite the value of follow-up studies and the concerns of environmental physicians about the potential long-term consequences of MCS, longitudinal data on MCS are scant. Terr[8] concluded that 96% of 50 subjects with MCS were unchanged or worse at a 2-year follow-up. More recently, Lax and Henneberger[11] reported on 35 persons diagnosed with MCS followed in an occupational health clinic for nearly 1.5 years. They reported that 46% of the subjects improved, even though they had a mean of 7.4 more symptoms than at their initial evaluation.

THE IOWA FOLLOW-UP STUDY

We recently reported findings from a 9-year follow-up of persons diagnosed with MCS.[12] The study began in 1988 with an intensive psychiatric assessment of 26 persons diagnosed "environmentally ill" by a clinical ecologist. They were recruited from support groups and clinic populations and by word of mouth. The study's purpose was to assess their symptoms, treatments, and attitudes towards both conventional medicine and chemical sensitivity. Black et al.[6,13] assessed subjects for both major mental (axis I) and personality (axis II) disorders and administered questionnaires to assess mood, personality, somatic concern, and hypochondriacal behavior. The data were contrasted to those of a group of persons from the general population approximately matched for age and gender. In brief, the subjects with MCS indicated a strong interest in their diagnosis, were mostly satisfied with their clinical ecologist's care, and were dissatisfied with conventional medicine. They reported varying treatments, including dietary restrictions, avoidance of offending agents, and physical treatments such as neutralizing injections. Using the Diagnostic Interview Schedule,[14] Black et al. reported that 65% met lifetime criteria for mood, anxiety, or somatoform disorders compared with 28% of 46 age- and gender-matched community controls. They assessed personality disorder using the Structured Interview for DSM-III Personality Disorders (SIDP) and found that 17 (74%) met criteria for at least one personality disorder, compared with 28% of a control group. Subjects with MCS also met criteria for a greater number of personality disorders (1.7 vs. 0.3) and a greater number of abnormal personality traits (16.8 vs. 10.7) than comparison sub-

TABLE 1. Characteristics of subjects with MCS followed up in 1997

Age, mean, years (SD)	60 (14)
% female	89
% married	83
Education, mean, years (SD)	14 (3)

jects. Of the 11 personality disorder types assessed, the schizotypal, histrionic, narcissistic, dependent, avoidant, and compulsive types were all overrepresented. When axis I and axis II conditions were combined, only 3 subjects (13%) failed to meet criteria for any disorder. Black *et al.* concluded that chemically sensitive persons frequently suffer from unrecognized psychological distress, which probably accounts for some or all of the symptoms attributed to environmental illness by their clinical ecologist.

In 1997, Black and colleagues reinterviewed 18 (69%) of the original subjects. By this time, their mean age was 60 years, with a range from 36 to 87 years (see TABLE 1). Seven subjects refused to participate and 1 could not be located, although she was still living. None of the subjects had died, despite their advanced age. All still believed that they were chemically sensitive, yet only 7 (39%) remained under a clinical ecologist's care. All but 2 subjects acknowledged that their diagnosis was controversial. In general, subjects used fewer treatments in 1997 than in 1998, in particular primrose oil, charcoal/cotton filter masks, or cleansing enemas. Fifteen subjects (83%) had modified their home to make it safer; more than half (56%) reported having received treatment in a special hospital for the environmentally ill. Subjects showed a strong interest in their condition; all acknowledged reading about MCS and 11 (62%) were currently attending support groups. All but 2 reported being pleased with their current MCS treatment program.

Case Example

The following case report from the Iowa cohort shows the continuity of illness belief over a 9-year period.

June, a 50-year-old homemaker, reported that she suffered from "environmental allergies", a diagnosis made 4 years earlier by a clinical ecologist and confirmed later at a clinic near Chicago specializing in the care of the chemically sensitive. June believed her problem started with farm chemicals 30 years earlier, when widespread spraying of the pesticide DDT took place. She reported a variety of symptoms, including weakness, fatigue, poor concentration, and memory impairment, which, she said, worsened when exposed to certain foods, perfumes, gasoline fumes, and cooking and other odors. To alleviate her symptoms, June minimized her contact with offending chemicals and, as a result, seldom left her home for fear of having a "reaction". She had recently given up her work as a schoolteacher and had applied for workers' compensation.

In addition to avoiding chemicals, her clinical ecologist had recommended a special rotation diet and had prescribed alkali salts and calcium carbonate. She was advised to take sublingual "neutralizing" drops following exposure to exhaust fumes, phenols, formaldehyde, or other chemicals. She was also diagnosed with "yeast" disease and took oral nystatin and received weekly injections to increase her defense against *C. albicans*. She turned her bedroom into a "safe" room that contained only her bed and special air purifiers. When reading newspapers, she wore a special air filter mask. June had serendipitously discovered that she could obtain significant relief by holding a pendulum that, when spinning clockwise, would counterbalance her excessive and abnormal internal magnetic forces.

June was pleased with her diagnosis of chemical sensitivity and had been unhappy with her conventional medical care practitioners. She had become very interested in her condition, joined support groups, and read widely about MCS. She was unhappy to have had to pay out of her own pocket a $15,000 bill for a 1-week stay at an "environmental control unit" at a special hospital.

June was a friendly woman who appeared her age and reported that her emotional adjustment was excellent. She acknowledged having been psychiatrically hospitalized 20 years earlier for unexplained left arm pain and underwent Sodium Amytal interviews for the apparent conversion disorder. She had been referred to our psychiatrists 3 years earlier to rule out agoraphobia because her lifestyle was severely restricted. She had presented the psychiatrists with a 12-page typed, single-spaced report on her medical condition. The psychiatrists diagnosed her with somatization disorder.

In 1997, we found June, now 59, living in the same home in a small Iowa town. She was friendly and neatly groomed. June explained that she continued to have significant problems with chemical sensitivity. Using the researcher's metal pen to sign the consent document reportedly gave her a toothache. She explained that she had extreme sensitivity to most metals and thus had all of her mercury amalgam dental filings removed. She used wooden utensils and cooked with Pyrex dishes. She also had the heating coils on her stove replaced with under-glass elements because she had felt that the direct contact with the elements caused "metal to pass through the glass cooking pots", thereby affecting the food.

June described her extensive in-hospital testing years earlier. Part of the procedure was to find out which foods she could eat so that a rotation diet could be designed specifically for her. She felt that she did well on the diet, but would occasionally find a food that would cause her to have symptoms. She reported how she had discovered that, if she would hang a glass ball from a cotton string and hang it over the food, the direction of the pendulum would indicate whether she would have a reaction. If the pendulum swung counterclockwise, it indicated that she would react adversely to the food. She gradually extended this practice to all items that would enter her home. For example, a clockwise spin over a couch would lead her to conclude that it was safe to purchase.

Using this tool and carefully avoiding fumes, June felt that she had been able to keep her symptoms at bay. She also felt that she had an excellent attitude and had decided that MCS "wasn't going to get the best of me".

In assigning a lifetime psychiatric diagnosis, we gathered interview data, questionnaires, and hospital records. We concluded that she met criteria for an ongoing somatization disorder because of her multiple physical symptoms beginning before age 30 that had no medical basis. She also met current criteria for panic disorder with agoraphobia as she still avoided places and situations for fear of having "chemical reactions". She used fewer treatments in general, but still used a special mask for reading the newspaper. She remained active in reading about MCS and continued to attend a support group. She currently received social security disability. Although June rated herself as "improved", since her 1988 interview we concluded that her condition was unchanged. She had the same complaints and remained socially and occupationally disabled.

Although Jane's outcome was worse than all but one of the other subjects, her vignette was selected because it vividly shows the illness conviction typical of MCS patients and its continuity over time. It also shows the extent to which subjects diagnosed with MCS will alter their lifestyle in their pursuit of what they believe will bring optimal symptomatic relief.

Psychiatric Diagnoses

The frequency of psychiatric diagnoses at follow-up was substantially higher than those originally reported. Using all source material, we diagnosed 15 subjects (83%) with a lifetime mood disorder, 10 (56%) with a lifetime anxiety disorder, and 10 (56%) with a lifetime somatoform disorder. While the original study diagnoses were based solely on the Diagnostic Interview Schedule results, the figures in the follow-up were based on a best estimate method in which all relevant data are taken into account. None of the subjects met current or lifetime criteria for a substance use disorder, a finding that other groups of investigators have also reported on subjects with MCS. The prevalence of somatization disorder was much higher than in 1988 (50% vs. 17%). Several subjects missed a diagnosis of somatization disorder in 1988 by 1 or 2 symptoms and now meet criteria. The additional time for symptoms to accumulate and be reported, combined with less stringent DSM-IV criteria for somatization disorder (requiring 8 symptoms rather than 13), and the use of the best estimate method[15] probably help explain the increased prevalence. The high rate of anxiety disorders, particularly panic disorder, probably reflects the fact that, for many subjects, their description of chemical reactions was nearly indistinguishable from that for panic attacks.

TABLE 2 shows results from the Personality Diagnostic Questionnaire-IV.[16] Seven (39%) subjects met criteria 1 or more personality disorder diagnoses. The most frequent diagnosis was schizotypal personality disorder in 4 subjects, followed by schizoid, histrionic, paranoid, narcissistic, and obsessive-compulsive types in 2 subjects each. Borderline, avoidant, dependent, and passive-aggressive personality types were found in 1 individual each. TABLE 3 lists symptoms reported by the 18 subjects that they attribute to MCS. The most frequently reported symptoms include headache, memory loss, forgetfulness, sore throat, joint aches, trouble thinking, shortness of breath, back pain, muscle aches, and nausea. All of these symptoms were found in more than 50% of the subjects.

Symptom Ratings

Subjects were rated for overall improvement: 2 (11%) were rated as having remitted, 5 (28%) as being "very much improved", 3 (17%) as "much" improved, 6 (33%) as improved, and 2 (11%) unchanged or worse. On the whole, most subjects were less outwardly symptomatic. They used fewer treatments, and fewer were under the care of a clinical ecologist. Nonetheless, most had modified their lives to conform to

TABLE 2. Current symptoms attributed to MCS by ≥50% of subjects

Symptom	n (%)
Headaches	14 (78)
Memory loss	14 (78)
Forgetfulness	14 (78)
Sore throat	13 (72)
Joint aches	12 (68)
Trouble thinking	12 (68)
Shortness of breath	11 (61)
Back pain	11 (61)
Muscle aches	11 (61)
Nausea	11 (61)
Heartburn	11 (61)
Joint pains	10 (56)
Eye discomfort	10 (56)
Skin rash	9 (50)
Skin dryness	9 (50)

TABLE 3. Personality disorder in subjects with MCS assessed in 1988 and 1997

Personality disorder	1988[a] n (%)	1997[b] n (%)
Schizoid	0	2 (13)
Schizotypal	3 (18)	4 (27)
Paranoid	2 (12)	2 (13)
Histrionic	7 (14)	2 (13)
Borderline	1 (6)	1 (7)
Narcissistic	1 (6)	2 (13)
Avoidant	3 (17)	1 (7)
Obsessive-compulsive	4 (22)	2 (13)
Dependent	2 (11)	1 (7)
Passive-aggressive	1 (6)	1 (7)
Any disorder	11 (65)	7 (39)

[a] $n = 17$; assessed with the Personality Diagnostic Questionnaire-Revised.
[b] $n = 18$; assessed with the Personality Diagnostic Questionnaire-IV.

the disorder. Avoidance was still a common coping device and most continued to be less social than before developing MCS. Despite the reported improvement, subjects remain virtually as symptomatic as when first assessed according to Symptom Checklist-90-Revised (SCL-90-R)[17] and Illness Behavior Questionnaire (IBQ)[18] results. For both these instruments, there were no statistically significant differences

TABLE 4. Mean scores on the Medical Outcome Survey in subjects with MCS and a U.S. population sample

Quality of life dimension	MCS ($n = 18$) mean (SD)	U.S. population ($n = 3474$)[a] mean (SD)	Difference in standard deviation units[b]
Physical functioning	60.9 (38.3)	84.2 (23.3)	−1.00
Bodily pain	30.5 (15.6)	75.2 (23.7)	−1.89
General health	62.2 (31.1)	72.0 (20.3)	−0.48
Social functioning	75.0 (30.6)	83.3 (22.7)	−0.37
Role-emotional	56.3 (47.9)	81.3 (33.0)	−0.70
Mental health	77.8 (24.1)	74.4 (18.1)	0.19

[a]Source: reference 10.
[b]Mean score for subjects with MCS minus mean score for the U.S. population divided by the SD of the U.S. population score.

for the results compared in 1988 and 1997. With both instruments, there were substantial differences from a comparison group. SCL-90-R results show that subjects differed from the comparison sample along the obsessive-compulsive, somatization, and general symptom dimensions. These data provide further confirmation of the diagnostic data showing high rates of both somatization and anxiety disorders. The IBQ confirmed that subjects remain preoccupied with their symptoms, reject responsibility for their illness, seek medical and not psychological treatments, and remain hypochondriacal.

As part of the follow-up study, we also inquired about the mental health of subjects' first-degree relatives.[19] In contrast to a comparison group, first-degree relatives of persons diagnosed with MCS were significantly more likely to have depression, alcoholism, panic disorder, or antisocial personality disorder. Suicide attempts and psychiatric care in general were also more commonly encountered among the relatives of the subjects with MCS. These results are consistent in part with those of Bell et al.,[7] who found high rates of alcohol and drug use disorders among the relatives of chemically sensitive persons not meeting criteria for MCS. We also found that nearly 10% of the relatives were believed to have MCS themselves.

The Medical Outcome Study 36-Item Short Form (SF-36)[10] was used to assess health-related quality of life. This instrument measures physical and mental dimensions of health, role limitation due to emotional health, social functioning, physical functioning, role limitation due to physical health, bodily pain, and general health and vitality. The instrument provides reliable and valid measures of health status and has been used in research on highly diverse groups. TABLE 4 lists the health-related quality-of-life data from the SF-36. (We had used an abbreviated version that yields only 6 dimensions.) Comparing the data to general U.S. population norms, the subjects were one standard deviation or greater from the U.S. population mean for physical functioning and bodily pain dimensions. General health, social functioning, and emotional role functioning were also worse than the U.S. population norms. The mental health dimension actually showed better functioning. Because we did not use age- and gender-matched controls and instead used published norms, these observed differences should be interpreted with caution.

The fact that mental health as measured by the SF-36 does not differ significantly from the general population mean merits comment in view of the high rate of lifetime psychiatric diagnoses. First, it is important to understand that the SF-36 is a cross-sectional measure; that is, it measures symptoms that a patient is experiencing at the time it is filled out. Half of our subjects had no current axis I (major mental) disorder, although 94% met lifetime criteria for the disorder; thus, many of our subjects had no current psychiatric complaints. This is not unexpected because the mood and anxiety disorders are remitting illnesses and, on the whole, subjects were globally improved. However, from a research perspective, it is the high *lifetime* frequency of disorders that is important and that separates them from the general population. As for those with somatization disorder, these individuals tend to minimize psychiatric symptoms; dimensional assessments such as the IBQ, however, confirm that many subjects continue to be symptomatic, yet remain resistant to psychological explanations of illness.

CONCLUSIONS

To our knowledge, ours is the longest follow-up study of persons with MCS reported in the literature. The two brief follow-up studies mentioned earlier both suggest that complaints of MCS are persistent in the short term. Our follow-up showed that persons diagnosed with MCS retain their illness belief and continue to endorse symptoms that contributed to their original diagnosis even after 9 years. Without exception, the subjects continued to believe that they had MCS and continued to report multiple somatic complaints. Even though they understood the controversial nature of their disorder, that knowledge had not undermined their confidence in the diagnosis and they remain satisfied with their medical care. Although most subjects reported improvement, most were symptomatic and continued to participate in treatment modalities originally recommended by their clinical ecologist, but not following as many. Subjects were highly likely to meet criteria for mood, anxiety, and somatoform disorders, but continue to be free of substance use disorders. Subjects' first-degree relatives are highly likely to have a psychiatric diagnosis themselves, which provides further validation for the psychiatric findings since most major psychiatric disorders are familial.

REFERENCES

1. AMERICAN COLLEGE OF PHYSICIANS. 1989. Clinical ecology: position statement. Ann. Intern. Med. **111:** 168–178.
2. AMERICAN COLLEGE OF OCCUPATIONAL AND ENVIRONMENTAL MEDICINE. 1993. Statement on multiple chemical sensitivities. Approved April 27, 1993.
3. AMERICAN MEDICAL ASSOCIATION. 1992. Report of the Council on Scientific Affairs: clinical ecology. JAMA **268:** 3465–3467.
4. INTERNATIONAL PROGRAM ON CHEMICAL SAFETY. 1996. Conclusions and recommendations of a workshop on multiple chemical sensitivities, February 21–23, 1996, Berlin, Germany. Regul. Toxicol. Pharmacol. **24:** S188–S189.

5. BLACK, D.W. 2000. The relationship of mental disorders and idiopathic environmental intolerance. Occup. Med. **15:** 557–570.
6. BLACK, D.W., A. RATHE & R.B. GOLDSTEIN. 1990. Environmental illness—a controlled study of 26 subjects with twentieth century disease. JAMA **264:** 3166–3170.
7. BELL, I.R., J.M. PETERSON & G.E. SCHWARTZ. 1995. Medical histories and psychological profiles of middle-aged women with and without self-reported illness from environmental chemicals. J. Clin. Psychiatry **56:** 151–160.
8. TERR, A.I. 1986. Environmental illness: a clinical review of 50 cases. Arch. Intern. Med. **146:** 145–149.
9. BLACK, D.W., B. DOEBBELING, M.D. VOELKER et al. 1999. Quality of life and health services utilization in a population-based sample of military personnel reporting multiple chemical sensitivities. J. Occup. Med. **41:** 928–933.
10. WARE, J. 1993. Appendix C: script for Personal Interview SF-36 administration. In SF-36 Health Survey Manuals: An Interpretation Guide. Nimrod Press. Boston.
11. LAX, M.B. & P.K. HENNEBERGER. 1995. Patients with multiple chemical sensitivities in an occupational health clinic: presentation and follow-up. Arch. Environ. Health **50:** 425–431.
12. BLACK, D.W., C. OKIISHI & S. SCHLOSSER. 2000. A 9-year follow-up of persons diagnosed with multiple chemical sensitivities. Psychosomatics **41:** 253–261.
13. BLACK, D.W., A. RATHE & R.B. GOLDSTEIN. 1983. Measures of distress in 26 "environmentally ill" subjects. Psychosomatics **34:** 131–138.
14. ROBINS, L.N., J.E. HELZER, J. CROUGHAN et al. 1981. The NIMH Diagnostic Interview Schedule, its history, characteristics, and validity. Arch. Gen. Psychiatry **38:** 381–389.
15. LECKMAN, J.F., S.D. SHOLOMSKA, W.D. THOMPSON et al. 1982. Best estimate of the Lifetime Psychiatric Diagnosis—a methodologic study. Arch. Gen. Psychiatry **39:** 879–883.
16. HYLER, S.E., R.O. REIDER & R.L. SPITZER. 1996. Personality Diagnostic Questionnaire-IV. New York State Psychiatric Institute. New York.
17. DEROGATIS, L.R. 1977. Symptom Checklist-90-R: Administration, Scoring, and Procedures Manual. Clinical Psychometric Research Division. Towson, MD.
18. PILOWSKY, I. & N.D. SPENSE. 1983. A Manual for the Illness Behavior Questionnaire. Second edition. Department of Psychiatry, University of Adelaide, Australia.
19. BLACK, D.W., C. OKIISHI, J. GABEL & S. SCHLOSSER. 1999. Psychiatric illness in the first-degree relatives of persons reporting multiple chemical sensitivities. Toxicol. Ind. Health **15:** 410–414.

Repeated Formaldehyde Effects in an Animal Model for Multiple Chemical Sensitivity

BARBARA A. SORG,[a] MATTHEW L. TSCHIRGI, SAMANTHA SWINDELL, LICHAO CHEN, AND JIDONG FANG

Program in Neuroscience, Washington State University, Pullman, Washington 99164, USA

ABSTRACT: Chemical intolerance is a phenomenon observed in multiple chemical sensitivity (MCS) syndrome, an ill-defined disorder in humans attributed to exposure to volatile organic compounds. Amplification of symptoms in individuals with MCS resembles the phenomenon of psychostimulant- and stress-induced sensitization in rodents. We have recently tested in rats the hypothesis that repeated chemical exposure produces sensitization of central nervous system (CNS) circuitry. A rat model of MCS in our laboratory has employed several endpoints of CNS function after repeated formaldehyde (Form) exposure (1 h/day × 5 days/week × 4 weeks). Repeated Form exposure produced behavioral sensitization to later cocaine injection, suggesting altered dopaminergic sensitivity in mesolimbic pathways. Rats given repeated Form also demonstrated increased fear conditioning to odor paired with footshock, implicating amplification of neural circuitry guiding fear responding to a conditioned odor cue. Recent studies examining the effects of repeated Form on locomotor activity during each daily exposure showed a decrease in rearing activity after 12–15 days of Form exposure compared to air-exposed controls. EEG recordings taken 1 week after withdrawal from daily Form revealed altered sleep architecture. Some of the differences in sleep disappeared after subsequent brief (15 min) challenge with Form the next day. Overall, the findings indicate that repeated low-level chemical exposure produces behavioral changes that may be akin to those observed in individuals with MCS, such as greater sensitivity to chemicals manifest as increased anxiety upon chemical exposure and altered sleep and/or fatigue. Study of the underlying CNS changes will provide a basis for mechanistically based animal models for MCS.

INTRODUCTION

An emerging issue in environmental health is the phenomenon of multiple chemical sensitivity (MCS). MCS is a controversial disorder characterized by multiorgan symptoms in response to low-level chemical exposures that are considered safe for the general population. The onset of MCS is often attributed to prior repeated chemical exposures in the home and/or workplace and, once initiated, symptoms are triggered by extremely low levels of many chemicals/foods. Some of the more common symptoms reported are extreme fatigue, headache, gastrointestinal problems, muscle

[a]Address for correspondence: Barbara A. Sorg, Ph.D., Program in Neuroscience, Department of VCAPP, Washington State University, Pullman, WA 99164-6520. Voice: 509-335-4709; fax: 509-335-4650.
 barbsorg@vetmed.wsu.edu

and joint pain, depression, memory and concentration difficulties, irritability, dizziness, anxiety, and upper airway irritation.[1-4]

Chemical intolerance (CI) has been used to describe a feeling of illness from low levels of environmental chemicals and is sometimes used interchangeably with MCS, although it is a symptom in a broader range of individuals who have been diagnosed with other conditions and (often ill-defined) illnesses. For example, new-onset food and chemical intolerance is reported in 80% of Gulf War veterans who have become chronically ill with Gulf War syndrome,[5] 60% of solvent-exposed workers,[6] approximately 30% of chronic fatigue syndrome patients, and 25–50% of fibromyalgia patients.[2] CI in these populations suggests some potential overlaps with these phenomena. Like MCS, up to 70–80% of those reporting CI are women.[7,8]

Recent and ongoing studies in our laboratory have focused on developing an animal model for MCS that is based upon the hypothesis that repeated chemical exposure produces amplification of central nervous system (CNS) circuitry that underlies changes in behavior and symptoms in MCS. This hypothesis was first proposed by Bell et al.[9] and posited that MCS, and possibly CI, is the result of a sensitization phenomenon occurring within certain CNS pathways, akin to sensitization observed in rodents after repeated stress or drugs of abuse.[10,11] The studies presented below support the possibility that long-term exposure to formaldehyde (Form) produces alterations in behaviors that are indicative of amplification or plasticity in CNS pathways.

SENSITIZATION OF COCAINE-INDUCED BEHAVIOR AFTER REPEATED FORMALDEHYDE EXPOSURE

Our earlier studies[12-14] focused on the hypothesis that repeated Form exposure would produce sensitization of cocaine-induced responses, similar to repeated psychostimulant- or stress-induced sensitization, as hypothesized by Bell et al.[9] If repeated inhalation of a chemical such as Form could produce sensitization of the CNS in the rat, this effect should be elicited by a psychostimulant (cocaine).

Sprague-Dawley rats, approximately 60–80 days of age, were obtained from Simonsen Laboratories (Gilroy, CA). For the first experiment, female rats were exposed to either ambient air or 11 ppm formalin vapor in inhalation chambers as previously described[12] for a 7-day period (1 h/day). For the second and third experiments, rats were exposed to approximately 1 ppm Form (from depolymerization of paraformaldehyde) as previously described[13] for either a 7-day period (1 h/day) or over a 1-month period (1 h/day × 5 days/week × 4 weeks). Horizontal and vertical activities were measured in photocell apparatus as previously described.[12,13]

TABLE 1 shows the results from these three experiments. Rats exposed to the higher dose of Form (11 ppm) demonstrated sensitized behavioral responding to a cocaine injection given within a few days after discontinuing daily Form exposure (early withdrawal). This augmented behavioral response was maintained 3–4 weeks later when examining vertical activity (late withdrawal). The lower dose of Form (1 ppm) exposure did not produce a significant change in the behavioral response (neither horizontal nor vertical activities) after only a 7-day exposure. However, longer duration of 1 ppm Form exposure produced a significant augmentation of vertical activity at both early and late withdrawal times. Behavioral responses to saline

TABLE 1. Effect of repeated formaldehyde exposure on cocaine-induced activity

	Early withdrawal		Late withdrawal	
	7-day exposure, 11 ppm			
	Horizontal	Vertical[a]	Horizontal	Vertical[a]
Air	24,459 ± 4291	133 ± 46	26,189 ± 3098	118 ± 15
Form	42,711 ± 6694*	189 ± 45	34,092 ± 4166	178 ± 26*
	7-day exposure, 1 ppm			
	Horizontal	Vertical[b]	Horizontal	Vertical[b]
Air	39,061 ± 4634	1170 ± 135	17,353 ± 2424	588 ± 121
Form	41,493 ± 4904	1102 ± 184	20,307 ± 2624	673 ± 97
	20-day exposure, 1 ppm			
	Horizontal	Vertical[b]	Horizontal	Vertical[b]
Air	51,417 ± 5019	1187 ± 224	59,522 ± 3218	1974 ± 328
Form	60,086 ± 4576	3412 ± 346*	56,493 ± 4364	3334 ± 308*

NOTE: Data taken from references 12 and 13.
[a]Number of vertical movements.
[b]Vertical activity.
*$p < 0.05$ compared to air controls.

injections were not different between control and Form groups in any of the experiments (not shown).

These results suggest that repeated Form exposure may produce alterations in the mesocorticolimbic dopamine system, which is known to at least partially mediate cocaine-induced locomotor responses.[15] The findings are in agreement with previous studies in animals and a recent study in humans linking repeated volatile organic compound exposure with altered dopaminergic function.[16–22] The present results are also in agreement with previous studies demonstrating enhanced physiological and behavioral sensitivity in mice after repeated exposure to Form.[23,24]

The observation that 20 days, but not 7 days, of the low-dose exposure (1 ppm) produced cross-sensitization to cocaine suggests that there is a relationship between duration of exposure and sensitization since the intensity of daily exposure was the same in both experiments. In some cases, horizontal activity was augmented; under other conditions, vertical activity was enhanced after repeated Form exposure. The reason for these differences is unknown, but may be related to the degree of sensitization.[25] The results speak to the possibility that low-level, long-term exposures may produce persistent sensitization of specific limbic circuitry.

ENHANCED CONDITIONED FEAR RESPONSE TO ODOR AFTER REPEATED FORMALDEHYDE EXPOSURE

Additional support for the hypothesis that MCS may occur by sensitization of CNS circuitry is provided by studies recently conducted in our laboratory examining conditioning to an odor in rats given repeated Form exposure[14] (unpublished results). Our previous studies focused on determining whether rats that had been previously exposed to repeated Form would demonstrate an increased ability to condition to an odor. To test this, a preliminary study[14] was done in which female Sprague-Dawley rats were administered daily air (control) or Form exposure for 20 days as described above. After an approximately 2- to 3-week withdrawal period, rats were presented with odor (pure orange extract) paired with footshock on the training day. One day later, rats were examined for their fear response (percent time spent freezing) to the context of the footshock in the absence of odor or footshock. No differences in the freezing response to the context of the footshock box were found,[14] and recent, more extensive studies in both male and female rats also showed no differences in the freezing response to the context (unpublished observations). One day later, rats were placed into a novel apparatus and presented first with a cotton swab containing water only (3 min) and then with a cotton swab containing the conditioned odor (3 min). Preliminary work[14] indicated that, in female rats, there was an increase in the fear response to odor in Form-pretreated rats when compared to animals that were also Form-pretreated, but not previously administered footshock. However, there were no significant differences between the Form and air control groups. One week later, these animals were again presented with water and conditioned odor and there was evidence, albeit preliminary, that female rats demonstrated a trend toward a decreased ability to extinguish the freezing response to the conditioned odor. In our more recent and extensive studies, there was clear evidence of a greater percent freezing in response to the conditioned odor, but not to water, after Form pretreatment in male rats, but not in female rats (unpublished observations). In this study, the response to water or conditioned odor presentation was examined for 5 days and the results suggest that, in male rats, there was a decreased ability to extinguish the fear response to odor after daily Form pretreatment as compared to controls.

The enhanced fear conditioning response in daily Form-pretreated rats suggests that multiple components of limbic circuitry may be sensitized. Most central to the formation of conditioned associations with aversive stimuli is the amygdaloid nuclear complex. The amygdala contributes significantly to autonomic, neuroendocrine, and behavioral responses to incoming stress.[26–28] Future studies will examine whether the conditioned response to the odor paired with footshock is accompanied by an alteration in amygdala function.

The conditioned fear results have implications for the involvement of conditioned responses to odors in at least a subset of individuals with MCS. Conditioning to odors as a critical contribution to MCS has been suggested by several investigators[29–35] (see also Van den Bergh, this volume). In the experiments described here, it is possible that increased airway irritation by prior daily Form exposure rendered the conditioned odor a more salient cue, producing a conditioned response that is not extinguished as readily as in air-exposed controls.

ALTERED SLEEP ARCHITECTURE AFTER REPEATED FORMALDEHYDE EXPOSURE

Among one of the more common complaints in MCS and individuals with other conditions in which CI has been reported, including chronic fatigue syndrome, fibromyalgia, and Gulf War syndrome, is overwhelming fatigue.[1,36,37] The first of two

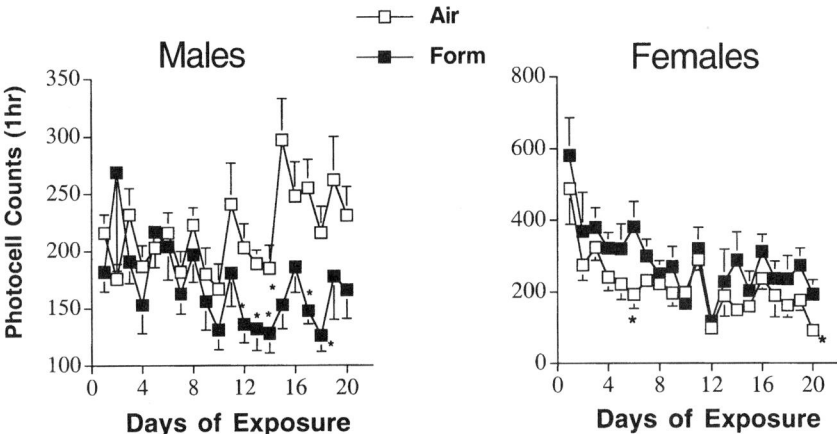

FIGURE 1. Vertical activity in male and female rats exposed to air or approximately 2 ppm Form as described. Rearing activity is shown as mean ± SEM. $N = 7-8$/group; $*p < 0.05$ compared to air controls as determined by Student's t test.

studies measured locomotor activity (rearing behavior) during each day of air or Form exposure in both male and female Sprague-Dawley rats. Vertical activity was measured as previously described[12] in cages measuring $20 \times 20 \times 20$ cm. The results from this set of experiments indicated that, in male rats, rearing behavior decreased in the presence of Form after 12 days of exposure compared to air controls (FIG. 1, left panel). This decrease was maintained for much of the remainder of the 20-day experiment. In contrast, females demonstrated a significant increase in rearing in Form animals at 5 and 20 days, with no changes in rearing between the two groups observed on any other days (FIG. 1, right panel). We have not previously observed decreases in rearing behavior after either saline or cocaine injections after daily Form pretreatment.[12,13] In fact, vertical activity is enhanced after cocaine challenge in Form-pretreated rats[13] (see above). Thus, the decreased activity in the *presence of Form* indicates that male rats may have a greater sensitivity to Form after long-term exposures (>12 days) and suggests that fatigue and/or alterations in sleep may be related to the decreased vertical activity that we observed.

The second study was therefore designed to test whether rats that had been repeatedly exposed to Form would demonstrate altered sleep patterns. Only male rats were chosen, based on the above-mentioned findings that rearing behavior was reduced in males, but not females, during Form exposure. Male Sprague-Dawley rats were surgically implanted with EEG and electromyogram (EMG) electrodes as previously described.[38] After a 1-week recovery, rats were exposed to air or Form for 20 days as described for TABLE 1, and vertical activity was measured during daily exposures as described above. After completion of daily exposures, animals were adapted to the recording cages and EEG/EMG recording cables for 6 days. The next day, baseline EEG and EMG recordings were collected for a 24-h period, beginning at dark onset (19:00 h). The next evening, at the beginning of dark onset, rats were exposed to a cotton swab saturated with 37% Form that was affixed to the side of their sleep

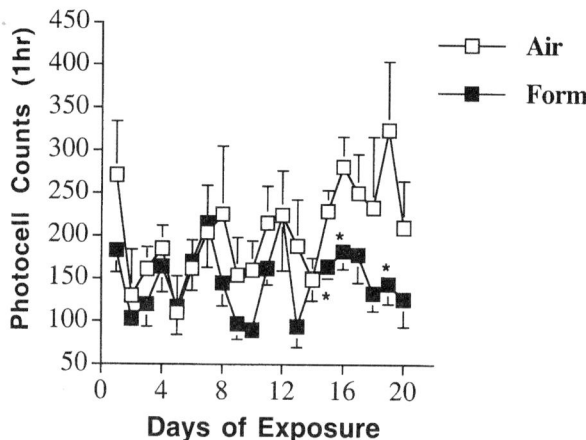

FIGURE 2. Vertical activity in male rats exposed to air or Form as before and used in the sleep studies shown in FIGURES 3 and 4 below. Rearing activity is shown as mean ± SEM. $N = 7$/group; $*p < 0.05$ compared to air controls as determined by Student's t test.

chambers for a 15-min period. Recordings were collected from the start of Form presentation and continued for a 24-h period.

The results shown in FIGURE 2 indicate that, similar to the previous experiment in males, rats preexposed to repeated Form demonstrated decreased rearing activity compared to controls, although this effect was not observed until day 15 (FIG. 2).

At baseline (before the 15-min Form reexposure), the pattern of sleep was significantly affected by repeated Form exposure (FIGS. 3A–F). The number of wakings and the number of NREMS were significantly attenuated in Form-pretreated rats, while the number of REMS was not different between Form and control groups (FIGS. 3A–C). The mean duration of waking episodes was significantly increased, while the mean duration of NREMS and REMS episodes was not significantly different between the two groups (FIGS. 3D–F).

After reexposure to a small amount of concentrated Form presented for a 15-min period the next day in the sleep chambers, the difference in sleep patterns that existed at baseline largely disappeared. No main effect of daily pretreatment was observed for any of the measures (FIGS. 4A–F). Although there was no significant treatment effect after Form challenge, post hoc analyses (t test using a Bonferroni correction) revealed that, at 13–18 h after Form reexposure, there was a significant decrease in number of waking episodes ($p = 0.028$) and number of NREMS episodes ($p = 0.02$), similar to what was found for the baseline condition. In addition, comparison between baseline and challenge within subjects revealed that Form-pretreated rats, but not air controls, demonstrated an initial decrease in duration of REMS episodes (1–6 h) (significant main effect of day, $p = 0.012$). The decrease in REMS episode duration at this time appeared to rebound within the next 7- to 12-h time period after Form challenge.

Overall, the sleep studies indicate that alterations in sleep architecture occur in Form-pretreated rats under baseline conditions after approximately 1 week of with-

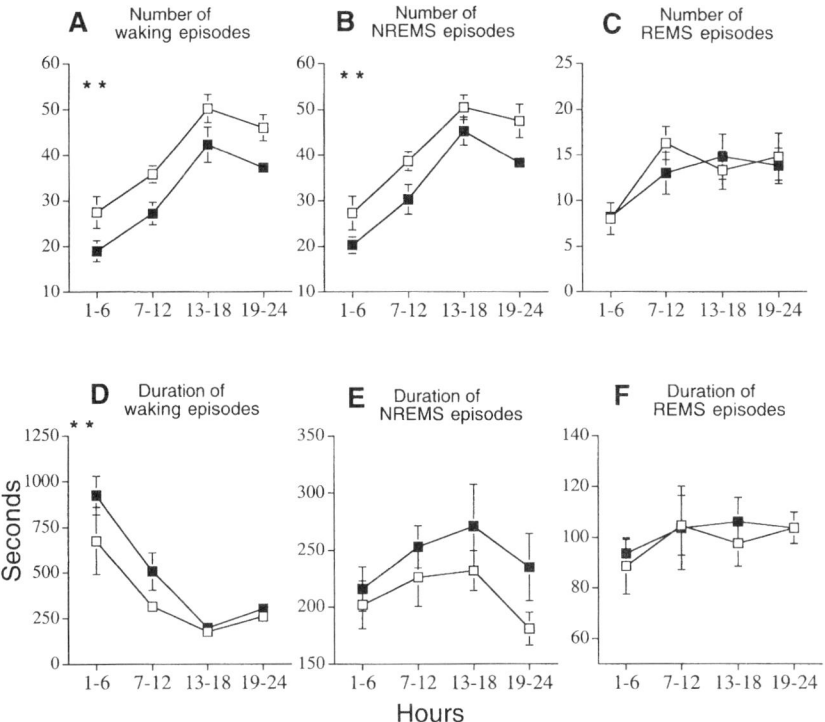

FIGURE 3. Mean ± SEM of number of episodes (**A–C**) or duration of episodes (**D–F**) for waking, NREMS, and REMS under baseline conditions. Male rats were exposed to air (□) or 2 ppm Form (■) as before and EEG/EMG activity was assessed 1 week later. The dark cycle is during the first 12-h period. **Indicates significant treatment effect as determined by a two-way ANOVA. $N = 6$/group (1 rat from each treatment group was excluded due to malfunction of sleep recording equipment).

drawal from daily Form exposures. However, this difference generally disappears after a short Form challenge. Together, the results suggest that there are time-dependent changes in sleep patterns during withdrawal that may be related to time of withdrawal and/or to alterations induced by Form exposure in the rates of adaptation to the EEG/EMG cable and novel cage. Any alterations in adaptation to novel situations may have importance for individuals reporting MCS. Future studies will examine the time dependence of the changes in sleep architecture found after repeated daily Form exposure.

Changes in sleep have been reported in humans with MCS or CI[39] and after organic solvent exposure.[40,41] In experimental animals, organic solvent exposure administered acutely[42–46] or chronically[43,44] also has been shown to alter sleep. Our results showed no effects of acute Form exposure in air controls, but it is possible that a 15-min exposure was too short and/or the dose was too low to detect any changes when evaluated over 6-h time blocks. There also was no effect of acute or

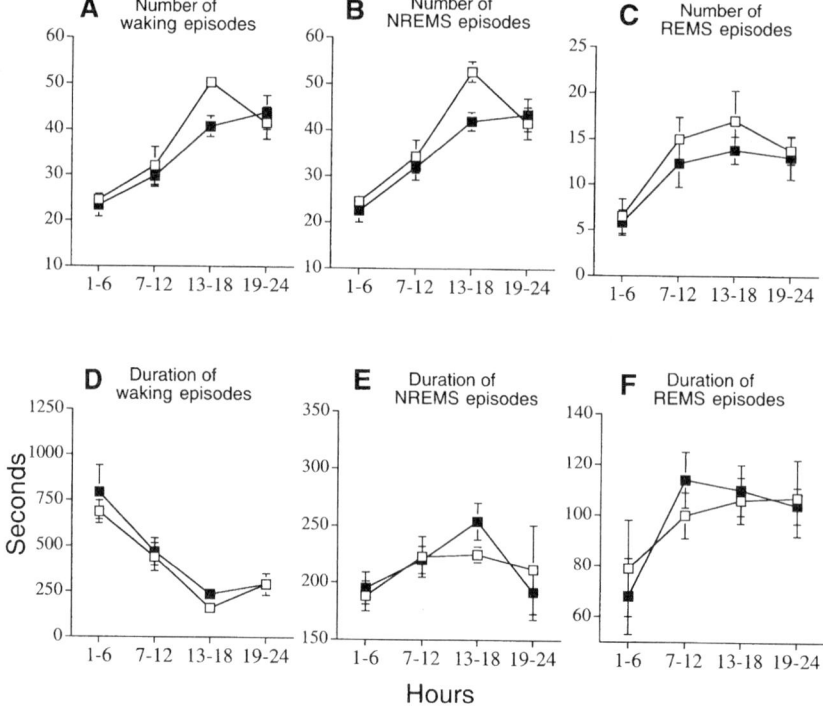

FIGURE 4. Mean ± SEM of number of episodes (**A–C**) or duration of episodes (**D–F**) for waking, NREMS, and REMS after a 15-min Form challenge in the sleep cages of rats shown in FIGURE 3. The dark cycle is during the first 12-h period. $N = 6$/group; (□) air; (■) Form.

repeated Form exposure on percent of total waking time and total time spent in NREMS or REMS. However, alterations in sleep architecture after repeated exposure to Form suggest the potential for enhanced fatigue states during waking.

CONCLUSIONS

Overall, the studies presented and discussed above demonstrate alterations in several behavioral endpoints after repeated Form exposure, including (1) increased cocaine-induced activity, (2) increased freezing response and/or decreased ability to extinguish a fear response to odor paired with an aversive event (footshock), and (3) decreased activity during Form exposure as well as altered sleep architecture after discontinuing Form exposure. These results suggest that Form may be acting as a chemical stressor. Current studies are under way to determine the levels of serum corticosterone, the major adrenal stress hormone in rats, after acute and repeated Form exposure. This interpretation is consistent with previous studies that have examined the effects of conventional stressors on the behaviors measured herein. For example, prior repeated stress has been shown in numerous laboratories to produce enhanced amphetamine- and cocaine-induced activity,[10,47–49] increases in fear conditioning,[50,51] and alterations in sleep.[52,53]

Specific limbic circuitry, including the amygdala and mesolimbic dopamine projections to the nucleus accumbens and prefrontal cortex, appears to be partly responsible for assigning relative salience to environmental stimuli.[54–56] Therefore, amplification of function within these brain regions may effect assignment of increased salience to multiple odors. Such findings may be of significance from the standpoint of the widely reported spreading phenomenon in MCS, in which individuals become intolerant to an increasing number of structurally unrelated chemicals in the environment. Additional research will need to address the specific neurotransmitters involved and the mechanisms for plasticity in these brain regions after repeated chemical exposure.

ACKNOWLEDGMENTS

We wish to thank Dr. James M. Krueger (Washington State University) for expert advice on the sleep studies. These studies were supported by Public Health Service Grant Nos. DA 11787 and ES 09135 (to B. A. Sorg).

REFERENCES

1. ASHFORD, N. & C. MILLER. 1998. Chemical Exposures: Low Levels and High Stakes. Wiley. New York.
2. BUCHWALD, D. & D. GARRITY. 1994. Comparison of patients with chronic fatigue syndrome, fibromyalgia, and multiple chemical sensitivities. Arch. Intern. Med. **154:** 2049–2053.
3. MILLER, C.S. 1994. Chemical sensitivity: history and phenomenology. Toxicol. Ind. Health **10:** 253–276.
4. MILLER, C.S. & H.C. MITZEL. 1995. Chemical sensitivity attributed to pesticide exposure versus remodeling. Arch. Environ. Health **50:** 119–129.
5. MILLER, C.S. 1996. Chemical sensitivity: symptom, syndrome, or mechanism for disease? Toxicology **111:** 69–86.
6. MORROW, L.A., C.M. RYAN, M.J. HODGSON & N. ROBIN. 1990. Alterations in cognitive and psychological functioning after organic solvent exposure. J. Occup. Med. **32:** 444–450.
7. FIEDLER, N., H.M. KIPEN, J. DELUCA et al. 1996. A controlled comparison of multiple chemical sensitivities and chronic fatigue syndrome. Psychosom. Med. **58:** 38–49.
8. BELL, I.R. 1998. Illness from low levels of environmental chemicals: relevance to chronic fatigue syndrome and fibromyalgia. Am. J. Med. **105:** 74S–82S.
9. BELL, I.R., C.S. MILLER & G.E. SCHWARTZ. 1992. An olfactory-limbic model of multiple chemical sensitivity syndrome: possible relationships to kindling and affective spectrum disorders. Biol. Psychiatry **32:** 218–242.
10. ANTELMAN, S.M., A.J. EICHLER, C.A. BLACK & D. KOCAN. 1980. Interchangeability of stress and amphetamine in sensitization. Science **207:** 329–331.
11. ROBINSON, T.E. & J.B. BECKER. 1986. Enduring changes in brain and behavior produced by chronic amphetamine administration: a review and evaluation of animal models of amphetamine psychosis. Brain Res. **396:** 157–198.
12. SORG, B.A., J.R. WILLIS, T.C. NOWATKA et al. 1996. A proposed animal neurosensitization model for MCS in studies with formaldehyde. Toxicology **111:** 135–145.
13. SORG, B.A., J.R. WILLIS, R.E. SEE et al. 1998. Repeated low-level formaldehyde exposure produces cross-sensitization to cocaine: possible relevance to chemical sensitivity in humans. Neuropsychopharmacology **18:** 385–394.

14. SORG, B.A. & T. HOCHSTATTER. 1999. Behavioral sensitization after repeated formaldehyde exposure in rats. Toxicol. Ind. Health **15:** 346–355.
15. KELLY, P.H. & S.D. IVERSEN. 1975. Selective 6-OHDA induced destruction of mesolimbic dopamine neurons: ablation of psychostimulant-induced locomotor activity in rats. Eur. J. Pharmacol. **40:** 45–56.
16. EDLING, C., B. HELLMAN, B. ARVIDSON et al. 1997. Do organic solvents induce changes in the dopaminergic system? Positron emission tomography studies of occupationally exposed subjects. Int. Arch. Occup. Environ. Health **70:** 180–186.
17. FUXE, K., K. ANDERSSON, O.G. NILSEN et al. 1982. Toluene and telencephalic dopamine: selective reduction of amine turnover in discrete DA nerve terminal systems of the anterior caudate nucleus by low concentrations of toluene. Toxicol. Lett. **12:** 115–123.
18. MUTTI, A., M. FALZOI, A. ROMANELLI et al. 1988. Brain dopamine as a target for solvent toxicity: effects of some monocyclic aromatic hydrocarbons. Toxicology **49:** 77–82.
19. VON EULER, G., K. FUXE & S.C. BONDY. 1990. Ganglioside GM1 prevents and reverses toluene-induced increases in membrane fluidity and calcium levels in rat brain synaptosomes. Brain Res. **508:** 210–214.
20. VON EULER, G., K. FUXE, F. BENFENATI et al. 1989. Neurotensin modulates the binding characteristics of dopamine D2 receptors in rat striatal membranes also following treatment with toluene. Acta Physiol. Scand. **35:** 443–448.
21. VON EULER, G., S-O. OGREN, S.C. BONDY et al. 1991. Subacute exposure to low concentrations of toluene affects dopamine-mediated locomotor activity in the rat. Toxicology **67:** 333–349.
22. VON EULER, G., S-O. OGREN, S.M. LI et al. 1993. Persistent effects of subchronic toluene exposure on spatial learning and memory, dopamine-mediated locomotor activity, and dopamine D2 agonist binding in the rat. Toxicology **77:** 223–232.
23. KANE, L.E. & Y. ALARIE. 1977. Sensory irritation to formaldehyde and acrolein during single and repeated exposures in mice. Am. Ind. Hyg. Assoc. J. **38:** 509–522.
24. WOOD, R.W. & J.B. COLEMAN. 1995. Behavioral evaluation of the irritant properties of formaldehyde. Toxicol. Appl. Pharmacol. **130:** 67–72.
25. LE MOAL, M. 1995. Mesocorticolimbic dopaminergic neurons. In Psychopharmacology: The Fourth Generation of Progress, pp. 283–294. Raven Press. New York.
26. BEAULIEU, S., T. DI PAOLO, J. COTE & N. BARDEN. 1987. Participation of the central amygdaloid nucleus in the response of adrenocorticotropin secretion to immobilization stress: opposing roles of the noradrenergic and dopaminergic systems. Neuroendocrinology **45:** 37–46.
27. BLANCHARD, D.C. & R.J. BLANCHARD. 1972. Innate and conditioned reactions to threat in rats with amygdaloid lesions. J. Comp. Physiol. Psychol. **81:** 281–290.
28. VAN DE KAR, L.D., R.A. PIECHOWSLI, P.A. RITTENHOUSE & T.S. GRAY. 1991. Amygdaloid lesions: differential effect on conditioned stress and immobilization-induced increases in corticosterone and renin secretion. Brain Res. **447:** 335–340.
29. SCHOTTENFELD, R.S. & M.R. CULLEN. 1986. Recognition of occupation-induced post-traumatic stress disorders. J. Occup. Med. **28:** 365–369.
30. BOLLA-WILSON, K., R.J. WILSON & M.L. BLEECKER. 1989. Conditioning of physical symptoms after neurotoxic exposure. J. Occup. Med. **31:** 684–686.
31. SCHUSTERMAN, D.J. & S.R. DAGER. 1991. Prevention of psychological disability after occupational respiratory exposures. Occup. Med. **6:** 11–27.
32. GUGLIELMI, R.S., D.J. COX & D.A. SPYKER. 1994. Behavioral treatment of phobic avoidance in multiple chemical sensitivity. J. Behav. Ther. Exp. Psychiatry **25:** 197–209.
33. SIEGEL, S. & R. KREUTZER. 1997. Pavlovian conditioning and multiple chemical sensitivity. Environ. Health Perspect. **105**(suppl. 2): 521–526.
34. VAN DEN BERGH, O., P.J. KEMPYNCK, K.P. VAN DE WOESTIJNE et al. 1995. Respiratory learning and somatic complaints: a conditioning approach using CO_2-enriched air inhalation. Behav. Res. Ther. **33:** 517–527.
35. VAN DEN BERGH, O., K. STEGEN & K.P. VAN DE WOESTIJNE. 1997. Learning to have psychosomatic complaints: conditioning of respiratory behavior and somatic complaints in psychosomatic patients. Psychosom. Med. **59:** 13–23.

36. CLAUW, D.J. & G.P. CHROUSOS. 1997. Chronic pain and fatigue syndromes: overlapping clinical and neuroendocrine features and potential pathogenic mechanisms. Neuroimmunomodulation **4:** 134–153.
37. HALEY, R.W., T.L. KURT & J. HOM. 1997. Is there a Gulf War syndrome? JAMA **277:** 215–222.
38. ZHANG, J., F. OBAL, JR., T. ZHENG et al. 1999. Intrapreoptic microinjection of GHRH or its antagonist alters sleep in rats. J. Neurosci. **19:** 2187–2194.
39. BELL, I.R., R.R. BOOTZIN, C. RITENBAUGH et al. 1996. A polysomnographic study of sleep disturbance in community elderly with self-reported environmental chemical odor intolerance. Biol. Psychiatry **40:** 123–133.
40. KILBURN, K.H., B.C. SEIDMAN & R. WARSHAW. 1985. Neurobehavioral and respiratory symptoms of formaldehyde and xylene exposure in histology technicians. Arch. Environ. Health **40:** 229–233.
41. INDULSKI, J.A., H. SINCZUK-WALCZAK, M. SZYMCZAK & W. WESOLOWSKI. 1996. Neurological and neurophysiological examinations of workers occupationally exposed to organic solvent mixtures used in the paint and varnish production. Int. J. Occup. Med. Environ. Health **9:** 235–244.
42. ARITO, H., H. TSURUTA & K. NAKAGAKI. 1984. Acute effects of toluene on circadian rhythms of sleep-wakefulness and brain monoamine metabolism in rats. Toxicology **33:** 291–301.
43. ARITO, H., H. TSURUTA & M. OGURI. 1988. Changes in sleep and wakefulness following single and repeated exposures to toluene vapor in rats. Arch. Toxicol. **62:** 76–80.
44. HISANAGA, N. & Y. TAKEUCHI. 1983. Changes in sleep cycle and EEG of rats exposed to 4000 ppm toluene for four weeks. Ind. Health **21:** 153–164.
45. TAKEUCHI, Y. & N. HISANAGA. 1977. The neurotoxicity of toluene: EEG changes in rats exposed to various concentrations. Br. J. Ind. Med. **34:** 314–324.
46. GHOSH, T.K., R.L. COPELAND, JR., J.C. GEAR & S.N. PRADHAN. 1989. Effects of toluene exposure on the spontaneous cortical activity in rats. Pharmacol. Biochem. Behav. **32:** 987–992.
47. KALIVAS, P.W. & J. STEWART. 1991. Dopamine transmission in the initiation and expression of drug- and stress-induced sensitization of motor activity. Brain Res. Rev. **16:** 223–244.
48. KALIVAS, P.W. & P. DUFFY. 1989. Similar effects of daily cocaine and stress on mesocorticolimbic dopamine neurotransmission in the rat. Biol. Psychiatry **25:** 913–928.
49. ROBINSON, T.E., A.L. ANGUS & J.B. BECKER. 1987. Sensitization to stress: the enduring effects of prior stress on amphetamine-induced rotational behavior. Life Sci. **37:** 1039–1042.
50. MAIER, S.F. & L.R. WATKINS. 1995. Intracerebroventricular interleukin-1 receptor antagonist blocks the enhancement of fear conditioning and interference with escape produced by inescapable shock. Brain Res. **695:** 279–282.
51. SHORS, T.J., C. WEISS & R.F. THOMPSON. 1992. Stress-induced facilitation of classical conditioning. Science **257:** 537–539.
52. BOUYER, J.J., M. VALEE, J.M. DEMINIERE et al. 1998. Reaction of sleep-wakefulness cycle to stress is related to differences in hypothalamo-pituitary-adrenal axis reactivity in rat. Brain Res. **804:** 114–124.
53. CHEETA, S., G. RUIGT, J. VAN PROOSDIJ & P. WILLNER. 1997. Changes in sleep architecture following chronic mild stress. Biol. Psychiatry **41:** 419–427.
54. BERRIDGE, K.C. & T.E. ROBINSON. 1998. What is the role of dopamine in reward: hedonic impact, reward learning, or incentive salience? Brain Res. Rev. **28:** 309–369.
55. AHN, S. & A.G. PHILLIPS. 1999. Dopaminergic correlates of sensory-specific satiety in the medial prefrontal cortex and nucleus accumbens of the rat. J. Neurosci. **19:** RC29.
56. WILKINSON, L., T. HUMBY, A. KILLCROSS et al. 1998. Dissociations in dopamine release in medial prefrontal cortex and ventral striatum during the acquisition and extinction of classical aversive conditioning in the rat. Eur. J. Neurosci. **10:** 1019–1026.

Does the Kindling Model of Epilepsy Contribute to Our Understanding of Multiple Chemical Sensitivity?

M. E. GILBERT[a]

Neurotoxicology Division, National Health and Environmental Effects Research Laboratory, United States Environmental Protection Agency, Research Triangle Park, North Carolina, and Department of Psychology, University of North Carolina, Chapel Hill, North Carolina, USA

> ABSTRACT: Multiple chemical sensitivity (MCS) is a phenomenon whereby individuals report an increased sensitivity to low levels of chemicals in the environment. Kindling is a model of synaptic plasticity whereby repeated low-level electrical stimulation to a number of brain sites leads to permanent increases in seizure susceptibility. Stimulation that is initially subthreshold for subclinical seizure provocation comes, over time, to elicit full-blown motor seizures. Kindling can also be induced by chemical stimulation, and repeated exposures to some pesticides have been shown to induce signs of behavioral seizure, facilitate subsequent electrical kindling, and induce subclinical electrographic signs of hyperexcitability in the amygdala. Many of the symptoms of MCS suggest that CNS limbic pathways involved in anxiety are altered in individuals reporting MCS. Limbic structures are among the most susceptible to kindling-induced seizures, and persistent cognitive and emotional sequelae have been associated with temporal lobe epilepsy (TLE) in humans and kindling in animals. Thus, a number of parallels exist between kindling and MCS phenomena, leading to initial speculations that MCS may occur via a kindling-like mechanism. However, kindling requires the activation of electrographic seizure discharge and has thus been primarily examined as a model for TLE. Events leading to the initial evocation of a subclinical electrographic seizure have been much less well studied. It is perhaps these events that may serve as a more appropriate model for the enhanced chemical responsiveness characteristic of MCS. Alternatively, kindling may be useful as a tool to selectively increase sensitivity in subcomponents of the neural fear circuit to address questions relating the role of anxiety in the development and expression of MCS.

Multiple chemical sensitivity (MCS) is a phenomenon whereby individuals present with increased sensitivity to low-level chemical exposures (see refs. 1 and 2 for recent reviews). The symptoms typically involve multiple organ systems, but a strong neurological component including cognitive and emotional sequelae is evident. A

---

[a]Address for correspondence: M. E. Gilbert, Ph.D., Neurotoxicology Division (MD-74B), National Health and Environmental Effects Research Laboratory, U.S. Environmental Protection Agency, Research Triangle Park, NC 27711. Voice: 919-541-4394; fax: 919-541-4849.
  gilbert.mary@epa.gov

neural sensitization model for MCS has received considerable attention in recent years and forms the focus of the present symposium on the role of neural plasticity in this disorder. In this paper, I will review briefly two plasticity models, long-term potentiation (LTP) and kindling, and attempt to formulate a working hypothesis of the potential role these plasticity processes may play in MCS.

LONG-TERM POTENTIATION (LTP)

LTP represents a long-lasting increase in synaptic strength in response to electrical stimulation of afferent pathways. It has been proposed, and fairly well accepted, that LTP reflects the activation of processes that are actually used in the encoding of a memory (see refs. 3–6 for review). LTP is typically assessed by measuring field potentials in the hippocampus before and after the application of a brief high-frequency train of electrical stimulation. Unlike kindling, described below, LTP does not require pathological electrographic seizures for its induction. Although it has been best characterized in the hippocampus, LTP appears to be a general property of many circuits in brain that are required for associative learning.[4,7–9]

The underlying neurobiological substrates of LTP have been intensively investigated. Briefly, calcium entry through voltage-sensitive N-methyl-D-aspartate (NMDA) channels is a critical step in the induction of LTP.[10,11] This rapid rise in intracellular calcium triggers a cascade of biochemical signaling events in a number of kinase systems, including protein kinase A (PKA), protein kinase C (PKC), calcium-calmodulin kinase II (CAMKII), and mitogen-activated protein kinase (MAPK).[12–14] The cascade and temporal sequence of kinase activation appear to be critical for the encoding of synaptic information and the formation of a memory. A variety of specific proteins are phosphorylated as a direct consequence of kinase activation and work in concert to produce both short-term and long-term modifications at the synapse.[12,14] Short-term modifications include the phosphorylation of additional receptors and ion channels that contribute to enhanced postsynaptic response amplitudes. Other proteins phosphorylated by kinase activation alter the cytoskeletal architecture presynaptically to facilitate release of transmitter, and postsynaptically to enhance responsiveness. Phosphorylation of additional kinase systems induces more enduring modifications in synaptic transmission through transcription of early and late effector genes that control synaptic growth and promote the persistence of LTP (hours/days/weeks) and presumably of memory.[4,14]

KINDLING

Electrical kindling refers to the gradual development of electrographic and behavioral seizures in response to the repeated application of brief, intermittent, low-intensity trains of electrical stimulation.[15,16] Like LTP, kindling is a model of synaptic plasticity, but one in which a progressive and permanent transsynaptic alteration in brain organization is induced. Kindling cannot be readily attributed to tissue damage resulting from either the stimulation or the subsequent seizure and has primarily been studied as a model of epilepsy. To initiate kindling, a forebrain site, typically the amygdala, is activated by direct electrical or chemical stimulation and results in the evocation of an epileptiform discharge or afterdischarge (AD). Although ADs must be evoked for kindling to proceed, repeated stimulation at subthreshold levels will eventually lower the threshold required to produce an AD.[17] Once an AD has been evoked, the target sites connected to the stimulated site receive aberrant input in response to that discharge. If the aberrant discharge is strong enough, reactive discharges may also be triggered in the target site itself. Kindling-induced potentiation, a process much like LTP, may facilitate the activation of these secondary sites (see below).

With once-daily repetition, the amygdala, pyriform, and perirhinal cortices eventually become actively recruited into the discharge. Once these regions become involved and begin to respond with independent reactive discharges, persistent changes occur in the electrical properties of the cells in these brain areas.[18] These changes involve increases in both sodium and calcium currents. One means whereby this is accomplished is through alterations in the kinetics of the NMDA subtype of glutamate receptors,[19] receptors that are strongly engaged during ictal discharges (i.e., electrographic seizures), but are generally silent during low-frequency synaptic transmission. As a result of ictal discharge, these receptors begin to contribute to normal synaptic transmission during ictal-free periods.[20] As the changes in cell-firing properties emerge in amygdala and pyriform regions, spontaneous interictal spikes (IIS) are generated within these structures at points in time remote from the epileptiform event. At the same time, more vigorous response from the cells during the ictal period triggers reactive ADs in additional synaptically connected sites until most of the forebrain is engaged upon activation of the primary kindled focus.[18]

The behavioral seizure itself at this point in the epileptogenic process is still focal in nature, manifesting as motor arrest, eye blink, chewing, and head nodding (Stages 1 and 2 of Racine).[21] Once the forebrain discharge reaches a critical level, the high-threshold brain stem structures that drive the skeletal motor response are activated and the convulsion itself is initiated. Behaviorally the animals engage in unilateral forelimb clonus (Stage 3), followed by rearing and bilateral clonus (Stage 4). With continued stimulation, the severity of seizure increases, the clonus spreads to the hindlimbs, and the animal loses postural control (Stage 5). With many stimulations, seizures will eventually be spontaneously evoked, appearing abruptly and fully generalized from the outset (see ref. 16 for review). It is likely that the changes in the biophysical properties of forebrain neurons that accompanied partial kindling (Stages 1 and 2) now occur in the more hardwired brain stem neurons and contribute to these spontaneous seizures.[18]

KINDLING HYPOTHESIS OF MCS

Kindling was suggested as a potential model of MCS by Bell *et al.*[22] Briefly, this hypothesis states that subconvulsive chemical kindling in the olfactory bulb, its primary afferent, the pyriform cortex, the amygdala, and hippocampus provides a neurobiological mechanism that serves to amplify reactivity to low-level chemical exposure. Certain analogies exist between kindling and MCS that make kindling an attractive model system to study in this context. (1) Kindling, like MCS, is progressive and its changes are long lasting, if not permanent. (2) Stimulus generalization occurs with kindling in the sense that once kindling has occurred, the organism maintains an increased sensitivity to a variety of seizuregenic agents with different modes of action. In MCS, an initiation stimulus may generalize to a number of different environmental chemical triggers, drugs, foods, and other exogenous stimuli. (3) Electrical kindling of the amygdala and pyriform cortex is robust, with both regions demonstrating a fairly rapid rate of kindling.[23] Alterations in these brain areas may be critical for progression of the kindling process.[18,23] Kindling, like MCS, results in a number of persistent alterations in affective and cognitive behavior that may be attributable to dysfunction in amygdala and pyriform regions (e.g., refs. 24 and 25).

A CONTINUUM OF PLASTICITY?

Despite the analogies between kindling and MCS, one of the biggest pitfalls of this hypothesis is that kindling is an epilepsy model—kindling requires the repeated evocation of subclinical electrographic seizures. Thus, a pathological electrographic seizure event is requisite to initiate and promote the progression of electrographic, biochemical, and behavioral manifestations that form the basis for the analogies outlined above. Without an AD, there can be no kindling. In contrast, MCS is clearly not an epilepsy-based disorder. Little evidence exists for an increased propensity of seizure disorders in MCS patients, nor is there evidence of increased incidence of MCS in temporal lobe epileptic patients (see refs. 1 and 2).

However, the two models of synaptic plasticity, LTP and kindling, may be viewed as divergent ends of a continuum of plasticity (FIG. 1). This continuum ranges from "normal" plastic processes exemplified by LTP and its role in learning and memory, to pathological processes in the case of kindling that underlie permanent predisposition to convulsive disorders. Although LTP is not likely the mechanism that underlies kindling, kindling and LTP share a number of common biochemical, physiological, and cellular properties. LTP is induced by kindling, may facilitate seizure spread and contribute to reductions in AD thresholds that occur in the absence of evoked ADs.[8,26,27] In addition, repeated induction of LTP, also in the absence of ADs, can facilitate subsequent kindling development.[28,29] MCS may lie somewhere along this continuum between the normal learning-based plasticity modeled by LTP and pathological seizure-based plasticity characteristic of kindling.

CHEMICAL KINDLING

There are many chemicals (toxicants as well as pharmaceutical agents) with a variety of primary actions on CNS function, that lead to convulsions with acute high-dose exposure.[30,31] Similarly, proconvulsant properties of many of these substances can be demonstrated by administration of subthreshold doses prior to the delivery of daily electrical stimulation in a standard kindling paradigm (see refs. 30 and 32 for review). Pesticides figure prominently among these and include lindane, endosulfan, chlordimeform, amitraz, and chlorpyrifos.[33-39] A subset of these chemicals, however, are also convulsant if delivered repeatedly at low concentrations and in the absence of electrical kindling stimulation.[39-41] Some may do this by means of cumulative toxicity, each successive dose increasing the body burden until a thresh-

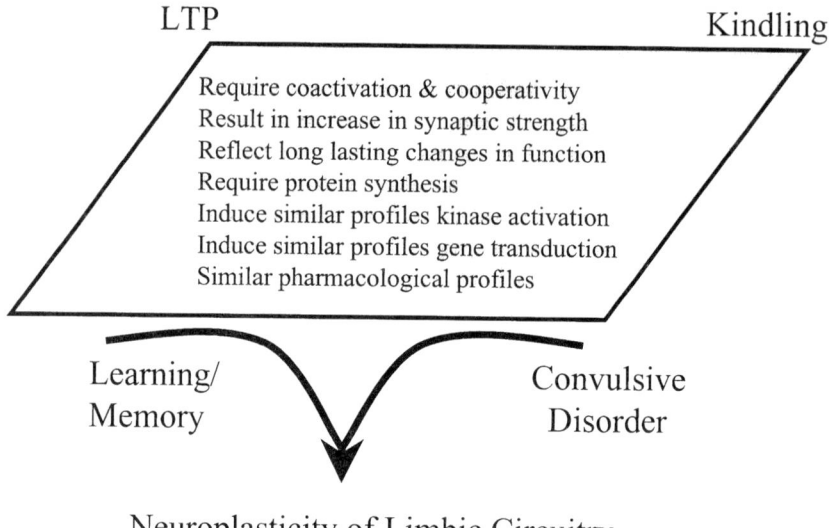

FIGURE 1. Continuum of neuroplasticity. Long-term potentiation (LTP) and kindling share many cellular, neurochemical, and neurophysiological substrates. MCS may occupy a place along the continuum between normal plastic processes that underlie learning and memory and those that lead to epileptic disorders.

old is passed and a convulsion ensues (see ref. 31). Other examples exist, however, whereby repeated administration of low concentrations of chemical leads to initially subclinical and then overt behavioral seizures (see refs. 39–43). In these situations, chemical kindling rather than cumulative toxicity drives the behavioral response, and unlike the cumulative acute convulsion, persistent neurological sequelae are likely to result. It appears that the chemical stimulus has merely substituted for the electrical stimulus and kindling progresses with each successive administration (see refs. 16, 30, 32, and 42). We have demonstrated evidence of chemical kindling with two pesticides of the cyclodiene class, endosulfan and lindane.

CHEMICAL KINDLING WITH CYCLODIENE PESTICIDES

Animals dosed daily or three times per week with endosulfan or lindane demonstrated an increase in the frequency of mild behavioral seizure signs.[39,40] The most common was myoclonic jerks, sometimes accompanied by very brief (2–3 s) bouts of forelimb clonus (FIG. 2A). After a rest period of 2–4 weeks to allow clearance from the body, subsequent administration led to behavioral and electrographic signs of focal seizure activity in a subset of animals (FIG. 2A, B). Electrical kindling of the amygdala 1–2 months later required many fewer stimulations in pesticide-treated subjects relative to controls. The facilitation of electrical kindling, however, was limited to the focal seizure stages. Positive transfer from lindane and endosulfan

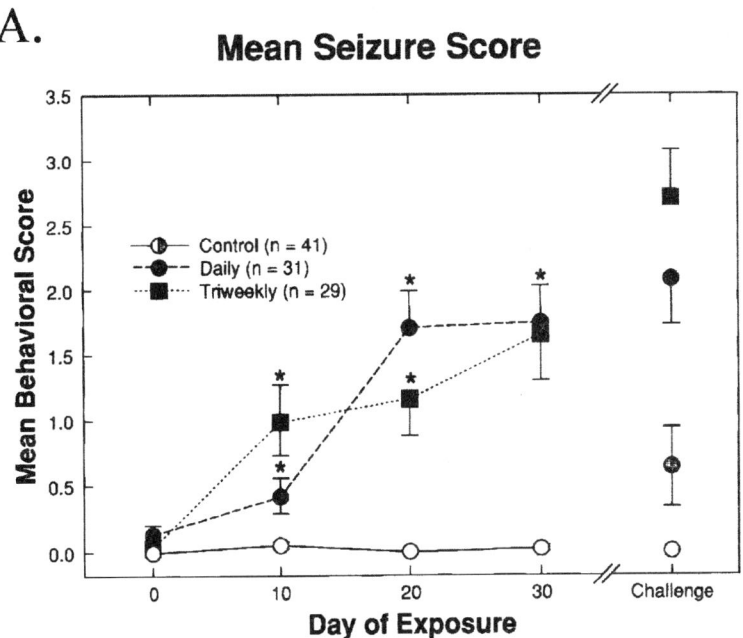

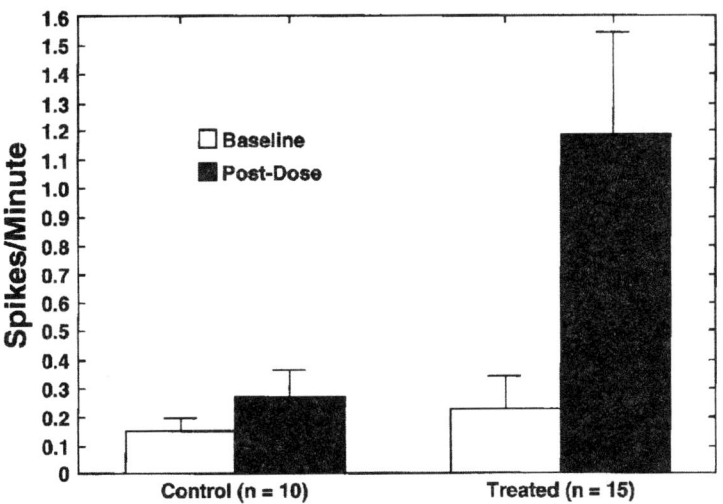

FIGURE 2. *See following page for caption.*

"chemical kindling" to "electrical kindling" induced by amygdala stimulation may be reflective of hyperreactive limbic focal seizure pathways. Furthermore, savings observed with electrical kindling following repeated low-level chemical exposure suggest that chemical kindling with these pesticides involves the same biological substrates as electrical kindling. Thus, it appears that repeated low-level exposure to pesticides can induce a persistent state of enhanced seizure susceptibility via a kindling mechanism.

Positive transfer from chemical to electrical kindling with lindane and endosulfan was bidirectional. Animals first kindled electrically to fully generalized seizures and challenged thereafter with low doses of lindane or endosulfan showed increased susceptibility to the seizure-inducing properties of these pesticides.[44] Behavioral and electrographic indices of seizure activity as well as reductions in AD thresholds were observed in kindled animals relative to nonstimulated controls upon challenge with subthreshold concentrations of endosulfan and lindane.

INTERICTAL EVENTS

Hyperexcitability of focal limbic circuits can be assessed by measuring spontaneous and evoked field potentials. Spontaneous IIS are a common marker of an epileptic brain and are used clinically to identify the region of focal epileptiform activity during seizure-free periods. IIS represent normal transients present in a nonepileptiform brain that become magnified in size and occur with a much higher probability in response to the epileptogenic process.[45] IIS are prominent in the amygdala and pyriform areas following electrical kindling (FIG. 3).

Alterations in synaptic and cellular responsiveness can also be investigated *in vivo* by evoking population events through direct stimulation of synaptic pathways. The lamellar structure of the hippocampus is ideally suited for this type of investigation. Single-pulse stimulation of perforant path fibers (the primary afferent to the hippocampus) and recording from the hilar region of the dentate gyrus reliably evoke

---

FIGURE 2. Behavioral and electrographic indices of hyperexcitability following repeated lindane exposure. (**A**) Mean behavioral seizure scores were progressively increased with successive doses of 10 mg/kg, po; vehicle: lindane in corn oil. Animals were treated with lindane once daily for 30 consecutive days (daily) or three times per week (Monday/Wednesday/Friday) for 10 weeks (*filled symbols*) or with corn oil (*open circles*). Seizure signs ranged from minor, motor arrest (Stage 1), myoclonic jerks (MCJ, Stage 2), multiple MCJ (Stage 3), prolonged MCJ with brief periods of clonus (2–3 s, Stage 4), to severe, clonic seizures (Stage 5), multiple clonic bouts (Stage 6). One month after the final dose, subjects were challenged with 10 mg/kg lindane, and seizure responsiveness was maintained. Control subjects were challenged with corn oil (*open circle*) or 10 mg/kg lindane (*gray circle*). The mean seizure stage was maintained at a higher level in treated groups, and one subject from the control group challenged with lindane responded with a clonic seizure, inflating the mean score. (**B**) The incidence of interictal spikes (IIS) recorded from indwelling electrodes in the amygdala was increased in animals with a 10-week history of lindane exposure as described above. Treated animals were drug-free for 4 weeks prior to challenge. Controls previously dosed with corn oil received lindane for the first time at challenge. Baseline is the mean number of EEG spikes in the 30-min predose period; postdose reflects the mean number of spikes in the 90-min postdosing period. (From ref. 40.)

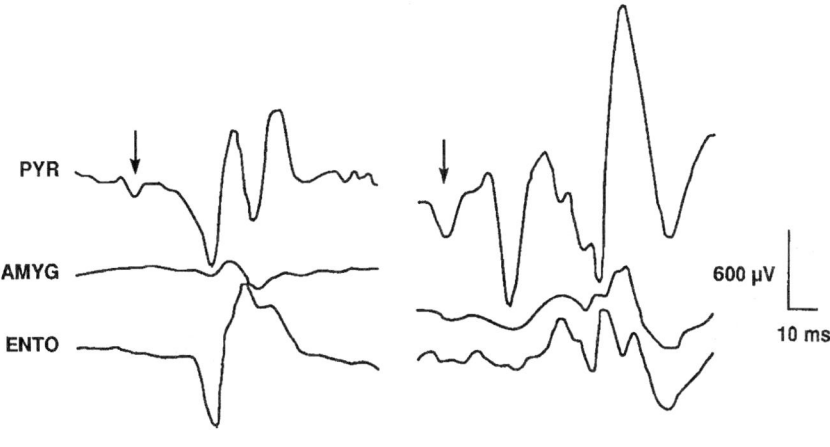

Pre-Kindling **Post-Kindling**

FIGURE 3. Spontaneous interictal spikes (IIS). Recordings taken before and after amygdala kindling. IIS are prominent in amygdala (AMYG) and pyriform cortex (PYR) after kindling. Spontaneous burst responses appear to evolve from normal population events observed in the naive animal prior to kindling, but are exaggerated in amplitude and occur at a much higher frequency after kindling. Onset latency (*arrow*) is shortest in pyriform suggesting that this region precipitates population events in other sites. Responses in the entorhinal cortex (ENTO) become more complex in morphology. (From ref. 45.)

a large-field potential reflecting population synaptic responses (excitatory postsynaptic potential, EPSP) and somatic excitability (population spike, action potential firing of granule cells of the dentate gyrus). Both the EPSP and population spike component of the evoked field potential are persistently enhanced as a result of kindling (FIG. 4A, B) in many forebrain sites.[8,9] This enhancement in synaptic strength appears within the first 1–2 ADs, does not require behavioral seizures, and looks similar to LTP.[8,27,46] However, the magnitude of the increase in synaptic response elicited by AD-inducing stimulation is much larger and persistent than that observed with conventional LTP-like stimulation.[8,9,27,46] Like LTP, kindling-induced potentiation is reduced by NMDA antagonists[46,47] (FIG. 4).

In addition to promoting increases in the amplitude of evoked field potentials, delivery of single-pulse stimulation in well-kindled animals can also lead to the elicitation of IIS. FIGURE 5 presents recordings from an animal before and 24 h after evoking 60 ADs. Prior to kindling, two-single pulse stimuli delivered 200 ms apart produced a typical evoked field potential in a naive animal (FIG. 5A). After many kindling stimulations, however, these single pulses produced the evoked potential as well as a series of spontaneous potentials (FIG. 5B). The spontaneous but not the evoked field potentials are readily blocked by the NMDA antagonist MK-801 (FIG. 5C).

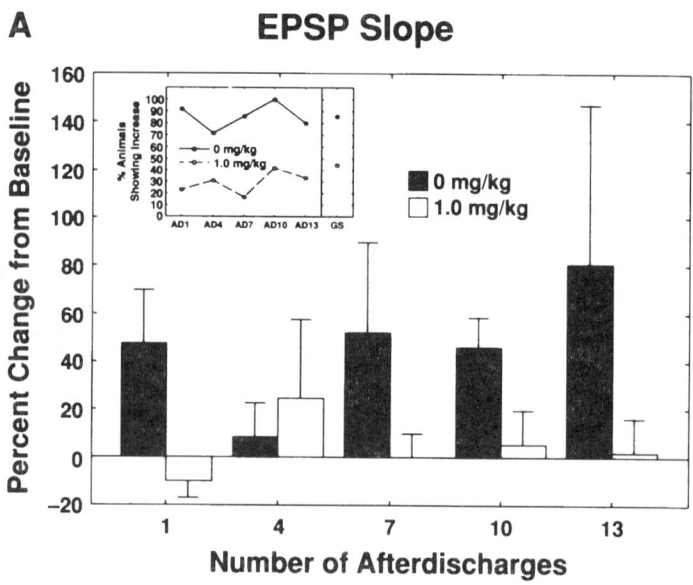
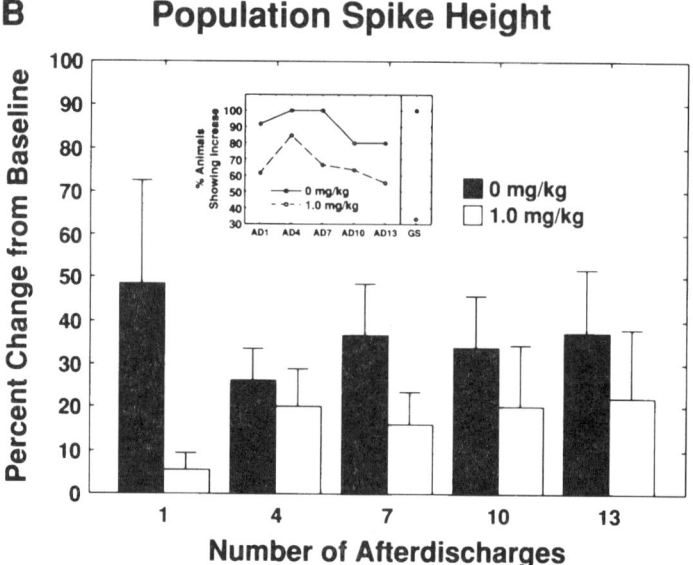

FIGURE 4. Potentiation induced by kindling and LTP *in vivo*. Percent increase in EPSP slope (**A**) and population spike (**B**) amplitude in dentate gyrus field potential 18–24 h after 1, 4, 7, 10, and 13 afterdischarges (AD) evoked by 2-s 60-Hz stimulation applied to the perforant path. Kindling-induced enhancement in field potential amplitude was reduced by 1.0 mg/kg, ip, MK-801 delivered 30 min prior to kindling stimulation. (**C**) LTP stimulation (50-ms 400-Hz train at 1000 µA) did not increase EPSP slope, but produced increases in PS amplitude measured 24 h after stimulation. LTP was blocked by 0.1 and 1.0 mg/kg MK-801 delivered 30 min prior to tetanus. See reference 46 for experimental details.

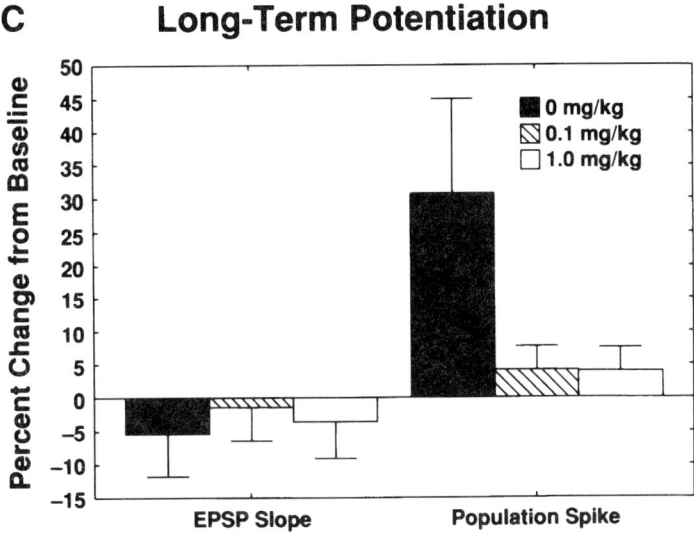

FIGURE 4. *Continued.*

INTERICTAL EVENTS INDUCED BY LINDANE

Electrographic events indicative of hyperexcitability in limbic sites, remote in time from the kindling treatment, have also been observed in animals repeatedly exposed to lindane. Rats administered lindane 30 times over a 10-week period (3 times/week) and challenged one month after termination of exposure, revealed significant alterations in waking EEG monitored from the amygdala.[40] Control animals with a history of vehicle treatment and subsequently challenged with lindane for the first time responded with a few EEG spikes, but not more than that seen under the predose condition. Animals with a history of lindane exposure, however, responded with a large increase in EEG spikes relative to both their predose baseline, and to control subjects receiving lindane for the first time. Some subjects displayed only electrographic signs of amygdala hyperexcitability, whereas in other subjects these electrographic events were accompanied by mild behavioral seizure signs (see FIG. 2). The half-life of lindane is estimated to be approximately 27 h.[48] Thus, the challenge dose delivered one month after the last exposure to lindane occurred at a time when body burdens had dissipated. These data, together with positive transfer to electrical kindling outlined above, clearly indicate that a history of low-level repeated exposure to lindane, much like kindling, produces a persistent state of hyperexcitability in forebrain sites. Consistent with behavioral alterations associated with electrical kindling (see below), Llorens *et al.*[49,50] have also reported alterations in locomotor activity and emotional behavior (as assessed on the elevated plus maze) following repeated dosing with lindane.

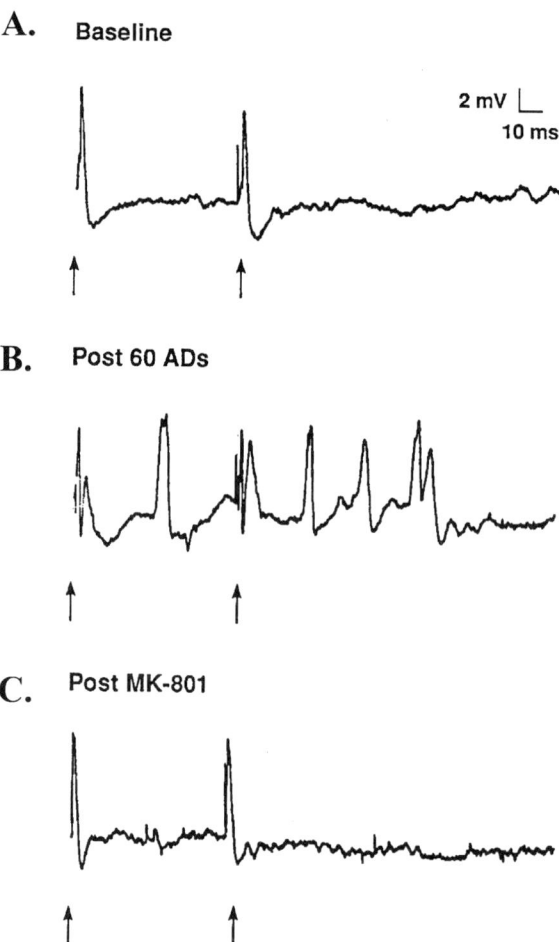

FIGURE 5. Interictal spikes are enhanced by kindling and reduced by NMDA antagonists. Potentials recorded from the dentate gyrus in response to two perforant path pulses delivered 200-ms apart are indicated by the arrows (**A**). After extensive kindling of the perforant path (60 ADs), evoked responses are increased in amplitude, and single-pulse stimulation induces a number of high-amplitude EEG spikes (**B**). These interictal events triggered as a result of single-pulse stimulation are blocked by MK-801 (**C**). (Burdette, unpublished observations.)

HOW COULD THIS STATE OF HYPEREXCITABILITY COME ABOUT?

The convulsant properties of lindane and related pesticides (endosulfan and dieldrin) in acute high dosages have been well established, and this action has been tied to effects on GABAergic inhibitory function in the CNS.[51–59] In rat brain, lindane binds to the t-[^{35}S]butylbicyclophosphorothionate (TBPS) site on the GABA receptor/ionophore complex and blocks GABA-mediated chloride flux.[51–56] In den-

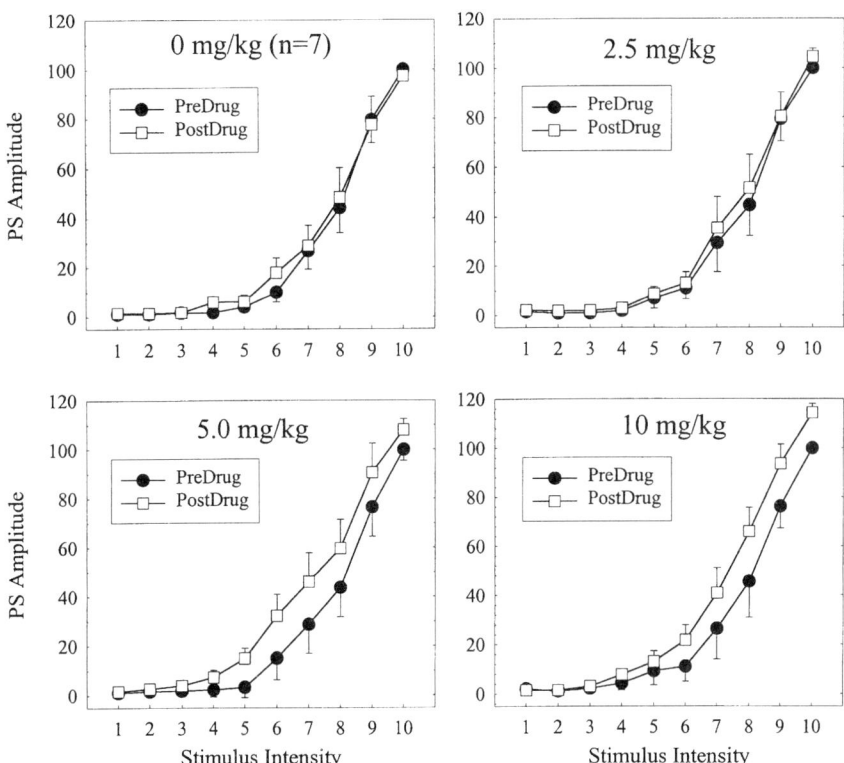

FIGURE 6. Lindane increases hippocampal excitability *in vivo*. Input/output functions taken before and 60 min after dosing with lindane (po in corn oil) in the dentate gyrus following perforant path stimulation *in vivo*. The 5- and 10-mg/kg dosages of lindane increased population spike (PS) amplitude (ANOVA, $p < 0.05$).

tate gyrus, field potential recordings in intact animals, lindane increases population spike amplitude at dosages well below electrographic seizure threshold (FIG. 6). Similarly, Joy and colleagues have demonstrated that acute exposure to lindane-induced decrements in GABA-mediated inhibition in the dentate gyrus *in vivo*[57] as well as in area CA1 of hippocampal slices[58,59] (see FIG. 7).

It is likely that the action of lindane and endosulfan in reducing GABA-mediated transmission contributes to the increases in limbic system excitability as reflected in (1) increases in excitatory synaptic transmission[58] (FIG. 6), (2) reductions in paired pulse depression[57-59] (FIG. 7), (3) facilitation of electrical kindling,[34,37] (4) behavioral sensitization observed during chemical kindling [39,40] (FIG. 2A), and (5) increased amygdala epileptiform spike activity following repeated lindane administration[40] (FIG. 2B). Reduction of GABA-mediated inhibition by selective GABA antagonists also facilitates the development of LTP.[60,61] Furthermore, repeated induction of LTP in hippocampal pathways may reduce AD thresholds and can

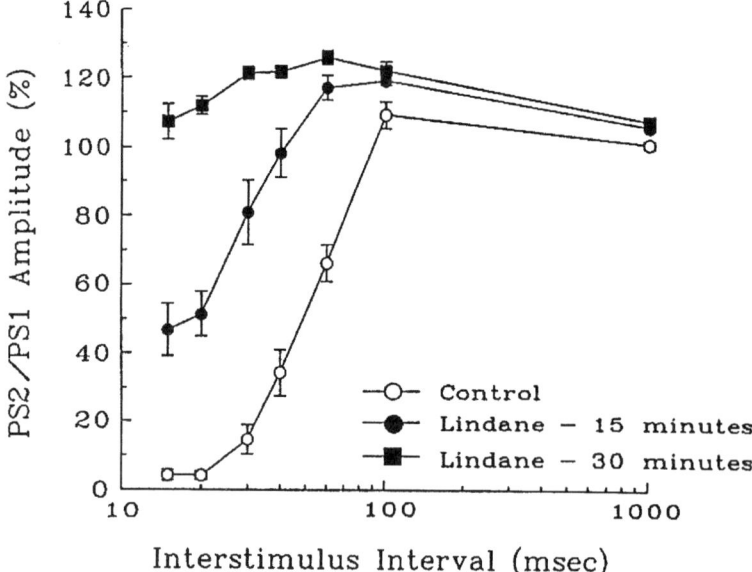

FIGURE 7. Lindane reduces GABA-mediated inhibition in hippocampus. When pairs of stimulus pulses are delivered at brief interstimulus intervals (10–100 ms), the population spike evoked by the second pulse of the pair (PS2) is reduced relative to the first (PS1) due to activation of GABA-mediated inhibitory circuits. These data are typically expressed as a ratio of the population spike amplitudes (PS2/PS1). GABA-mediated recurrent collateral inhibition is antagonized by 25 µmol lindane in area CA1 of hippocampus *in vitro*. (From ref. 58.)

promote strong facilitation of kindling development.[29] Thus, in the absence of electrographic seizure activation (i.e., ADs), increased excitation coupled with reduced inhibitory tone evoked by repeated administration of lindane may induce or facilitate LTP-like changes in certain synaptic circuits. In this way, and perhaps in the case of MCS, pesticides of this class may lead to persistent changes in limbic excitability and facilitate kindling in the absence of electrographic seizure discharge.

COGNITIVE AND EMOTIONAL CONSEQUENCES OF KINDLING

One of the properties that makes kindling an attractive model for both temporal lobe epilepsy and MCS is the behavioral sequelae that persist well beyond the ictal episodes and overlap those seen in affected patients of these disorders.[1,2,62-65] Alterations in both cognitive and emotional status have been reported by sufferers of MCS (see recent reviews: refs. 1 and 2). In animal models, electrographic seizure activity, discretely induced either chemically or electrically in limbic brain sites during task acquisition, clearly disrupts cognitive performance on a variety of learning and memory tasks.[66-71] However, deficits in learning and memory are also evident in epileptic patients during seizure-free periods, far removed from the acute ictal event.[63-65,72,73] In a similar fashion, a history of kindling, in the absence of overt behavioral or electrographic seizure manifestations at the time of testing, has also been shown to have persistent deleterious effects upon cognitive performance.[71,74–81]

Recently, attention has turned from primarily the cognitive realm to include disturbances of affective behavior that accompany kindling. Clear differences in performance on a number of emotionally motivated tasks were observed in animals selectively bred as fast versus slow kindlers.[82] Long-term disruption of behavioral indices of anxiety has been repeatedly demonstrated in fully kindled animals.[25,83–87] Several laboratories using a number of different behavioral paradigms have also observed increases in emotional responsiveness after partial kindling, that is, in animals that are not displaying overt signs of behavioral seizure.[24,88–91]

MCS AS AN ANXIETY DISORDER

In a recent review on MCS, Sorg[2] suggested that the wide variety of trigger compounds in MCS argues for an anxiety-associated mechanism. Peripheral infusion of sodium lactate is commonly used clinically to trigger attacks in panic-disorder patients.[92] In a small group of MCS patients, Binkley and Kutcher[93] reported that all patients responded with a panic-like state that reproduced many of their MCS symptoms under sodium lactate infusion but not under placebo control conditions. These findings and additional data (reviewed in refs. 1, 2, and 62) support the notion that the CNS pathways involved in anxiety are altered in individuals reporting MCS.

The amygdala is critical for the perception of many types of fear-provoking or aversive stimuli in humans and is necessary for the behavioral expression of fear.[94–98] Downstream outputs from the amygdala drive the different behaviors indicative of fear and anxiety (see FIG. 8). Many of these behaviors (i.e., freezing, heart rate, and star-

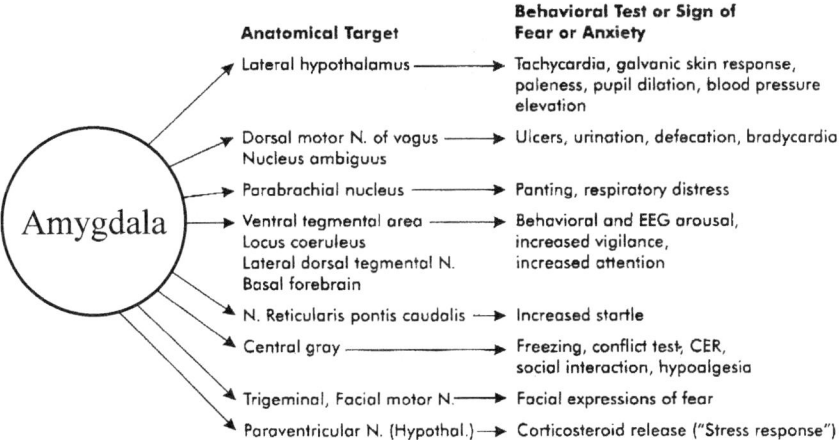

FIGURE 8. Amygdala controls expression of fear behavior. Direct connections between the central nucleus of the amygdala and a variety of hypothalamic and brain stem target areas involved in various indices of fear and anxiety. CER: conditioned emotional response. (Modified from ref. 94.)

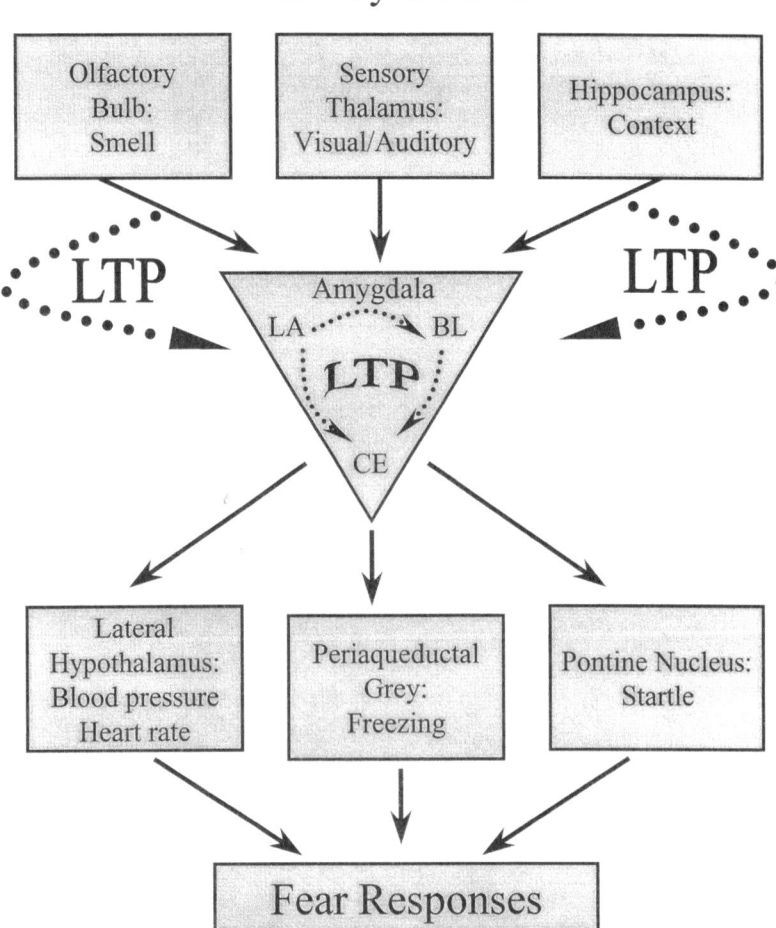

FIGURE 9. Role of synaptic plasticity in fear conditioning. Stimuli enter the amygdala from cortical and subcortical relays conveying information about the sensory and contextual milieu. Projections from these sensory relays target the lateral (LA) and basolateral (BL) nuclei of the amygdala, which in turn project to the central amygdala nucleus (CE). The CE innervates brain structures involved in the generation of fear responses, for example, hypothalamus, periaqueductal gray, and pontine nucleus (see also FIG. 8). Long-term potentiation (LTP) can occur at the synaptic connection between sensory inputs and the amygdala, and within the nuclei of the amygdala itself to augment activation of fear-related behavior. (Modified from ref. 99.)

tle) can be conditioned to neutral stimuli using classical conditioning techniques.[5,7,94–96,99,100] Recent advances elucidating the anatomical substrates and physiology of fear-related circuitry have provided additional credence to and support for the role of neuroplasticity in behavioral indices of fear and anxiety. LTP in the amygdala is not only critical for fear conditioning, but is induced endogenously in the amygdala during fear conditioning.[7,99] Modifications of a model (FIG. 9)

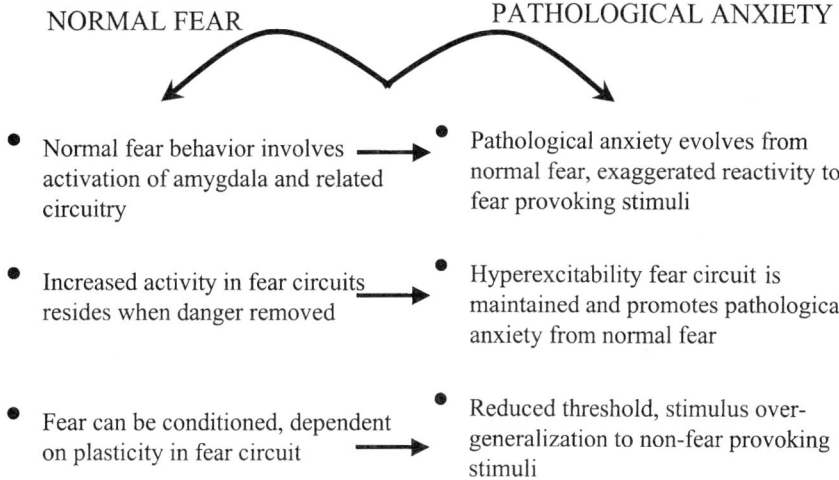

FIGURE 10. Relationship between normal fear and pathological anxiety. Anxiety may represent exaggerated fear responsiveness as described by Davis,[94–96] LeDoux,[97,98] and Rosen and Schulkin.[107]

proposed by Maren and Fanselow[99] depict how LTP occurring in sensory pathways carrying information about conditioned stimuli into the amygdala, and LTP between nuclei within the amygdala itself, induces the behavioral correlates of fear upon presentation of a previously neutral stimulus (see refs. 7, 95, and 99).

AMYGDALA HYPEREXCITABILITY AND ANXIETY

It has been hypothesized that pathological anxiety evolves from normal adaptive fear responses due to hyperexcitability within the neuronal circuitry subserving normal fear (FIG. 10). Kindling stimulation was used by Rosen et al.[91] to induce a state of hyperexcitability in the amygdala and examine its effects on "anxiety" using the fear potentiated startle (FPS) paradigm. In response to an abrupt unanticipated auditory stimulus (eliciting stimulus), rodents display a reflexive startle response. In the FPS paradigm, a light conditioned stimulus (CS) is paired with a shock unconditioned stimulus (US). Response to the tone eliciting stimulus, when presented in combination with the light CS, induces a much larger startle response relative to the tone alone, and is dependent upon plasticity within the amygdala.[95] Stimulation of the amygdala to evoke as few as two ADs leads to an augmentation in the fear-potentiated response with no change in baseline startle amplitude (FIG. 11). Interestingly, similar stimulation to the hippocampus did not alter FPS, indicating that hyperexcitability within specific limbic sites was a necessary condition for enhanced fear responsiveness. These data also clearly demonstrate that emotional lability does not require a chronic, long-term, severe, convulsive state, but is evident with minimal seizure activation.

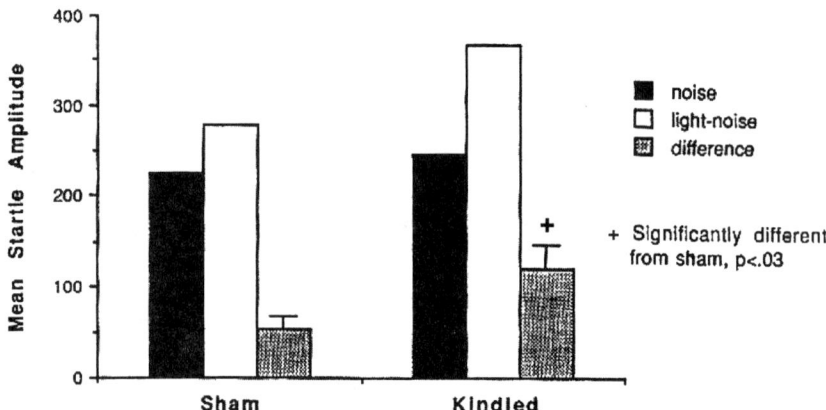

FIGURE 11. Minimal kindling increases fear behavior. Fear-potentiated startle was enhanced in animals given as few as two afterdischarges (mean duration ~17 s) to each amygdala. No change in baseline startle response was observed. (From ref. 91.)

In a different experimental procedure, Sanders et al.[101] delivered daily administrations of subthreshold concentrations of the GABA antagonist, bicuculline, directly into the amygdala over a period of several days. The authors reported progressive augmentation of physiological indices of fear, that is, blood pressure and heart rate (FIG. 12A). Although similar treatment can lead to chemical kindling,[102–105] increases in the physiological fear responses were evident prior to the elicitation of seizure activity, which was confirmed by monitoring EEG from indwelling amygdala electrodes (FIG. 12B). These findings are significant because they indicate that repeated blockade of GABA receptors in the amygdala leads to progressive increases in the excitability of the fear circuitry. This enhanced excitability alone, in the absence of a pathological seizure discharge, is sufficient to promote progressive and persistent increases in fear behavior.

MODEL OF CYCLODIENE PESTICIDES, KINDLING, AND ANXIETY

The relationship between pesticide exposure, neuronal excitability and plasticity, and behavioral change as discussed above is summarized in FIGURE 13. It is well established that kindling increases excitability in fear circuits and that this augmentation leads to persistent changes in affective behavior.[25,83–91] Patients with anxiety disorders may have a lower threshold for anxiety-provoking stimuli.[92,106,107] Kindling may induce emotional lability by both augmenting excitability in fear circuitry and lowering the threshold for anxiety-provoking stimuli. The work of Sanders et al.[101] indicates that kindling per se may not be necessary for this behavioral change. Both non-AD-inducing chemical[101] and non-AD-inducing electrical stimulation[5,96,99,108,109] of amygdala circuitry are sufficient to promote potentiation of synaptic transmission in the amygdala and to increase fear behavior[7,100,109] in experimental animals. Acute exposure to some chemicals, most notably those with

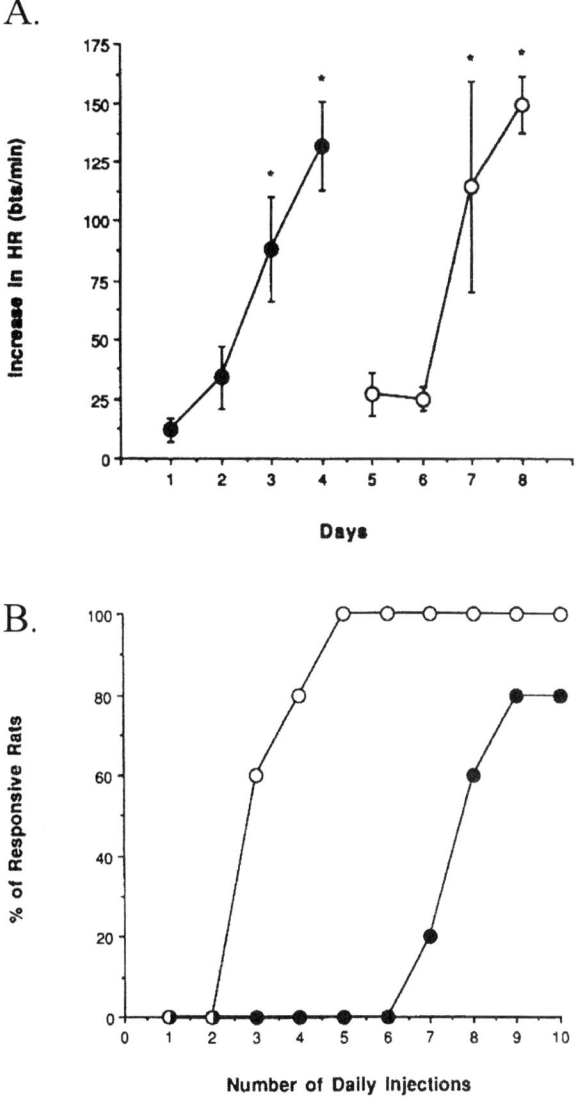

FIGURE 12. Cardiovascular effects of GABA antagonism in the absence of afterdischarges. (**A**) Repeated intra-amygdala administration of 6 pmol bicuculline methiodide (BMI) produced progressive increases in fear behavior as assessed by heart rate (*filled circles*). *Open circles* reflect response of animals previously treated with saline (during which no change in heart rate or other physiological indicators of fear was observed; data not shown), and subsequently administered BMI for four consecutive days. (**B**) Percent of animals responding to intra-amygdala BMI injection with increases in heart rate and blood pressure (*open circles*). Clear increases in these physiological indices were evident prior to any indication of electrographic seizure activity measured from electrodes in the amygdala (*filled circles*). (From ref. 101.)

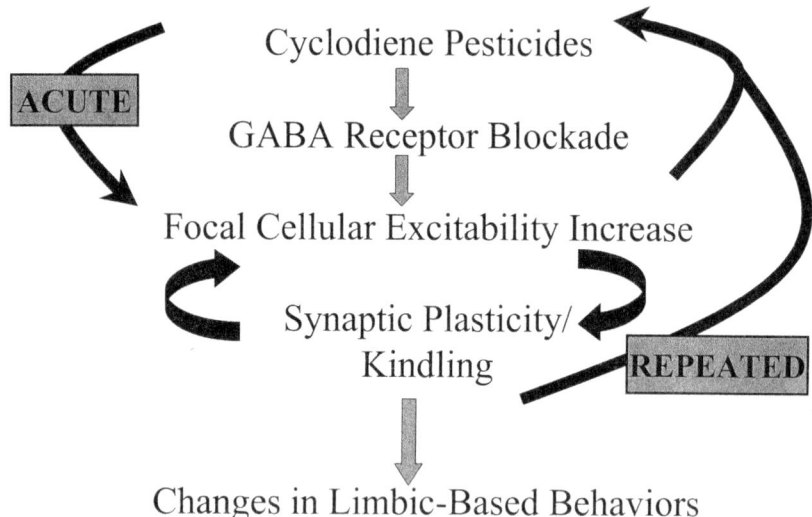

FIGURE 13. Plasticity-induced changes in affective behavior. Kindling increases excitability in fear circuits and leads to persistent changes in affective behavior. Acute exposure to some xenobiotics, most notably those with GABAergic-blocking properties, causes focal cellular excitability increases in limbic sites. With repetition, these chemically induced acute excitatory events may induce plasticity on their own, or secondarily facilitate the induction of naturally occurring LTP. Exposure to some environmental contaminants may contribute to the symptomatology of MCS by increasing lability of the limbic system through neuroplastic mechanisms.

GABAergic-blocking properties, leads to focal cellular excitability increases in limbic sites[57–59] (FIG. 6). Pesticides such as lindane, endosulfan, amitraz, and members of the pyrethroid class have all been demonstrated to alter limbic excitability at subconvulsive doses.[30,32–44,57–59,110,111] With repetition, chemically induced acute excitatory events may induce plasticity on their own, or secondarily facilitate the induction of naturally occurring LTP. In this way, in addition to genetic, experiential, and organismal factors such as age, trauma, and disease, exposure to some environmental contaminants may contribute to the symptomatology of MCS involving cognitive and emotional dysfunction.

Characterization of the clinical etiology of chemical intolerance remains a hotly debated issue. This symposium is significant in focusing on potential mechanisms of MCS, and has served to move the discussion beyond arguments over its authenticity. Participating scientists considered the phenomenon in light of their own expertise and in so doing offered instructive glimpses into potential mechanisms and further theorizing. Although this may have done little to resolve the controversy over the veracity of MCS, it has promoted a healthy dialogue regarding potential neurobiological substrates for this and related clinical syndromes. Neuroplasticity, as characterized by the LTP and kindling models, may provide a plausible mechanism underlying the syndrome of chemical intolerance.

ACKNOWLEDGMENTS

The information in this document has been funded by the U.S. Environmental Protection Agency. It has been subjected to review by the National Health and Environmental Effects Research Laboratory and approved for publication. Approval does not signify that the contents reflect the views of the Agency, nor does mention of trade names or commercial products constitute endorsement or recommendation for use.

REFERENCES

1. BELL, I.R., C.M. BALDWIN, M. FERNANDEZ et al. 1999. Neural sensitization model of multiple chemical sensitivity: overview of theory and empirical evidence. Toxicol. Ind. Health **14:** 295–304.
2. SORG, B.A. 1999. Multiple chemical sensitivity: potential role for neural sensitization. Crit. Rev. Neurobiol. **13:** 283–316.
3. BLISS, T.V.P. & G.L. COLLINGRIDGE, 1993. A synaptic model of memory: long-term potentiation in the hippocampus. Nature **361:** 31–39.
4. MALENKA, R.C. & R.A. NICOLL. 1999. Long-term potentiation—a decade of progress? Science **285:** 1870–1874.
5. MAREN, S. 1996. Synaptic transmission and plasticity in the amygdala: an emerging physiology of fear conditioning circuits. Mol. Neurobiol. **13:** 1–22.
6. MARTINEZ, J.L. & B.E. DERRICK. 1996. Long-term potentiation and learning. Annu. Rev. Psychol. **47:** 173–203.
7. MAREN, S. 1999. Long-term potentiation in the amygdala: a mechanism for emotional learning and memory. Trends Neurosci. **22:** 561–567.
8. RACINE, R.J., N.W. MILGRAM & S. HAFNER. 1983. Long-term potentiation phenomena in the rat limbic forebrain. Brain Res. **260:** 217–231.
9. RACINE, R.J., K.A. MOORE & C. EVANS. 1991. Kindling-induced potentiation in the pyriform cortex. Brain Res. **556:** 218–225.
10. COLLINGRIDGE, G.L. 1992. The mechanism of induction of NMDA receptor-dependent long-term potentiation in the hippocampus. Exp. Physiol. **77:** 771–797.
11. MALENKA, R.C. 1992. The role of postsynaptic calcium in the induction of long-term potentiation. Mol. Neurobiol. **5:** 289–295.
12. ROBERSON, E.D., J.D. ENGLISH & J.D. SWEATT. 1996. A biochemist's view of long-term potentiation. Learn. Memory **3:** 1–24.
13. SODERLING, T.R. & V.A. DERKACH. 2000. Postsynaptic protein phosphorylation and LTP. Trends Neurosci. **23:** 75–80.
14. SWEATT, J.D. 1999. Towards a molecular explanation for long-term potentiation. Learn. Memory **6:** 399–416.
15. GODDARD, G.V., D.C. MCINTYRE & C.K. LEECH. 1969. A permanent change in brain function resulting from daily electrical stimulation. Exp. Neurol. **25:** 295–330.
16. RACINE, R.J. 1978. Kindling: the first decade. Neurosurgery **3:** 234–252.
17. RACINE, R.J. 1972. Modification of seizure activity by electrical stimulation: I. After-discharge threshold. Electroencephalogr. Clin. Neurophysiol. **32:** 269–279.
18. RACINE, R.J., W.M. BURNHAM, M.E. GILBERT et al. 1986. Kindling mechanisms: I. Electrophysiological studies. In Kindling 3, pp. 263–279. Raven Press. New York.
19. MODY, I., P.K. STANTON & U. HEINEMANN. 1988. Activation of N-methyl-D-aspartate receptors parallels changes in cellular and synaptic properties of dentate granule cells after kindling. J. Neurophysiol. **59:** 1033–1054.
20. MODY, I. & U. HEINEMANN. 1987. NMDA receptors of dentate gyrus granule cells participate in synaptic transmission following kindling. Nature **326:** 701–704.
21. RACINE, R.J. 1972. Modification of seizure activity by electrical stimulation: II. Motor seizures. Electroencephalogr. Clin. Neurophysiol. **32:** 281–294.

22. BELL, I.R., C.S. MILLER & G.E.R. SCHWARTZ. 1992. An olfactory-limbic model of multiple chemical sensitivity syndrome: possible relationships to kindling and affective spectrum disorders. Biol. Psychiatry **32:** 218–242.
23. MCINTYRE, D.C. & M.E. KELLY. 1998. The perirhinal cortex and kindled motor seizures. *In* Kindling 5, pp. 167–176. Plenum. New York.
24. ADAMEC, R.E. 1990. Does kindling model anything clinically relevant? Biol. Psychiatry **27:** 249–279.
25. KALYNCHUK, L.E., J.P.J. PINEL, D. TREIT *et al.* 1998. Persistence of the interictal emotionality produced by long-term amygdala kindling in rats. Neuroscience **85:** 1311–1319.
26. RACINE, R.J., E. KAIRISS & G. SMITH. 1981. Kindling mechanisms: the evolution of the burst response versus enhancement. *In* Kindling 2, pp. 15–27. Raven Press. New York.
27. SUTULA, T. & O. STEWARD. 1986. Quantitative analysis of synaptic potentiation during kindling of the perforant path. J. Neurophysiol. **56:** 732–746.
28. RACINE, R.J., F. NEWBERRY & W.M. BURNHAM. 1975. Postactivation potentiation and the kindling phenomenon. Electroencephalogr. Clin. Neurophysiol. **39:** 261–271.
29. SUTULA, T. & O. STEWARD. 1987. Facilitation of kindling by prior induction of long-term potentiation in the perforant path. Brain Res. **420:** 109–117.
30. GILBERT, M.E. 1992. Neurotoxicants and limbic kindling. *In* The Vulnerable Brain and Environmental Risks. Vol. 1: Malnutrition and Hazard Assessment, pp. 173–192. Plenum. New York.
31. HAYES, W.J. & E.R. LAWS. 1991. Handbook of Pesticide Toxicology. Academic Press. New York.
32. GILBERT, M.E. 1994. The phenomenology of limbic kindling: symposium on low level chemical sensitivity. Toxicol. Ind. Health **10:** 343–358.
33. GILBERT, M.E. 1988. Formamidine pesticides enhance susceptibility to kindled seizures in amygdala and hippocampus of the rat. Neurotoxicol. Teratol. **10:** 221–227.
34. GILBERT, M.E. 1992. Proconvulsant activity of endosulfan in amygdala kindling. Neurotoxicol. Teratol. **14:** 143–149.
35. GILBERT, M.E., S.K. ACHESON, C.M. MACK *et al.* 1990. An examination of the proconvulsant actions of pyrethroid insecticides using pentylenetetrazol and kindling seizure models. Neurotoxicology **11:** 73–86.
36. GILBERT, M.E. & C.M. MACK. 1989. Enhanced susceptibility to kindling by chlordimeform is mediated by a local anesthetic action. Psychopharmacology **99:** 163–167.
37. JOY, R.M., L.G. STARK & T.E. ALBERTSON. 1983. Proconvulsant actions of lindane: effects on afterdischarge thresholds and durations during amygdaloid kindling in rats. Neurotoxicology **2:** 211–220.
38. WURPEL, J.N.D., P.C. HIRT & J.H. BIDANSET. 1993. Amygdala kindling in immature rats: proconvulsant effect of the organophosphate insecticide—chlorpyrifos. Neurotoxicology **14:** 429–436.
39. GILBERT, M.E. 1992. A characterization of chemical kindling with the pesticide endosulfan. Neurotoxicol. Teratol. **14:** 151–158.
40. GILBERT, M.E. 1995. Repeated low level exposure to lindane leads to behavioral sensitization and facilitates electrical kindling. Neurotoxicol. Teratol. **17:** 131–142.
41. JOY, R.M., L.G. STARK, S.L. PETERSON *et al.* 1980. The kindled seizure: production of and modification by dieldrin in rats. Neurobehav. Toxicol. **2:** 117–124.
42. CAIN, D.P. 1986. The transfer phenomenon in kindling. *In* Kindling 3, pp. 231–248. Raven Press. New York.
43. WASTERLAIN, C.G., A. MORIN, D.G. FUJIKAWA *et al.* 1983. Chemical kindling. *In* The Clinical Relevance of Kindling, pp. 35–53. Wiley. New York.
44. GILBERT, M.E. & C.M. MACK. 1995. Seizure thresholds for the pesticides lindane and endosulfan are reduced in kindled animals. Neurotoxicol. Teratol. **17:** 143–150.
45. RACINE, R.J., M. MOSHER & E.W. KAIRISS. 1988. The role of the pyriform cortex in the generation of interictal spikes in the kindled preparation. Brain Res. **454:** 251–263.
46. GILBERT, M.E. & C.M. MACK. 1990. The NMDA antagonist, MK-801, suppresses long-term potentiation, kindling, and kindling-induced potentiation in the perforant path of the unanesthetized rat. Brain Res. **519:** 89–96.

47. ROBINSON, G.B. & G.D. REED. 1992. Effects of MK-801 on the induction and subsequent decay of long-term potentiation in the unanesthetized rabbit hippocampal dentate gyrus. Brain Res. **569:** 78–85.
48. TUSELL, J.M., C. SUNOL, E. GELPI *et al.* 1987. Relationship between lindane concentration in blood and brain and convulsant response in rats after oral or intraperitoneal administration. Arch. Toxicol. **60:** 432–437.
49. LLORENS, J., J.M. TUSELL, C. SUNOL *et al.* 1992. Repeated lindane exposure in the rat results in changes in spontaneous motor activity at 2 weeks post-exposure. Toxicol. Lett. **61:** 265–274.
50. LLORENS, J., J.M. TUSELL, C. SUNOL *et al.* 1990. On the effects of lindane on the plus-maze model of anxiety. Neurotoxicol. Teratol. **12:** 643–647.
51. ABALIS, I.M., M.E. ELDEFRAWI & A.T. ELDEFRAWI. 1985. High-affinity stereospecific binding of cyclodiene insecticides and gamma-hexachlorocyclohexane to gamma-aminobutyric acid receptors of rat brain. Pestic. Biochem. Physiol. **24:** 95–102.
52. CATTABENI, F., M.C. PASTORELLO & M. ELI. 1983. Convulsions induced by lindane and the involvement of the GABAergic system. Arch. Toxicol. (Suppl.) **6:** 244–249.
53. ELDEFRAWI, M.E., S.M. SHERBY, I.M. ABALIS *et al.* 1985. Interactions of pyrethroid and cyclodiene insecticides with nicotinic acetylcholine and GABA receptors. Neurotoxicology **6:** 47–62.
54. LAWRENCE, L.J. & J.E. CASIDA. 1984. Interaction of lindane, toxephine cyclodienes with brain specific *t*-butylbicyclophophorothionate receptor. Life Sci. **35:** 171–178.
55. LLORENS, J., C. SUNOL, J.M. TUSELL *et al.* 1990. Lindane inhibition of [^{35}S]TBPS binding to the GABA$_A$ receptor in rat brain. Neurotoxicol. Teratol. **12:** 607–610.
56. ABALIS, I.M., M.E. ELDEFRAWI & A.T. ELDEFRAWI. 1986. Effects of insecticides on GABA-induced chloride influx into rat brain microsacs. J. Toxicol. Environ. Health **18:** 13–23.
57. JOY, R.M. & T.E. ALBERTSON. 1987. Interactions of lindane with synaptically mediated inhibition and facilitation in the dentate gyrus. Neurotoxicology **8:** 529–542.
58. JOY, R.M., W.F. WALBY, L.G. STARK *et al.* 1995. Lindane blocks GABA$_A$-mediated inhibition and modulates pyramidal cell excitability in the rat hippocampal slice. Neurotoxicology **16:** 217–228.
59. STARK, L.G., R.M. JOY, W.F. WALBY *et al.* 1998. Interactions between convulsants at low-dose and phenobarbital in the hippocampal slice preparation. *In* Kindling 5, pp. 451–463. Plenum. New York.
60. CHAPMAN, C.A., Y. PEREZ & J.C. LACAILLE. 1998. Effects of GABA$_A$ inhibition on the expression of long-term potentiation in CA1 pyramidal cells are dependent on tetanization parameters. Hippocampus **8:** 289–298.
61. WIGSTROM, H. & B. GUSTAFSSON. 1983. Large long-term potentiation in the dentate gyrus *in vitro* during blockade of inhibition. Brain Res. **275:** 153–158.
62. BELL, I.R. 1992. Neuropsychiatric and biopsychosocial mechanisms in multiple chemical sensitivity: an olfactory-limbic system model. *In* National Research Council Report: Multiple Chemical Sensitivities. Addendum to Biologic Markers in Immunotoxicology, pp. 89–108. National Academy Press. Washington, D.C.
63. FLOR-HENRY, P. 1976. Epilepsy and psychopathology. *In* Recent Advances in Clinical Psychiatry, pp. 262–294. Churchill Livingstone. New York.
64. GLOOR, P., O. OLIVIER, L.F. QUESNEY *et al.* 1982. The role of the limbic system in experiential phenomena of temporal lobe epilepsy. Ann. Neurol. **12:** 129–144.
65. GALLASSI, R., A. MORREALE, S. LORUSSO *et al.* 1988. Epilepsy presenting as memory disturbance. Epilepsia **29:** 624–629.
66. KESNER, R.P. 1982. Brain stimulation: effects on memory. Behav. Neural Biol. **36:** 315–367.
67. KNOWLTON, B.J., M.L. SHAPIRO & D.S. OLTON. 1989. Hippocampal seizures disrupt working memory performance but not reference memory acquisition. Behav. Neurosci. **103:** 1144–1147.
68. LEPAINE, F.G. & A.G. PHILLIPS. 1978. Differential effects of electrical stimulation of amygdala, caudate-putamen, or substantia nigra pars compacta on taste aversion and passive avoidance in rats. Physiol. Behav. **21:** 979–985.

69. MCNAMARA, R.K., R.D. KIRKBY, G.E. DEPAPE *et al.* 1992. Limbic seizures, but not kindling, reversibly impair place learning in the Morris water maze. Behav. Brain Res. **50:** 167–175.
70. MILKULKA, P.J. & F.G. FREEMAN. 1984. The effect of amygdala-kindled seizures on the acquisition of taste and odor aversions. Physiol. Behav. **32:** 967–972.
71. PEELE, D.B. & M.E. GILBERT. 1992. Functional dissociation of acute and persistent cognitive deficits accompanying amygdala-kindled seizures. Behav. Brain Res. **48:** 65–76.
72. HALGREN, E. & C.L. WILSON. 1985. Recall deficits produced by afterdischarges in the human hippocampal formation and amygdala. Electroencephalogr. Clin. Neurophysiol. **61:** 375–380.
73. HERMANN, B.P., A.R. WYLER, E.T. RICHEY *et al.* 1987. Memory function and verbal learning ability in patients with complex partial seizures of temporal lobe origin. Epilepsia **28:** 547–554.
74. BELDHUIS, H.J.A., H.G.J. EVERTS, E.A. VAN DER ZEE *et al.* 1992. Amygdala kindling-induced seizures selectively impair spatial memory. 1. Behavioral characteristics and effects on hippocampal neuronal protein kinase C isoforms. Hippocampus **2:** 397–410.
75. BOAST, C. & D.C. MCINTYRE. 1977. Bilateral kindled amygdala foci and inhibitory avoidance behavior in rats: a functional lesion effect. Physiol. Behav. **18:** 25–28.
76. FEASEY-TRUGER, K.J., L. KARGL & G. TEN BRUGGENCATE. 1993. Differential effects of dentate kindling on working and reference spatial memory in the rat. Neurosci. Lett. **151:** 25–28.
77. LEUNG, L.S., K. BOON, T. KAIBARA *et al.* 1990. Radial maze performance following hippocampal kindling. Behav. Brain Res. **40:** 119–129.
78. LEUNG, L.S. & B. SHEN. 1991. Hippocampal CA1 evoked response and radial 8-arm maze performance after hippocampal kindling. Brain Res. **555:** 353–357.
79. LOPES DA SILVA, F.H., J.A. GORTER & W.J. WADMAN. 1986. Kindling of the hippocampus induces spatial memory deficits in the rat. Neurosci. Lett. **63:** 115–120.
80. NIEMINEN, S.A., J. SIRVIO, K. TEITTINEN *et al.* 1992. Amygdala kindling increased fear-response, but did not impair spatial memory in rats. Physiol. Behav. **51:** 845–849.
81. ROBINSON, G.B. 1992. Reversal learning of the rabbit nictitating membrane response following kindling-induced potentiation within the hippocampal dentate gyrus. Behav. Brain Res. **50:** 185–192.
82. MOHAPEL, P. & D.C. MCINTYRE. 1998. Amygdala kindling-resistant (SLOW) or -prone (FAST) rat strains show differential fear responses. Behav. Neurosci. **112:** 1402–1413.
83. ADAMEC, R.E. & D. MCKAY. 1993. Amygdala kindling, anxiety, and corticotrophin releasing factor (CRF). Physiol. Behav. **54:** 423–431.
84. DEPAULIS, A., V. HELFER, C. DERANSART *et al.* 1997. Anxiogenic-like consequences in animal models of complex partial seizures. Neurosci. Biobehav. Rev. **21:** 767–774.
85. HELFER, V., C. DERANSART, C. MARESCAUX *et al.* 1996. Amygdala kindling in the rat: anxiogenic-like consequences. Neuroscience **74:** 971–978.
86. HENKE, P.G. & R.M. SULLIVAN. 1985. Kindling in the amygdala and susceptibility to stress ulcers. Brain Res. Bull. **14:** 5–8.
87. KALYNCHUK, L.E., J.P.J. PINEL & D.TREIT. 1998. Long-term kindling and interictal emotionality in rats: effect of stimulation site. Brain Res. **779:** 149–157.
88. ADAMEC, R.E. 1999. Evidence that limbic neural plasticity in the right hemisphere mediates partial kindling induced lasting increases in anxiety-like behavior: effects of low frequency stimulation (quenching?) on long-term potentiation of amygdala efferents and behavior following kindling. Brain Res. **839:** 133–152.
89. ADAMEC, R.E. & C. STARK-ADAMEC. 1983. Partial kindling and emotional bias in the cat: lasting aftereffects of partial kindling of the ventral hippocampus. I. Behavioral changes. Behav. Neural Biol. **38:** 205–222.
90. ADAMEC, R.E. & C. STARK-ADAMEC. 1983. Partial kindling and emotional bias in the cat: lasting aftereffects of partial kindling of the ventral hippocampus. II. Physiological changes. Behav. Neural Biol. **38:** 223–239.
91. ROSEN, J.B., E. HAMERMAN, J.R. GLOWA *et al.* 1996. Hyperexcitability: exaggerated fear-potentiated startle produced by partial amygdala kindling. Behav. Neurosci. **110:** 43–50.

92. REIMAN, E.M., M.J. FUSSELMAN, P.J. FOX et al. 1991. Neuroanatomical correlates of anticipatory anxiety. Science **243:** 1071–1074.
93. BINKLEY, K.E. & S. KUTCHER. 1997. Panic response to sodium lactate infusion in patients with multiple chemical sensitivity syndrome. J. Allergy Clin. Immunol. **99:** 570–574.
94. DAVIS, M. 1992. The role of the amygdala in fear-potentiated startle: implications for animal models of anxiety. Trends Pharmacology **13:** 35–41.
95. DAVIS, M. 1997. Neurobiology of fear responses: the role of the amygdala. J. Neuropsychiatr. Clin. Neurosci. **9:** 382–402.
96. DAVIS, M., W.A. FALLS, S. CAMPEAU & M. KIM. 1993. Fear-potentiated startle: a neural and pharmacological analysis. Behav. Brain Res. **58:** 175–198.
97. LEDOUX, J.E. 1996. The Emotional Brain. Simon & Schuster. New York.
98. LEDOUX, J.E. 1992. Emotion and the amygdala. *In* The Amygdala: Neurobiological Aspects of Emotion, Memory, and Mental Dysfunction, pp. 339–351. Wiley–Liss. New York.
99. MAREN, S. & M.S. FANSELOW. 1996. The amygdala and fear conditioning: has the nut been cracked? Neuron **16:** 237–240.
100. ROGAN, M.T., U.V. STAUBLI & J. LEDOUX. 1997. Fear conditioning induces associative long-term potentiation in the amygdala. Nature **390:** 604–607.
101. SANDERS, S.K., S.L. MORZORATI & A. SHEKHAR. 1995. Priming of experimental anxiety by repeated subthreshold GABA blockade in the rat amygdala. Brain Res. **699:** 250–259.
102. CAIN, D.P. 1987. Kindling by repeated intraperitoneal or intracerebral injection of picrotoxin transfers to electrical kindling. Exp. Neurol. **97:** 243–254.
103. NUTT, D.J., P.J. COWEN, C.C. BATTS et al. 1982. Repeated administration of subconvulsant doses of GABA antagonist drugs. I. Effects on seizure threshold (kindling). Psychopharmacology **76:** 84–87.
104. UEMURA, S. & H. KIMURA. 1988. Amygdaloid kindling with bicuculline methiodide in rats. Exp. Neurol. **102:** 346–353.
105. UEMURA, S. & H. KIMURA. 1990. Common epileptic pathway in amygdaloid bicuculline and electrical kindling demonstrated by transferability. Brain Res. **537:** 315–317.
106. MARKS, I.M. 1987. Fears Phobias and Rituals. Oxford University Press. London/New York.
107. ROSEN, J.B. & J. SCHULKIN. 1998. From normal fear to pathological anxiety. Psychol. Rev. **105:** 325–350.
108. CLUGNET, M.C. & J.E. LEDOUX. 1990. Synaptic plasticity in fear conditioning circuits: induction of LTP in the lateral nucleus of the amygdala by stimulation of the media geniculate body. J. Neurosci. **10:** 2818–2824.
109. ROGAN, M.T. & J.E. LEDOUX. 1995. LTP is accompanied by commensurate enhancement of auditory-evoked responses in a fear-conditioning circuit. Neuron **15:** 127–136.
110. GILBERT, M.E. & R.S. DYER. 1988. Increased hippocampus excitability produced by amitraz. Neurotoxicol. Teratol. **10:** 229–235.
111. GILBERT, M.E., C.M. MACK & K.M. CROFTON. 1989. Pyrethroids and enhanced inhibition in the hippocampus of the rat. Brain Res. **477:** 314–321.

A Genetic Rat Model of Cholinergic Hypersensitivity: Implications for Chemical Intolerance, Chronic Fatigue, and Asthma

DAVID H. OVERSTREET[a,b] AND VELJKO DJURIC[c]

[b]*Department of Psychiatry and Center for Alcohol Studies, University of North Carolina at Chapel Hill, Chapel Hill, North Carolina 27599-7178, USA*

[c]*McMaster Psychiatric Unit, St. Joseph's Hospital, Hamilton, Ontario L8N 4A6, Canada*

ABSTRACT: The fact that only some individuals exposed to environmental chemicals develop chemical intolerance raises the possibility that genetic factors could be contributing factors. The present communication summarizes evidence from a genetic animal model of cholinergic supersensitivity that suggests that an abnormal cholinergic system could be one predisposing genetic factor. The Flinders Sensitive Line (FSL) rats were established by selective breeding for increased responses to an organophosphate. It was subsequently found that these FSL rats were also more sensitive to direct-acting muscarinic agonists and had elevated muscarinic receptors compared to the selectively bred parallel group, the Flinders Resistant Line (FRL) rats, or randomly bred control rats. Increased sensitivity to cholinergic agents has also been observed in several human populations, including individuals suffering from chemical intolerance. Indeed, the FSL rats exhibit certain behavioral characteristics such as abnormal sleep, activity, and appetite that are similar to those reported in these human populations. In addition, the FSL rats have been reported to exhibit increased sensitivity to a variety of other chemical agents. Peripheral tissues, such as intestinal and airway smooth muscle, appear to be more sensitive to both cholinergic agonists and an antigen, ovalbumin. Hypothermia, a centrally mediated response, is more pronounced in the FSL rats after nicotine and alcohol, as well as agents that are selective for the dopaminergic and serotonergic systems. In some cases, the increased sensitivity has been detected in the absence of any changes in the receptors with which the drugs interact (dopamine receptors), while receptor changes have been seen in other cases (nicotine receptors). Therefore, there may be multiple mechanisms underlying the multiple chemical sensitivity-chemical intolerance of the FSL rats. An elucidation of these mechanisms may provide useful clues to those involved in chemical intolerance in humans.

INTRODUCTION

Patients suffering from multiple chemical sensitivity (MCS) or chemical intolerance (CI) frequently report symptoms that overlap with those reported by patients suffering from chronic fatigue syndrome and/or asthma.[1–4] The overlap in the prev-

[a]Address for correspondence: David H. Overstreet, Ph.D., Bowles Center for Alcohol Studies, CB 7178, 3011 Thurston-Bowles Building, University of North Carolina at Chapel Hill, Chapel Hill, NC 27599-7178. Voice: 919-966-1159; fax: 919-966-5679.
dhover@med.unc.edu

alence of these conditions suggests that there might be some underlying common mechanism. This brief review considers the hypothesis that a hyperresponsive cholinergic system might provide a link between asthma, chemical intolerance, and chronic fatigue by considering evidence obtained in a genetic animal model of cholinergic hyperresponsiveness.[5,6]

The cholinergic nervous system, which uses acetylcholine at its nerve terminals, is very pervasive.[7,8] Not only does it innervate voluntary skeletal muscles (acting upon nicotinic receptors) and involuntary smooth muscles and the heart (acting upon muscarinic receptors), but it also sends fibers into many regions of the brain from basal forebrain and midbrain nuclei.[8] Stimulation of cholinergic pathways by pesticides and other agents may produce a variety of peripheral and central symptoms which are reminiscent of the complaints of people suffering from asthma and/or MCS, including respiratory, gastrointestinal, and CNS symptoms. Indeed, a patient's hyperresponsiveness to the cholinergic agonist methacholine is commonly used to confirm a diagnosis of asthma. Therefore, the pervasiveness of the cholinergic system makes it a likely candidate to be involved in the multi-organ complaints frequently reported by individuals with CI, including difficulties in concentration, irritable bowel, and asthma.[1,3]

The hypothesis that a hyperresponsive cholinergic system participates in the symptoms reported by individuals with CI or chronic fatigue will be examined by reviewing some findings from a genetic animal model of cholinergic hypersensitivity. Specifically, the increased sensitivity of this animal model to hypothermia induced by drugs acting upon multiple neurotransmitter systems and its increased sensitivity to breathing difficulties induced by an allergen will be summarized. Previous reports[5,6] may be consulted for details.

AN ANIMAL MODEL OF CHOLINERGIC HYPERSENSITIVITY

This year marks the twenty-fifth anniversary of the first studies on the Flinders Line rats, developed at Flinders University in Australia, by selective breeding for differential responses to the anticholinesterase agent, diisopropyl fluorophosphate.[9,10] The Flinders Sensitive Line (FSL) rats also are more sensitive to directly acting muscarinic and nicotinic agonists than the Flinders Resistant Line (FRL) rats.[5,11] Consistent with this hyperresponsivity, the FSL rats also have elevated brain muscarinic and nicotinic receptors in selected brain regions.[12,13] The cholinergic hyperresponsiveness of the FSL rat appears to be an innate trait because it can be observed as soon as a functional response can be recorded.[14,15] As illustrated in TABLE 1, the FSL rats clearly have greater hypothermic responses following treatment with cholinergic agonists than do the FRL rats. In the most recent investigation, temperature was recorded in undisturbed animals by telemetry and a reference group of Sprague-Dawley rats obtained from Harlan was included. After a challenge dose of 0.2 mg/kg oxotremorine, the peak responses of the FSL and FRL rats were very different, −3.2 and −0.3°C, respectively. The response of the Sprague-Dawley rats was almost exactly in the middle: −1.6.[16] Thus, the FSL and the FRL rats are, respectively, sensitive and resistant to oxotremorine compared to this reference population of Sprague-Dawley rats.

TABLE 1. Hyperresponsiveness of hypothermic response to cholinergic agonists in FSL rats

	Mean change from baseline (°C)		
Compound	FSL rats	FRL rats	Reference
Arecoline (2 mg/kg)	−3.2 ± 0.2	−1.4 ± 0.1[a]	26
Oxotremorine (0.2 mg/kg)	−2.3 ± 0.1	−1.2 ± 0.1[a]	26
Pilocarpine (20 mg/kg)	−1.5 ± 0.1	−0.5 ± 0.1[a]	56
Nicotine (0.4 mg/kg)	−1.5 ± 0.1	−0.5 ± 0.1[a]	43

[a]Significantly different from FSL rats, $p < 0.05$, Student's t test.

Because the cholinergic system plays a role in many behavioral functions and, in particular, because individuals with depressive disorders are also more sensitive to cholinergic agents,[17] the FSL and FRL rats were subjected to a battery of behavioral and physiological tests. In most respects, the FSL rats exhibited behaviors that were similar to the symptoms expressed by depressed individuals, including reduced appetite and body weight, reduced activity in novel environments, increased REM sleep, and increased inhibitory responses upon exposure to stressors.[11,18] The FSL rats also satisfy the key criterion of predictive validity because their exaggerated immobility in the forced swim test is reduced by chronic (but not acute) treatment with antidepressants.[11,19–21]

People suffering from CI, chronic fatigue, and/or asthma may also periodically experience symptoms of depression. It is not usually clear, however, whether these symptoms are to be regarded merely as secondary to the primary disease state or whether they reflect an underlying depressive disorder. Nevertheless, there are some indications that these three disorders may be overlapping with each other as well as with depressive disorders. Moreover, some studies have suggested that a cholinergic hypersensitivity might underlie each of these conditions as well.[5,6,22]

CHEMICAL INTOLERANCE (CI)/MULTIPLE CHEMICAL SENSITIVITY (MCS)

Evidence supporting the FSL rat as a model for MCS has been previously reviewed in some detail,[6] so only a few key points will be made here. FSL rats resemble MCS patients for several behavioral characteristics, including fatigue, sleep disturbances, and reduced activity.[6]

Clinical observations suggest that CI/MCS can be precipitated by acute or chronic exposure to diverse chemical agents.[23] There is no evidence for precipitating exposures in the FSL rats, but they do exhibit increased sensitivity to anticholinesterase agents and muscarinic agonists.[24–26] Importantly, MCS patients also appear to exhibit increased sensitivity to anticholinesterases.[23,27,28] Whether patients with CI/MCS are more sensitive to direct cholinergic agonists is currently unknown, but such agents are among those which many MCS patients say they cannot tolerate. Thus, there is limited information to suggest that both FSL rats and CI/MCS patients exhibit cholinergic hyperresponsiveness.

TABLE 2. Increased hypothermic responses to multiple drugs in FSL rats

Compound	Mean change from baseline (°C)		Reference
	FSL rats	FRL rats	
Dopaminergic agents			
Apomorphine			
0.6 µmol/kg	−1.9 ± 0.1	−0.6 ± 0.2[a]	29
1.0 µmol/kg	−3.5 ± 0.2	−2.6 ± 0.3[a]	29
Quinpirole (0.6 µmol/kg)	−1.9 ± 0.2	−1.2 ± 0.2[a]	29
Serotonergic agents			
MCPP (2 mg/kg)	−1.9 ± 0.1	−1.1 ± 0.3[a]	31
8-OH-DPAT			
0.1 mg/kg	−1.5 ± 0.1	−0.8 ± 0.1[a]	25
0.5 mg/kg	−5.1 ± 0.2	−2.3 ± 0.1[a]	38
Ethanol (3 g/kg)	−2.8 ± 0.5	−1.6 ± 0.5[a]	6

[a]Significantly different from FSL rats, $p < 0.05$, Student's t test.

One of the key features of individuals with CI/MCS is their sensitivity/intolerance to a variety of chemically unrelated compounds, whose mechanisms of action are not known.[3] The FSL rat is also more sensitive to a variety of chemically diverse compounds, so it shares a superficial resemblance to individuals with CI/MCS. However, unlike the case with the human data, most of the compounds given to the FSL rats have well-defined mechanisms of action. Thus, a possibility exists that the basis for the multiple chemical sensitivity of the FSL rats can be determined. Such information may provide clues as to what may be happening in CI/MCS patients.

As illustrated in TABLE 2, the FSL rats are also more sensitive to the hypothermic effects of a variety of agents, some of which are selective for specific neurotransmitter systems. The FSL rats are supersensitive to the hypothermic[29] and aggression-promoting[30] effects of apomorphine, a mixed D1/D2 agonist, and quinpirole, a selective D2 agonist. However, there were no detectable differences in dopamine D2 receptors between FSL and FRL rats.[29] Therefore, the increased hypothermic effects of dopamine agonists in the FSL rats cannot be simply explained by elevated D2 receptors. Other mechanisms to account for these differences will be discussed in a later section.

The FSL rats also exhibit increased hypothermic responses to serotonergic agents (TABLE 2).[25,31,32] As yet, no data exist on the effects of selective serotonergic agents in MCS patients, so the similarity between the FSL rats and MCS patients for this parameter cannot be evaluated at present. Schiller[33] has reported in preliminary investigations that the FSL rats have elevated 5-HT receptors, but this observation needs to be followed up. It remains unclear at present whether the increased sensitivity of FSL rats to the 5-HT1A agonist, 8-OH-DPAT, can be accounted for by an increased number of 5-HT1A receptors.

In addition to the above drugs that interact selectively with specific neurotransmitter receptors, the FSL and FRL rats are differentially sensitive to the effects of several other pharmacological agents. However, the differential effects are observed only for some, not for all, actions of the drugs. For example, ethanol induces a greater hypothermia in the FSL rats, but not a greater intoxication.[34] Similarly, diazepam produces greater behavioral suppressant effects in the FSL rats,[35] but the anxiolytic effects of diazepam in the two lines are comparable.[36]

The FSL and FRL rats do not exhibit differential responses to every drug tested. Their hypothermic response to salbutamol, a β-adrenergic agonist, and clonidine, an α-noradrenergic agonist, were similar.[11,18]

In summary, it is quite clear that the FSL rat is more sensitive to a variety of chemical agents in addition to the anticholinesterase for which they were selectively bred. In this regard, the FSL rat is, in part, analogous to MCS patients who become more sensitive to a range of agents following exposure to organophosphate anticholinesterases.[23,27] However, the reactions of the rats following exposure to solvents and other chemicals to which MCS patients are exquisitely sensitive have yet to be tested. Similarly, the reactions of MCS patients to direct cholinergic and serotonergic agonists, to which FSL rats are hyperresponsive, have not been tested.

CHRONIC FATIGUE

Reduced activity, sleep abnormality, and disturbed appetite are behavioral characteristics of the FSL rats that resemble some of the symptoms expressed by individuals with chronic fatigue syndrome. However, it has recently been demonstrated that individuals suffering from chronic fatigue exhibit exaggerated hormonal responses following challenge with a cholinergic agent.[22] Thus, these individuals have a cholinergic hyperresponsivity just like the FSL rats. It should be stressed that the cholinergic hyperresponsivity in the FSL rats is not confined only to hypothermic responses, as illustrated in TABLE 1, but it is also seen for behavioral and hormonal responses.[16,24,37] In particular, the FSL rats exhibit greater increases in growth hormone after the same challenge agent, pyridostigmine, that was used in the individuals with chronic fatigue.[16,22] Very recently, it has been shown that the FSL rats exhibit increased prolactin responses to the 5-HT1A partial agonist, buspirone,[39] than do FRL rats. This serotonergic supersensitivity has also been observed in individuals with chronic fatigue.[40] In contrast, depressed individuals often exhibit blunted hormonal responses to serotonergic challenges.[41] Thus, the FSL rat appears to be a more appropriate model for chronic fatigue syndrome than for depression, at least for these hormonal challenge data.

EXPERIMENTAL ASTHMA

The FSL and FRL rats were selectively bred for differential responses to an anticholinesterase that has both central and peripheral effects. However, much of the early work with these rats focused on changes in the brain and responses to centrally acting drugs.[11] Collaborations with Canadian colleagues interested in the potential involvement of cholinergic mechanisms in conditions such as irritable bowel and asthma were initiated in the early 1990s.

In the first study, isolated intestinal strips from FSL rats were found to be more responsive to the muscarinic agonist bethanechol than were strips from the FRL rats.[42] In this study, the indices of systemic and intestinal allergy were also investigated. Following sensitization to ovalbumin (OA), rats of both lines were challenged *in vivo* with 3 mg OA or saline. The FSL rats were more susceptible to allergy than were the FRL rats, as evidenced by more pronounced mast cell degranulation, more intense hypothermic reaction, higher hematocrit values, and increases in the transport tone and permeability of isolated small intestinal tissues.[42] Since no difference existed between the two lines in levels of circulating IgE antibodies, we concluded that other factors, neuroendocrine ones are responsible for the greater susceptibility of the FSL rat.

The study above suggested that the hyperresponsiveness of intestinal tissues to cholinergic agonists in the FSL rats might be a contributory factor to their greater response to the antigen challenge. To determine whether the peripheral cholinergic hypersensitivity is pervasive in the FSL rats, we turned our attention to another model system: experimental asthma. The details of this study have recently been published,[5] so a summary of the findings will be reported here.

The FSL rats were found to be supersensitive to the breathing difficulties induced by the cholinergic agonist methacholine, but they were also more sensitive to the effects of the antigen ovalbumin.[5] In one experiment, a group of randomly bred rats was included and it was found that the FRL rats were very similar to the randomly bred rats, while the FSL rats were again much more afffected by methacholine and the antigen. The bronchoalveolar lavage fluids from the FSL rats had greater numbers of white blood cells and higher relative proportions of neutrophils and eosinophils, indicating a more pronounced inflammation of the airways.[5] These findings clearly establish that the FSL rat is exhibiting abnormal, heightened responses to the antigen challenge. Therefore, a hyperresponsive cholinergic system may contribute to asthma.

MECHANISMS UNDERLYING MCS IN FSL RATS

The papers reviewed in this communication are consistent with the hypothesis that cholinergic hyperresponsiveness may contribute to asthma, chronic fatigue, and CI/MCS. Below, we consider this hypothesis in greater detail and then consider two other potential mechanisms underlying MCS in the Flinders rats.

Increased Muscarinic Receptors

The mechanisms underlying the postsynaptic cholinergic hyperresponsiveness of the FSL rat have not been elucidated. Certainly, there are elevated muscarinic receptors in the brain of the FSL rats.[12] However, the increased responsiveness of the FSL rats to the hypothermic effects of oxotremorine is observed prior to there being any evidence of elevated muscarinic receptors.[14,15,38] The peripheral hyperresponsiveness of FSL rats has been studied only recently, so receptor-binding studies have yet to be performed. Because muscarinic receptors are key in the airways,[7] studies of these receptors could be informative. Thus, it is unclear whether the increases in muscarinic receptor binding that have been reported are responsible for the increased cholinergic responses, so it is even less likely that they underlie the multiple chemical sensitivity of the FSL rats.

In fact, there are two pharmacological studies and two genetic studies that provide inconclusive findings on this hypothesis. It was reported that the hypothermic effects of nicotine could be substantially reduced by pretreating the rats with scopolamine, a muscarinic antagonist,[43] suggesting that nicotine may be producing hypothermia by stimulating the release of acetylcholine, which then induces hypothermia by interacting with muscarinic receptors. However, there were still differences between the FSL and FRL rats in the scopolamine-pretreated groups,[43] as well as differences in nicotinic receptors.[13] In contrast with nicotine, the hypothermic effects of 8-OH-DPAT, a selective 5-HT1A receptor agonist, were not affected by pretreatment with scopolamine.[38] In a genetic study involving the cross-breeding of the FSL and FRL rats, the hypothermic responses to 8-OH-DPAT and oxotremorine segregated separately in the F2 population, suggesting an independence of the two responses.[32] However, a short-term selective breeding study for oxotremorine-induced hypothermia indicated that 8-OH-DPAT-induced hypothermia also changed.[38] No definite conclusions can be made from these data.

Balance between Systems

Because the FSL rats are more sensitive to the hypothermic effects of dopamine agonists than are the FRL rats (TABLE 2) without any changes in dopamine receptors,[29] a balance model might be appropriate. Both cholinergic and dopaminergic stimulation promote hypothermic and aggressive responses.[44–46] On the other hand, the FSL rats are subsensitive to the stereotypy-inducing effects of apomorphine and quinpirole at similar doses where supersensitivity to the hypothermic effects are seen.[29] Cholinergic stimulation has the opposite effects to dopaminergic stimulation in the modulation of activity and stereotypy.[47,48] Thus, the opposite changes in dopamine sensitivity in the various functions could be related to the way the cholinergic and dopaminergic systems interact to modulate these functions. According to this model, the FSL rats would also be more sensitive to the hypothermic effects of 5-HT1A receptor agonists because both cholinergic and 5-HT1A stimulation produces hypothermia. To date, no instance of a subsensitive response to 5-HT1A agonists in FSL rats has been observed, but it is well known that 5-HT1A and cholinergic mechanisms are differentially involved in slow wave and REM sleep.[49] Therefore, a study of cholinergic and 5-HT1A agonists on sleep parameters could provide data to evaluate this model.

Second Messengers

The balance model described above is a conceptual model that does not imply any specific biochemical mechanisms other than rejecting a simple change in neurotransmitter receptors. Potential mechanisms that might underlie the cholinergic hyperresponsiveness are alterations in some component(s) of the second messenger cascade that occur following the interaction of acetylcholine with the muscarinic receptor. Changes in G-protein function, cyclic AMP, and/or phosphatidyl inositol are just a few of the candidates. The attractiveness of this hypothesis is that it might also account for the increased sensitivity of the FSL rats to some of the noncholinergic drugs and thus provide a biochemical mechanism underpinning the balance model. Serotonergic agonists that stimulate the 5-HT1A receptor subtype may use the same second messenger pathway and the same G proteins as cholinergic agonists.[38] Determining the mechanisms underlying the hyperresponsiveness of the FSL rats to drug-induced hypothermia and bronchoconstriction may be useful in better understanding asthma, chronic fatigue, and CI/MCS.

Altered second messengers in CI/MCS patients may not only account for their increased sensitivity to cholinergic agents; they may also account, in part, for their increased sensitivity to specific odors. It has been reported that symptoms in these patients can be triggered by fragrances,[50] as well as gasoline and pesticides. These odors are transmitted to cortical smell-receiving areas by pathways traversing the olfactory bulb, which also receives input from the locus coeruleus noradrenergic neurons and the basal forebrain cholinergic neurons.[51] There is evidence that these cholinergic neurons positively modulate neural activity in this area.[52] There is also evidence that the cholinergic system can modulate the release of norepinephrine by the noradrenergc neurons.[53] Thus, if the neural pathways transmitting information about smell utilize the same second messenger systems as does the cholinergic system, then supersensitive responses to the odors would be predicted in animals/individuals with a hyperresponsive cholinergic system.

CONCLUSIONS/FURTHER DIRECTIONS

The FSL rats are clearly more sensitive to cholinergic agonists, both centrally and peripherally.[5,10,12] They are also more sensitive to the effects of a variety of other drugs influencing other neurotransmitter systems (TABLE 2), suggesting responses similar to MCS patients.[23,27] However, as indicated above, solvents, perfumes, and other exotic odors that have been known to trigger responses in patients with MCS have not been tested in the Flinders rats. Because these diverse substances may use the same afferent smell pathways, we predict that the FSL rat will be supersensitive to these agents. The whole-body plethysmography technique may be suitably adapted to test these compounds. Because the FSL rats are more sensitive to the bronchoconstriction induced by both the cholinergic agonist methacholine and the relatively nonspecific antigen ovalbumin, it is likely that they may also be hyperresponsive to these odors as well.

Allergies have been commonly reported in depressed patients as well as those with MCS.[2,54] Depression is also a commonly reported symptom of MCS patients, and the similarities between depression, MCS, and behavioral symptoms in the FSL rats have recently been reviewed.[6] Others have suggested that a cholinergic hyperresponsiveness may be the common link between depression and allergies.[54] Thus, a group of conditions with overlapping symptoms, including depressive disorders,[17] irritable bowel syndrome,[55] asthma,[5] chronic fatigue syndrome,[22] and CI/MCS,[6] may be influenced by a pathological, hyperresponsive cholinergic system.

ACKNOWLEDGMENTS

We thank the following colleagues who have contributed to the work reported herein: John Bienenstock, Gerard Cox, Alina Dragomir, Mary H. Perdue, Lesley Smith, Meir Steiner, Roger Russell, Claudia Miller, David Janowsky, Grant Schiller, Ann Crocker, Lynette Daws, Joe Orbach, Kjell Fuxe, Olgierd Pucilowski, Anders Lehmann, Gal Yadid, Abraham Zangen, Laura Caberlotto, Yasmin Hurd, Aleksander Mathe, Amir H. Rezvani, and Ying Yang. The experiments reviewed in this paper have been supported by funding from the Australian Research Grants Scheme, the National Health and Medical Research Council, the U.S. Army, the University of North Carolina, and the UNC Bowles Center for Alcohol Studies.

REFERENCES

1. LEVY, F. 1997. Clinical features of multiple chemical sensitivity. Scand. J. Work Environ. Health **23**(S3): 69–73.
2. MEGGS, W.J., K.A. DUNN, N.M. BLOCH et al. 1996. Prevalence and nature of allergy and chemical sensitivity in a general population. Arch. Environ. Health **51**: 275–282.
3. ROSS, G.H. 1997. Clinical characteristics of chemical sensitivity, an illustrative case history of asthma and MCS. Environ. Health Perspect. **105**(S2): 437–441.
4. ZIEM, G. & J. MCTANNEY. 1997. Profile of patients with chemical injury and sensitivity. Environ. Health Perspect. **105**(S2): 417–436.
5. DJURIC, V.J., G. COX, D.H. OVERSTREET et al. 1998. Genetically transmitted cholinergic hyperresponsiveness predisposes to experimental asthma. Brain Behav. Immun. **12**: 272–284.
6. OVERSTREET, D.H., C.S. MILLER, D.S. JANOWSKY et al. 1996. Potential animal model of multiple chemical sensitivity with cholinergic supersensitivity. Toxicology **111**: 119–134.
7. BARNES, P.J. 1992. Modulation of neurotransmission in airways. Physiol. Rev. **72**: 699–729.
8. MESULAM, M-M. 1995. Structure and function of cholinergic pathways in the cerebral cortex, limbic system, basal ganglia, and thalamus of the human brain. In Neuropsychopharmacology: The Fourth Generation of Progress, pp. 135–146. Raven Press. New York.
9. OVERSTREET, D.H., R.W. RUSSELL, S.C. HELPS et al. 1979. Selective breeding for sensitivity to the anticholinesterase, DFP. Psychopharmacology **65**: 15–20.
10. RUSSELL, R.W., D.H. OVERSTREET, M. MESSENGER et al. 1982. Selective breeding for sensitivity to DFP: generalization of effects beyond criterion variables. Pharmacol. Biochem. Behav. **17**: 885–891.
11. OVERSTREET, D.H., P. PUCILOWSKI, A.H. REZVANI et al. 1995. Administration of antidepressants, diazepam, and psychomotor stimulants further confirms the utility of Flinders Sensitive Line rats as an animal model of depression. Psychopharmacology **121**: 27–37.
12. OVERSTREET, D.H., R.W. RUSSELL, A.D. CROCKER et al. 1984. Selective breeding for differences in cholinergic function: pre- and post-synaptic mechanisms involved in sensitivity to the anticholinesterase, DFP. Brain Res. **294**: 327–332.
13. TIZABI, Y., D.H. OVERSTREET, A.H. REZVANI et al. 1999. Antidepressant effects of nicotine in an animal model of depression. Psychopharmacology **142**: 193–199.
14. DAWS, L.C., G.D. SCHILLER, D.H. OVERSTREET et al. 1991. Early development of muscarinic supersensitivity in a genetic animal model of depression. Neuropsychopharmacology **4**: 207–217.
15. DAWS, L.C. & D.H. OVERSTREET. 1999. Ontogeny of muscarinic cholinergic hypersensitivity in the Flinders Sensitive Line rat. Pharmacol. Biochem. Behav. **62**: 367–380.

16. OVERSTREET, D.H., G.A. MASON, Y. YANG et al. 1998. Supersensitive growth hormone responses following pyridostigmine challenge in a genetic animal model of depression. Presented at the Twenty-eighth Annual Meeting of the Society for Neuroscience, Los Angeles, November 7–12, 1998. Abstr. no. 189.10.
17. JANOWSKY, D.S., D.H. OVERSTREET & J.I. NURNBERGER, JR. 1994. Is cholinergic sensitivity a genetic marker for the affective disorders? Am. J. Med. Genet. Neuropsychiatr. Genet. **54:** 335–344.
18. OVERSTREET, D.H. 1993. The Flinders Sensitive Line rats: a genetic animal model of depression. Neurosci. Biobehav. Rev. **17:** 51–68.
19. CABERLOTTO, L., K. FUXE, D.H. OVERSTREET et al. 1998. Alterations in neuropeptide Y and Y1 receptor mRNA expression in brains of an animal model of depression: region-specific adaptation after fluoxetine treatment. Mol. Brain Res. **59:** 58–65.
20. ZANGEN, A., D.H. OVERSTREET & G. YADID. 1997. High serotonin and 5-hydroxyindoleacetic acid levels in limbic regions of a rat model of depression: normalization by chronic antidepressant treatment. J. Neurochem. **69:** 2477–2483.
21. ZANGEN, A., D.H. OVERSTREET & G. YADID. 1999. Increased catecholamine levels in specific brain regions of a rat model of depression: normalization by chronic antidepressant treatment. Brain Res. **824:** 243–250.
22. CHAUDHURI, A., T. MAJEED, T. DINAN et al. 1997. Chronic fatigue syndrome: a disorder of central cholinergic transmission. J. Chronic Fatigue **3:** 3–16.
23. MILLER, C.S. & H.C. MITZEL. 1995. Chemical sensitivity attributed to pesticide exposure versus remodeling. Arch. Environ. Health **50:** 119–129.
24. OVERSTREET, D.H. & R.W. RUSSELL. 1982. Selective breeding for sensitivity to DFP: effects of cholinergic agonists and antagonists. Psychopharmacology **78:** 150–154.
25. OVERSTREET, D.H., A.H. REZVANI & D.S. JANOWSKY. 1992. Genetic animal models of depression and ethanol preference provide support for cholinergic and serotonergic involvement in depression and alcoholism. Biol. Psychiatry **31:** 919–936.
26. OVERSTREET, D.H., R.W. RUSSELL, D.A. HAY et al. 1992. Selective breeding for increased cholinergic function. Biometrical genetic analysis of muscarinic responses. Neuropsychopharmacology **5:** 197–204.
27. CONE, J.E. & T.A. SULT. 1992. Acquired intolerance to solvents following pesticide/solvent exposure in a building: a new group of workers at risk for multiple chemical sensitivities? Toxicol. Indust. Health **8:** 29–39.
28. ROSENTHAL, N. & C.L. CAMERON. 1991. Exaggerated sensitivity to an organophosphate pesticide (letter). Am. J. Psychiatry **148:** 270.
29. CROCKER, A.D. & D.H. OVERSTREET. 1991. Changes in dopamine sensitivity in rats selectively bred for differences in cholinergic function. Pharmacol. Biochem. Behav. **38:** 105–108.
30. PUCILOWSKI, O., B.S. EICHELMAN, D.H. OVERSTREET et al. 1991. Enhanced affective aggression in genetically bred hypercholinergic rats. Neuropsychobiology **24:** 37–41.
31. WALLIS, E., D.H. OVERSTREET & A.D. CROCKER. 1988. Selective breeding for increased cholinergic function: increased serotonergic sensitivity. Pharmacol. Biochem. Behav. **31:** 345–350.
32. OVERSTREET, D.H., D.S. JANOWSKY, O. PUCILOWSKI et al. 1994. Swim test immobility cosegregates with serotonergic, but not cholinergic sensitivity in cross breeds of Flinders Line rats. Psychiatr. Genet. **4:** 101–107.
33. SCHILLER, G.D. 1990. Altered behavioral sensitivity to serotonergic agonists in an animal model of depressive disorders: receptor binding correlates and cholinergic-serotonergic systems interaction. J. Neurochem. **57:** S138.
34. OVERSTREET, D.H., A.H. REZVANI & D.S. JANOWSKY. 1990. Increased hypothermic responses to ethanol in rats selectively bred for cholinergic supersensitivity. Alcohol Alcohol. **25:** 59–65.
35. PEPE, S., D.H. OVERSTREET & A.D. CROCKER. 1988. Enhanced benzodiazepine responsiveness in rats with increased cholinergic function. Pharmacol. Biochem. Behav. **31:** 15–20.
36. SCHILLER, G.D., L.C. DAWS, D.H. OVERSTREET et al. 1991. Absence of anxiety in an animal model of depression with cholinergic supersensitivity. Brain Res. Bull. **26:** 443–447.

37. OVERSTREET, D.H., R.A. BOOTH, R. DANA et al. 1986. Enhanced elevation of corticosterone following arecoline administration to rats selectively bred for increased cholinergic function. Psychopharmacology **88**: 129–130.
38. OVERSTREET, D.H., L.C. DAWS, G.D. SCHILLER et al. 1998. Cholinergic/serotonergic interactions in hypothermia: implications for rat models of depression. Pharmacol. Biochem. Behav. **59**: 777–785.
39. LEHMANN, A. & G. SVANTESSON. 2000. Altered neuroendocrine response and motility in the Flinders Sensitive Line rat. Presented at Digestive Diseases Week, May 21–24, 2000, San Diego.
40. CLEARE, A.J., BEARN, J.T. ALLAIN et al. 1995. Contrasting neuroendocrine responses in depression and chronic fatigue syndrome. J. Affect. Dis. **34**: 283–289.
41. MAES, M. & H.Y. MELTZER. 1995. The serotonin hypothesis of major depression. In Psychopharmacology: The Fourth Generation of Progress, pp. 933–944. Raven Press. New York.
42. DJURIC, V.J., D.H. OVERSTREET, J. BIENENSTOCK et al. 1995. Immediate hypersensitivity in the Flinders rat: further evidence for a possible link between susceptibility to allergies and depression. Brain Behav. Immun. **9**: 196–206.
43. SCHILLER, G.D. & D.H. OVERSTREET. 1993. Selective breeding for increased cholinergic function: preliminary study of nicotinic mechanisms. Med. Chem. Res. **2**: 578–583.
44. COX, B., R.W. KERWIN, T.F. LEE et al. 1980. A dopamine-5-hydroxytryptamine link in the hypothalamic pathways which mediate heat loss in the rat. J. Physiol. **303**: 9–21.
45. PUCILOWSKI, O. 1987. Monoaminergic control of affective aggression. Acta Neurobiol. Exp. **47**: 25–50.
46. RAY, A., P. SEN & M. ALKONDON. 1989. Biochemical and pharmacological evidence for central cholinergic regulation of shock-induced aggression. Pharmacol. Biochem. Behav. **32**: 867–871.
47. FIBIGER, H.C., L.D. LYTLE & B.A. CAMPBELL. 1970. Cholinergic modulation of adrenergic arousal in the developing rat. J. Comp. Physiol. Psychol. **3**: 384–389.
48. KLEMM, W.R. 1989. Drug effects on active immobility responses: what they tell us about neurotransmitter systems and motor function. Prog. Neurobiol. **32**: 403–422.
49. JONES, B.E. 1991. Paradoxical sleep and its chemical/structural substrates in the brain. Neuroscience **40**: 637–656.
50. ROSS, P.M., J. WHYSNER, V.T. VOVELLO et al. 1999. Olfaction and symptoms in the multiple chemical sensitivites syndrome. Prevent. Med. **28**: 467–480.
51. ICHIKAWA, T., K. AJIKI, J. MATSUURA et al. 1997. Localization of two cholinergic markers, choline acetyltransferase and vesicular acetylcholine transporter in the central nervous system of the rat: in situ hybridization histochemistry and immunohistochemistry. J. Chem. Neuroanat. **13**: 23–29.
52. ELAAGOUBY, A., N. RAVEL & R. GERVAIS. 1991. Cholinergic modulation of excitability in the rat olfactory bulb: effect of local application of cholinergic agents on evoked field potentials. Neuroscience **45**: 653–662.
53. EL-ETRI, M.M., M. ENNIS, E.R. GRIFF et al. 1999. Evidence for cholinergic regulation of basal norepinephrine release in the rat olfactory bulb. Neuroscience **93**: 611–617.
54. MARSHALL, P.S. 1993. Allergy and depression: a neurochemical threshold model of the relation between the illnesses. Psychol. Bull. **113**: 23–43.
55. WHITE, A.M., W.H. STEVENS, A.R. UPTON et al. 1991. Airway responsiveness to inhaled methacholine in patients with irritable bowel syndrome. Gastroenterology **100**: 69–74.
56. MILLAN, M.H., O. PUCILOWSKI & D.H. OVERSTREET. 1995. Susceptibility of Flinders Sensitive and Resistant rats to pharmacologically induced convulsions. Pharmacol. Biochem. Behav. **50**: 504–508.

Episodic Exposures to Chemicals
What Relevance to Chemical Intolerance?

R. C. MACPHAIL

Neurotoxicology Division, National Health and Environmental Effects Research Laboratory, United States Environmental Protection Agency, Research Triangle Park, North Carolina 27711, USA

ABSTRACT: Episodic exposures refer to intermittent acute exposures to chemicals that ordinarily have a rapid onset and short duration of effect. There has been a long tradition in preclinical behavioral pharmacology of using episodic-exposure paradigms in order to establish dose-response functions in individual organisms. In these experiments, stable baselines of behavior are first established and then followed by administering varying doses of a drug intermittently, for example, once or twice a week. The power of this approach is well established; the within-subjects design reduces error variance, allows exploration of the entire range of effective doses, and can be used to identify individual differences in drug sensitivity. Of course, the approach is only applicable to reversibly acting compounds, and checks need to be included to insure effects of one dose are not influenced by prior exposure to another dose. We have used baseline approaches to evaluate the effects of pesticides and solvents on the behavior of adult male rats and mice. Moreover, a novel probabilistic dose-tolerance analysis applied to the data suggests substantial individual differences in chemical sensitivity, often spanning orders of magnitude. These results suggest that individual differences in chemical sensitivity may be much greater than previously acknowledged.

This conference has been organized to explore the scientific basis of potential mechanisms underlying the phenomenon of chemical intolerance. Numerous reports have now appeared that suggest certain individuals may be highly sensitive (intolerant) to low levels of chemical exposure. While the vast majority of this conference's presentations outline possible biochemical and physiological processes that may lead to chemical sensitivity, speculation is hampered by the profound lack of data on the range and distribution of chemical sensitivity in the population. This paper focuses on an approach to empirically determining, in laboratory animals, the range of susceptibility to chemical intoxication that is based upon intensive investigations of the responses of individual organisms.

In theory, the fundamental unit of analysis in toxicology is the individual organism, but one would be hard-pressed to glean this principle from the literature. Scientists in many fields seem to have an almost exclusive preoccupation with measures of central tendency (means or medians). From this perspective, variability in responses between organisms is viewed mainly as a nuisance rather than a topic of investigation in its own right. Variability can be minimized most straightforwardly by gaining firm control over the variables that influence the response. Instead, most seem content to minimize variability artificially by increasing sample sizes and calculating standard errors of the mean (or worse, pooled standard errors). While the result may be a more aesthetic presentation of dose-response plots, the tradition severely obfuscates our appreciation of individual differences in susceptibility to chemical exposures.

There are several factors that may confer susceptibility to chemical intoxication in an individual. Risk factors include age, gender, genetics, and health status. There is currently much interest in age as a risk factor, especially the susceptibility of infants and children to environmental pollutants.[1] There is also increasing interest that the elderly may be a special subpopulation at risk, and this interest will most assuredly grow with the shifting age demographics in our society. Evidence also exists for gender differences in susceptibility,[2] although the evidence isn't as strong as for age-related susceptibility. One's genetic makeup can be another risk factor, as is evident from growing concerns over cancer caused in some individuals by polymorphisms in their genes responsible for certain metabolic enzymes. Recent evidence also suggests a genetic basis for the neurotoxic effects of cholinesterase-inhibiting insecticides and related agents.[3] Finally, the health status of an individual may influence susceptibility due to poor nutrition, existing disease, and/or exposure to other toxic substances. It should be clear that an adequate understanding of these risk factors is essential for estimating susceptibility in the population.

Episodic exposures refer to intermittent acute exposures of organisms to chemicals that ordinarily have a rapid onset and brief duration of action. There has been a long tradition in preclinical behavioral pharmacology of using episodic-exposure paradigms in order to establish dose-response functions, in individual organisms, for both therapeutic drugs and drugs of abuse.[4] In these experiments, stable baselines of behavior are first established and then followed by administering varying doses of a drug, for example, once or twice a week. Doses are administered according to an ascending, descending, or (more typically) scrambled sequence. The drug vehicle is also given intermittently and additional doses may be included to determine the reliability of prior dose effects or to characterize more fully the function. The power of this approach is well established: the within-subjects design significantly reduces error variance (as do all repeated-measures designs), allows exploration of the entire range of effective doses, and can be used to identify individual differences in drug sensitivity. Of course, the approach is only applicable to reversibly acting compounds, and checks need to be included to insure the effects of one dose are not influenced by prior exposure to another dose (as may occur with increasing or decreasing doses). Further, while the baseline approach offers the distinct possibility of identifying individual differences in susceptibility, an intense characterization of those differences is generally lacking, at least for decision-making purposes regarding the risk (or benefits) of chemical exposures.

The U.S. EPA has the formidable responsibility of setting standards of exposure for the populace to a wide variety of environmental chemicals in order to insure safety and/or minimize the risk of adverse health effects. Two general approaches are used: one for agents that cause cancer and the other for agents that damage specific organ systems (see refs. 5 and 6). It is beyond the scope of this paper to detail these approaches to risk assessment. Briefly, however, cancer risk assessment involves extrapolating data on effects (usually from laboratory animals) to extremely low exposure levels likely to produce a small (viz., 1 in 1,000,000) increase in cancer in the population. Cancer risk assessments rely on mathematical models for low-dose extrapolation, and the resulting estimates can vary by several orders of magnitude depending on the model.[6,7] Risk assessment for systemic (noncancer) toxicity entails calculating a reference dose (RfD) or a reference concentration (RfC), which differ only in the details: that is, RfDs are established for orally and dermally applied compounds, whereas RfCs are established for inhaled compounds. An RfD is calculated by dividing a dose that produces no effect, ordinarily derived from an experiment on laboratory animals, by a series of uncertainty factors (UFs). UFs are included to make conservative estimates of "safe" exposure levels and are usually assigned values of 10. The inclusion of UFs specifically recognizes our incomplete knowledge of how chemicals produce adverse effects. One UF is included to compensate for individual differences in chemical sensitivity. In other words, it is generally accepted science policy that susceptibility in the population varies by no more than 1 or 2 orders of magnitude. However, how realistic is this policy? Moreover, how can we attempt to empirically determine ranges and distributions of sensitivity at the level of the population?

The vast majority of studies in toxicology use groups (between-subjects) designs in which individuals are assigned to a single dose group. Groups designs, however, can tell us little, if anything, about individual differences in sensitivity. Consider, for example, the hypothetical data in FIGURE 1. The upper panel shows the effect of a single dose of a toxicant in an experimental group of organisms. The dose produced an average 10% reduction in behavioral function. With a sufficient number of subjects, the distribution of sensitivity can be determined, from which the most sensitive and the least sensitive individual can be identified. However, how reliable are these differences? If the same dose were given again, would the least and most sensitive individuals still be the least and most sensitive? This type of replication is rarely (if ever) done and therefore answers to these questions are speculative at best. Moreover, if additional doses were included, would relative sensitivity be preserved over that dose range? The two lower panels of FIGURE 1 present opposing outcomes, neither of which can be supported by data derived from experiments using groups designs.

Baseline designs are needed to accurately (i.e., quantitatively) evaluate individual differences in chemical sensitivity. We shall next describe our approach to quantifying individual differences, but it is acknowledged that there is much interest in better characterizing dose-response relationships due to many of the shortcomings of the RfD approach (see ref. 8 for details). In general, these newer approaches use all (or most) of the data from an experiment rather than just the no-effect dose, which is a point estimate. They also identify a benchmark effect (usually a 10% change from control) that is conceivably on the cusp of our ability to empirically determine. The dose-effect function is then mathematically characterized, and variance is specifically incorporated into the resulting risk estimates. It is important to note, however, that there are theoretically two sources of variability in dose-response functions: (1) variability in the effect of a fixed dose and (2) variability in the dose producing a fixed effect. Most toxicologists view variability from the former perspective because of the broad use of between-groups designs. As was apparent from discussion of FIGURE 1, however, this type of variability is insufficient for measuring individual differences in susceptibility.

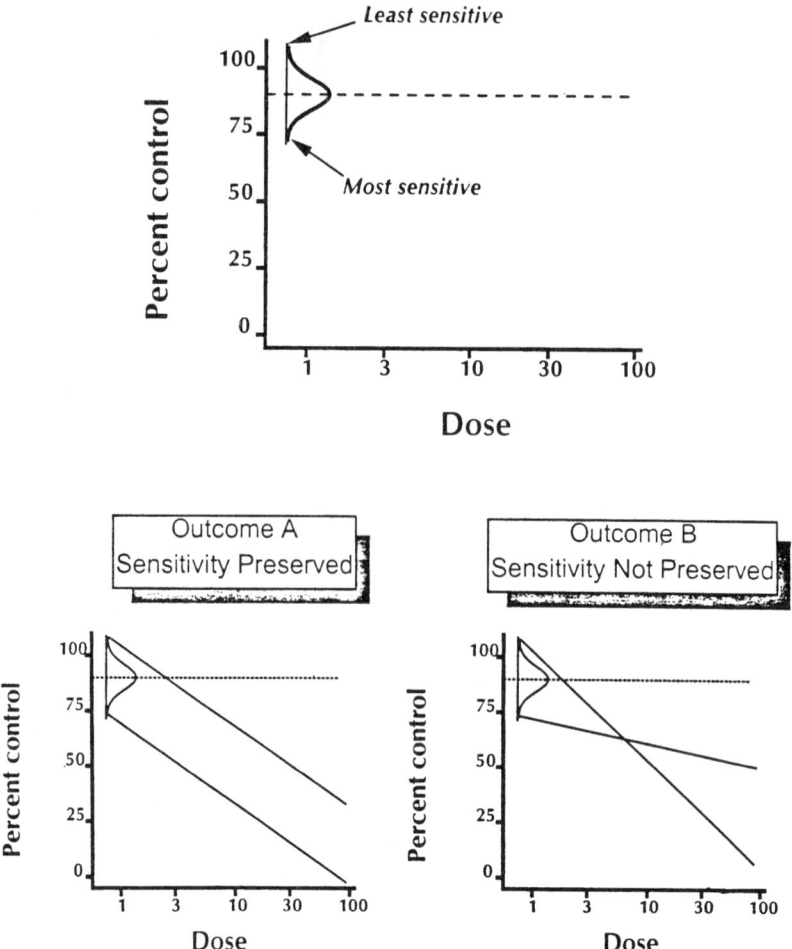

FIGURE 1. Hypothetical data showing a distribution of effects of a single dose of a toxicant in a group of organisms (upper panel). The distribution can be used to identify the most and the least sensitive organisms. Lower panels show possible outcomes of relative sensitivity over the dose range of the toxicant.

We have used a dose-tolerance approach that focuses on the second type of variability to determine the effects of solvents and pesticides on the behavior of mice and rats, respectively. Solvent experiments[9] involved cumulative dosing of a group of 12 mice while they were responding in an operant chamber for milk reinforcement. By this procedure, cycles were sequentially arranged in which the opportunity to respond alternated with time-out periods. Concentrations of a solvent were increased

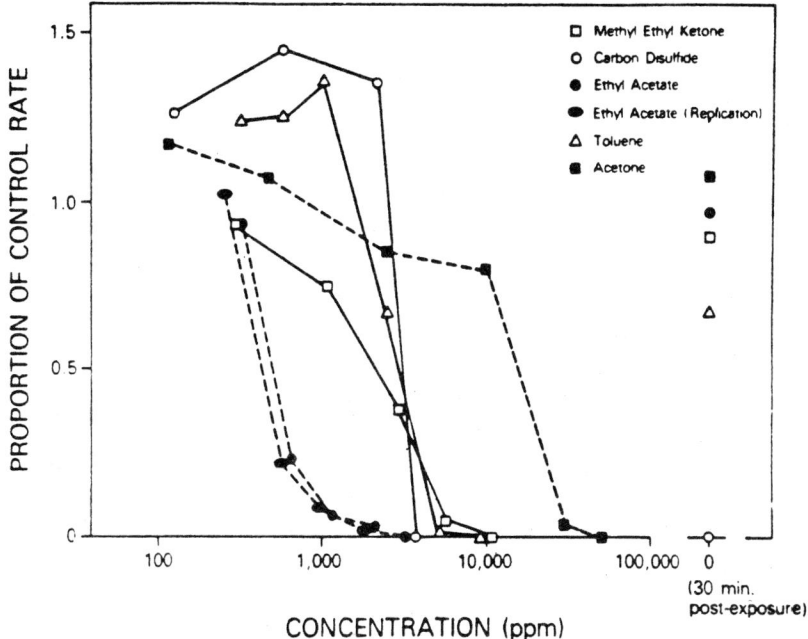

FIGURE 2. Effects of solvents on the operant (reinforced) behavior of mice ($N = 12$). Low concentrations had either no effect or increased responding. Higher concentrations uniformly decreased responding. Reproduced from reference 9 with permission.

systematically during the time-outs, with the effects of each increment on performance determined during the next period of reinforcement availability. Low concentrations generally did not affect performance, intermediate concentrations increased performance (depending on the solvent), and higher concentrations uniformly decreased performance. For all solvents, the highest concentrations completely eliminated milk-reinforced responding (FIG. 2). Quantitative analysis involved fitting a linear function to the descending limb of the concentration-effect function for each mouse, with effects transformed to a proportion of the baseline control value and concentrations transformed to natural logarithms. The concentration estimated to produce a 10% decrease in performance was determined for each mouse and then averaged across mice to arrive at the mean and standard deviation (SD) concentration producing the 10% effect (i.e., an EC10). The distribution of EC10 values was normal (ln-normal) and therefore tables of z scores (or t scores) could be used to estimate the concentration producing a 10% decrement in successively smaller proportions of the "population" (e.g., 1 in 100 mice, 1 in 1000 mice, etc.). These results are presented in TABLE 1.

We also determined the effect of the carbamate insecticide, carbaryl, and the triazole fungicide, triadimefon, on the motor activity of rats, but by using a slightly different experimental design. Adult male Long-Evans rats were first adapted to the testing routine, during 30-min sessions in a photocell device, in order to establish

TABLE 1. Estimated concentrations (ppm) of solvents decreasing operant responding by 10% in successively smaller portions of a population of mice

Solvent	$p = 0.1$	$p = 0.01$	$p = 0.001$
Acetone	495	71	13
Ethyl acetate	176	89	49
Methyl ethyl ketone	300	66	17
Toluene	322	97	34
Carbon disulfide	555	204	84

NOTE: Modified from reference 9 and based on data shown in FIGURE 2: $p = 0.1$, 1 in 10 mice; $p = 0.01$, 1 in 100 mice; $p = 0.001$, 1 in 1000 mice.

stable baselines of motor activity. For each pesticide, rats were then divided into four groups of nine, which determined the order that they received doses of carbaryl or triadimefon (and vehicle). Each dose was given weekly in order to avoid any possible carryover effects, but in each week the pesticide dose-effect functions were established between groups. In the end, each rat received every dose of a pesticide plus pesticide vehicle. FIGURE 3 shows the effects of carbaryl on activity at the level of group assignment. Carbaryl produced dose-related decreases in motor activity. These effects were also evident in the initial (group-defined) dose-effect determina-

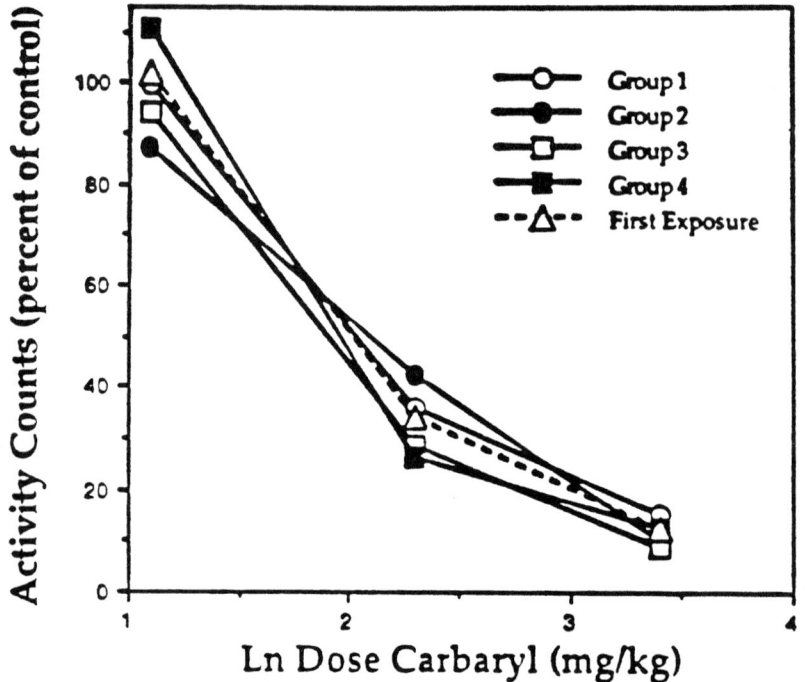

FIGURE 3. Effect of carbaryl on the motor activity of four groups of rats ($N = 9$ each). Carbaryl produced dose-related decreases in motor activity. From reference 8.

TABLE 2. Estimated doses of carbaryl (mg/kg) decreasing motor activity by 10% in successively smaller portions of a population of rats

$p = 0.1$	$p = 0.01$	$p = 0.001$
0.92	0.40	0.18

NOTE: Modified from reference 8 and based on data shown in FIGURE 3: $p = 0.1$, 1 in 10 rats; $p = 0.01$, 1 in 100 rats; $p = 0.001$, 1 in 1000 rats.

TABLE 3. Estimated ranges of individual susceptibility to chemical intoxication

	Minimum (ppm)	Maximum (ppm)	Ratio
Solvent			
Acetone	56	184,647	3297
Ethyl acetate	82	1389	17
Methyl ethyl ketone	55	30,315	551
Toluene	84	12,352	147
Carbon disulfide	180	11,766	65
Pesticide			
Carbaryl	0.24	29.2	122

NOTE: From reference 10. Minimum = mean EC10 or ED10 − 3SD. Maximum = mean EC10 or ED10 + 3SD. Ratio = maximum ÷ minimum.

tion. Similar results were obtained for triadimefon, although this pesticide increased motor activity in a dose-related fashion. Quantitative analysis of the dose-effect data then proceeded as described above for the mouse solvent data. The results of this analysis are shown in TABLE 2.

We next estimated the "range" of individual differences in sensitivity to solvents and pesticides by dividing the mean concentration (or dose) + 3 SD by the mean concentration − 3 SD producing 10% changes in behavior. These results are presented in TABLE 3. Individual differences in sensitivity spanned 1.25 to 3.5 orders of magnitude, depending on the toxicant. In other words, variability in sensitivity was in many cases much greater than the 1 order of magnitude typically assumed in calculating RfDs or RfCs. Moreover, our experiments used adult, healthy, male, outbred rats and mice. As a consequence, none of the variables described earlier that could affect susceptibility was included in these experiments. Therefore, these results can only be considered lower-bound estimates on the range of susceptibility likely to occur in the population. Nevertheless, these results provide empirical support for the notion that some individuals in the population may be remarkably sensitive to chemical intoxication.

Designing an experiment to determine chemical sensitivity in the population requires enormous resources. For example, say the design included three ages of organism, both genders, and both healthy and compromised organisms. The design would therefore include 12 groups and, with 30 organisms in each group, a total of 360 organisms. The time required to carry out the experiment could easily span months of effort and yet the experiment would characterize population-level sensi-

TABLE 4. Estimated doses (mg/kg) of triadimefon producing a 10% increase in the motor activity of successively smaller portions of a population of rats

Analysis	$p = 0.1$	$p = 0.01$	$p = 0.001$
Empirical	4.88	2.96	2.01
Modeled	8.56	6.29	4.88

NOTE: Modified from reference 11: $p = 0.1$, 1 in 10 rats; $p = 0.01$, 1 in 100 rats; $p = 0.001$, 1 in 1000 rats. Empirical entries indicate estimates based on data from a group of 36 rats. Modeled entries indicate estimates based on 4 groups of 9 rats using randomization analyses.

tivity for only one chemical. It is clear, however, that this is exactly what is needed if we are ever to understand the range of chemical sensitivity across individuals.

While we have shown the importance of within-subjects (baseline) designs in assessing individual differences and the potential implications for sensitivity in the population, the problem still remains of the widespread use of between-groups designs especially in toxicology. We have thus developed a modification of the dose-tolerance approach to make it applicable to groups-design data.[11] Randomization analyses permute a data set, typically exhaustively, in order to calculate the exact probability of occurrence of the effect in that data set. Our approach has been the following: The initial group-defined dose-response function for triadimefon was permuted by taking the effect of the lowest dose of the pesticide in one randomly selected rat and combining the effect with that of a randomly selected rat from the second "group", and so on for the highest dose. A linear function was fit to these dose-effect data from which an ED10 was calculated. The data were next replaced in the data set and the process was repeated until all possible combinations (and dose-effect functions) were exhausted. The grand distribution of ED10s was then used to calculate the risk figures, and these values were compared with those derived from the empirical (or "true") distributions established in the rats. The results of this comparison (TABLE 4) show a close correspondence between the risk of figures derived from the two methods of analysis. Although estimates were consistently higher for the modeling approach, these differences were relatively small (i.e., considerably less than an order of magnitude). Differences in dose estimates using the two approaches did, however, increase as probability of the effect in the population decreased, as would be expected when moving further into the tails of different probability distributions.

In summary, the observation of chemical intolerance raises the possibility that differences in chemical susceptibility in the population may be substantial. This possibility is empirically supported by laboratory data and novel approaches to quantifying the range of susceptibility in a population.

ACKNOWLEDGMENTS

This manuscript has been reviewed by the National Health and Environmental Effects Research Laboratory, U.S. Environmental Protection Agency, and approved for publication. Mention of trade names or commercial products does not constitute endorsement or recommendation for use.

REFERENCES

1. NATIONAL RESEARCH COUNCIL. 1993. Pesticides in the Diets of Infants and Children. National Academy Press. Washington, D.C.
2. MOSER, V.C., S.M. CHANDA, S.P. MORTENSEN & S. PADILLA. 1998. Age- and gender-related differences in sensitivity to chlorpyrifos in the rat reflect developmental profiles of esterase activities. Toxicol. Sci. **46:** 211–222.
3. DAVIES, H.G., R.L. RICHTER, M. KEIFER *et al.* 1996. The effect of serum paraoxonase is reversed with diazoxon, soman, and sarin. Nat. Genet. **14:** 334–336.
4. KELLEHER, R.T. & W.H. MORSE. 1968. Determinants of the specificity of behavioral effects of drugs. Rev. Physiol. Biochem. Exp. Pharmacol. **60:** 1–56.
5. BARNES, D.G. & M. DOURSON. 1988. Reference dose (RfD): description and use in health risk assessments. Regul. Toxicol. Pharmacol. **8:** 471–486.
6. KREWSKI, D., C. BROWN & D. MURDOCH. 1984. Determining "safe" levels of exposure: safety factors or mathematical models? Fundam. Appl. Toxicol. **4:** S383–S394.
7. CORTRUVO, J. 1988. Drinking water standards and risk assessment. Regul. Toxicol. Pharmacol. **8:** 288–299.
8. GLOWA, J.R. & R.C. MACPHAIL. 1995. Quantitative approaches to risk assessment in neurotoxicology. *In* Neurotoxicology: Approaches and Methods, pp. 777–787. Academic Press. New York.
9. GLOWA, J.R. & P.B. DEWS. 1987. Behavioral toxicology of volatile organic solvents. IV. Comparisons of the rate-decreasing effects of acetone, ethyl acetate, methyl ethyl ketone, toluene, and carbon disulfide on schedule-controlled behavior of mice. J. Am. Coll. Toxicol. **6:** 461–469.
10. MACPHAIL, R.C. & J.R. GLOWA. 1999. Quantitative risk assessment in neurotoxicology: past, present, and future. *In* Neurotoxicology, pp. 367–382. Taylor & Francis. London/New York.
11. BOGDAN, M.A., R.C. MACPHAIL & J.R. GLOWA. 2001. A randomization test-based method for risk assessment in neurotoxicology. Risk Anal. **21:** 107–116.

Environmental Risks and Public Health

BERNARD D. GOLDSTEIN[a]

Environmental and Occupational Health Sciences Institute (EOHSI), Piscataway, New Jersey 08854, USA

ABSTRACT: There are currently a number of initiatives aimed at considering and redefining the role of environmental health. These include an effort under the auspices of the Institute of Medicine Roundtable on Environmental Health and another under the auspices of the American Schools of Public Health. Both will result in conferences to be held in the same month of the New York Academy of Sciences (NYAS) conference on "The Role of Neural Plasticity in Chemical Intolerance", for which this paper is being prepared. This questioning of our definition and of our approach to the field of environmental health is an instructive background on which to consider the issue of environmental risks and public health—the topic given to me by the organizers of the NYAS conference. My approach will be to touch on those issues related to the nervous system and to unexplained symptoms in keeping with the subject of the conference, as well as to discuss some of the broader issues surrounding environmental health.

INTRODUCTION

Environmental health is a subset of public health. A classic definition of health is given by the World Health Organization:

> HEALTH is a state of COMPLETE physical, mental, and social well-being and not merely the ABSENCE of disease or infirmity.

I stress that this definition does not restrict public health only to disease. There has been much debate as to whether individuals with unexplained symptoms that fall into categories such as multiple chemical sensitivities (MCS), chronic fatigue syndrome, Gulf War syndrome, etc., are in fact suffering from a disease. While a legitimate question, a negative answer cannot and should not absolve the field of environmental health from its responsibilities in responding to the many individuals in our society with unexplained symptoms. There is no question that these individuals are not healthy whether or not we can fully classify them into a specific disease.

Allow me to indulge in two personal anecdotes that color my perception of the issue of the role of the nervous system and of behavioral factors as the basis for adverse health experiences related to medically unexplained symptoms. While a second-year medical student in 1959, my classmates and I were told by the faculty that we could ignore a relatively large section of our required textbook of physical diagnosis. This was the section having to do with the physical findings differentiat-

---

[a]Address for correspondence: Bernard D. Goldstein, Director, Environmental and Occupational Health Sciences Institute (EOHSI), 170 Frelinghuysen Road, Piscataway, NJ 08854. Voice: 732-445-0205; fax: 732-445-0131.
bgold@eohsi.rutgers.edu

ing "true" paralysis from hysterical paralysis, as we were no longer likely to observe the latter disease whose incidence had dropped dramatically. I actually did see two cases of hysterical paralysis as a house officer and as a ward attending at Bellevue Hospital. Both were treated as extreme curiosities, leading to visits by all available students, ward staff, and attending physicians, and both raised among us some degree of consternation by physical findings that were seemingly inexplicable and irrational. A second personal anecdote concerns being an intern at Bellevue Hospital covering the female psychomedical ward the night after Marilyn Monroe committed suicide. Our usual one or two attempted suicides requiring gastric intubation were replaced by a virtual deluge of cases of young women who were admitted to the ward because of an alleged or actual overdose of pills.

Both hysterical paralysis and failed attempted suicides are phenomena whose incidence has occurred in waves over time and that have a female preponderance during these outbreaks. Both were recognized by the medical profession as disorders that fell under the purview of psychiatrists. They differ in that hysterical paralysis represents a dramatic change in body function manifested through an alteration in the nervous system, while attempted suicide is manifested to the medical profession as a consequence of an overt personal action, such as ingesting a toxic chemical.

I bring up these two anecdotes for a purpose, and the purpose is not at all to belittle the suffering or concerns of those with unexplained symptoms. Recently, the U.S. government established a Presidential/Congressional Commission on Risk Assessment and Risk Management.[1] It developed a six-step framework (FIG. 1) that makes two important statements particularly relevant to the problem being addressed at this meeting. One is that environmental health issues are best dealt with in cooperation with all stakeholders—in this case, clearly including those whose health has been affected. We need to pay much more attention to those who are suffering. To really be effective, though, we need to include government agencies, the broad scientific community, and even the private sector in our deliberations. Another relevant aspect of the framework is that its very first step is to consider the context of the problem being addressed. I suggest that a critically important context for unexplained symptoms is our society and its environment.

The relation of external chemicals to mass behavior conditioned by societal mores has been suggested in a number of instances. A notable example is the conjecture that the Salem witch trial episode in seventeenth-century New England was due to weather-related growth of molds producing ergot alkaloids in the grain.[2] There are other episodes, considered to be mass hysteria, for which thorough study has revealed no basis for the symptoms that were alleged to be due to exposure to chemicals, for example, the CDC investigation of a wave of symptoms among female Palestinian teenagers based upon the rumor that Israelis were subjecting them to chemical poisoning.

DEFINING ENVIRONMENTAL HEALTH

The definition of environmental health is a moving target—even if we restrict the term to just referring to human health, not the general environment.[3] From different vantage points, there are different views of what is meant by the environment in terms of its impact on human health. The broadest definition of the environment is

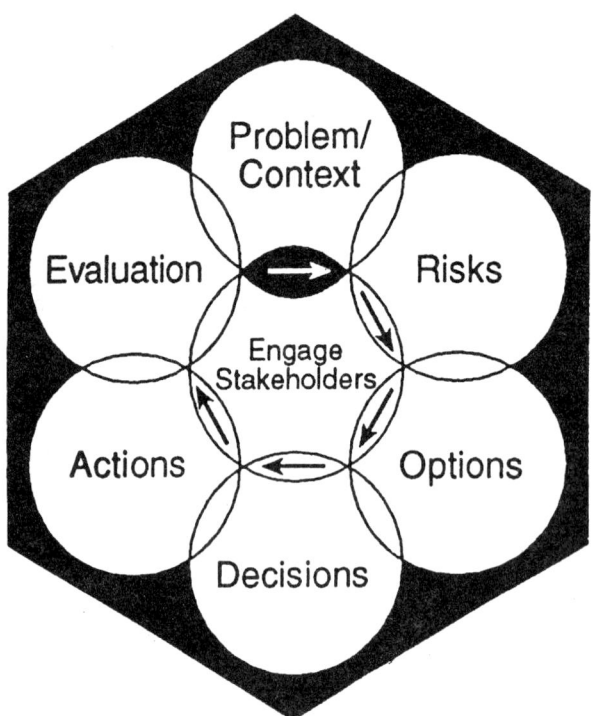

FIGURE 1. The six-step framework recommended by the Presidential/Congressional Commission on Risk Assessment and Risk Management.

everything that is not genetic. More narrower definitions are based on such criteria as governmental mandates for the boundaries between academic disciplines. For example, using the broadest definition of the term, cigarette smoking is the major environmental cause of cancer and is the subject of much needed attention by public health authorities and health agencies. A more narrow definition of environmental health is that which restricts the U.S. Environmental Protection Agency to deal solely with cigarettes in terms of environmental tobacco smoke. Note that defining secondhand smoking as "environmental" implies that mainstream smoking is somehow not environmental.

Even the simple definition of environment, everything not covered by genetics, is becoming clouded. The unraveling of the human genome has taken us well past simple Mendelian genetics in which genetic inheritance can readily be identified as sufficient to cause disease. This simple approach is not generalizable to our rapidly increasing understanding of the genetic basis for human disease. What we are finding is that there are families of susceptibility genes that may each have a small impact on the possibility that an individual will develop a specific disease—for example, over a dozen genes have been identified as being involved in adult-onset diabetes mellitus. While these genes may be necessary for the development of a given disease, they are not sufficient. Sufficiency comes from the environmental factors responsible for disease. Also of importance is that the majority of high-incidence human diseases fit into the category of having such sensitivity genes. A major goal of environmental health will be to obtain an understanding of the external factors that convert a genetic propensity into human disease. Identification of such environmental factors will allow primary prevention to be appropriately targeted.

Before this understanding of the human genome can be converted into prevention strategies, targeted research to identify gene environment interactions will be necessary. The good news is that having basic genetic information provides an opportunity for facilitating research approaches to identify these environmental factors. For example, limiting studies of potential cause-and-effect relationships to individuals who have specific genetic risk factors greatly increases the power of epidemiological studies to demonstrate such relationships. Of particular pertinence to the present symposium is the value of exploring genetic specificity as a means to establish that a specific disorder actually exists. I personally will find it very convincing that MCS truly exists as a distinct disorder if a specific genetic pattern is found in a well-characterized series of individuals with this alleged disorder. Further, of particular interest would be a finding that such individuals had specificity in genes related to absorption, distribution, metabolism, or excretion of chemicals. On the other hand, the absence of a discernible pattern could be interpreted as a point against there being a true disorder. A similar argument could be made about the protein expressing of genetic characteristics as it is proteins that are responsible for cellular activity.

ROLE OF ENVIRONMENTAL HEALTH SCIENCE

Central to advances in environmental health have been the rapid and notable advances in environmental health sciences. The three core disciplines of environmental health are toxicology, epidemiology, and exposure assessment. Toxicology is particularly relevant to issues being discussed at this conference. The gap between usual dose-response characteristics of chemicals and the complaints of individuals with chemical sensitivities is profound. Central to bridging this gap is to develop the mechanistic understanding of the relationship between exposure and effects in affected individuals. With such an understanding, acceptance of the legitimacy of the relation between chemicals and effects in MCS and related disorders can be gained, and insight into effective prevention and treatment measures achieved. However, this must be subject to the full rigors of scientific enquiry rather than the hand waving and borderline paranoia that have characterized many of the approaches to theoretical understanding of the cause-and-effect relationships in MCS and related disorders.

It is not appropriate for us to turn our backs on the suffering of individuals because our toxicological science does not know how to link the potential cause to the reported effects. However, it is even more inappropriate to mislead these sufferers by unvalidated claims of scientific truth. We must rigorously subject any of our ideas about the etiology and pathogenesis of unexplained symptoms to full scientific study. The scientific method can be described as going up alleys to see if they are blind. In this field, we need a little more humility from those who are willing to identify these alleys, but who are unwilling to engage in the hard work necessary to enter the alley and see where it goes.

TABLE 1. Risk assessment

(1) Hazard identification

(2) Dose-response evaluation

(3) Exposure assessment

(4) Risk characterization

TABLE 2. The three laws of toxicology

(1) The dose makes the poison.

(2) Chemicals have specific effects.

(3) Humans are animals.

Both epidemiology and exposure assessment are also important to increasing knowledge about individuals with unexplained symptoms. Careful case identification, surveillance, and evaluation of intervention strategies are hallmarks of public health epidemiology. Finding associations that can provide insights into cause-and-effect relationships will also be necessary. However, this is not possible without very carefully developed case definitions.[4,5] The challenge is to not define the putative disorder so broadly as to obscure true cause-and-effect relationships or too narrowly so as to not have enough statistical power to make observations. Surveillance also depends upon clear case definitions that allow ascertainment of trends over time and location.

For epidemiological studies to be successful will require close cooperation with the relatively new discipline of exposure assessment, particularly in relation to discovering possible etiologies due to exposure to chemical or physical agents. Understanding exposure is central to determining risk—without exposure, there is no risk. Understanding exposure pathways also enables preventive actions to be aimed at interdicting risk.

Advances in environmental health sciences have been the basis for the development of environmental risk assessment. Risk assessment consists of four steps: hazard identification, dose-response assessment, exposure assessment, and risk characterization (TABLE 1).[6] These steps in part are based on the "laws" of toxicology (TABLE 2). That the dose makes the poison is a central concept in toxicology and underlies the role of dose-response assessment. With the exception of agents that cause mutations, such as genotoxic carcinogens, it is believed that there is a threshold for the effects of chemicals such that lower doses produce no adverse effects. To a toxicologist, a major issue in understanding the symptoms of individuals with MCS is the apparent relation of these nonspecific symptoms to levels of chemicals far below those that are known to produce such symptoms. What is needed, and what will be discussed at this conference, is a testable model that would explain why certain individuals are at risk at these lower levels, while the bulk of the population is nonresponsive.

Some individuals with MCS present another problem to the science of toxicology—the gap in apparent understanding includes the issue of hazard identification. Another toxicological "law" is that chemicals have specific effects, reflecting both their chemistry and the biology of the receptor. Benzene causes bone marrow toxicity, not peptic ulcer; and asbestos causes lung cancers, not macular degeneration. The complex symptomatology exhibited by some individuals identified as having MCS does not always fit the known hazards of the substances that elicit the symptoms. This suggests a generic mechanism of effect that is divorced from the toxicological specificity of the identified hazard.

Pertinent to the problem addressed at this conference is the goal of identifying barriers blocking performance of the needed research. One of these barriers is our academic culture. Those of us in academic environmental research have found it difficult to learn to listen to the community. As academics, we tend to have a high opinion of our own skills and often find it difficult to condescend to listen to those without advanced degrees and peer-reviewed publications. In our program at the Environmental and Occupational Health Sciences Institute in New Jersey, we think of community-based research as occurring at three levels.[7] The most superficial is to simply inform the affected community about our research. A more appropriate approach is, whenever possible, to engage the community in the research activity, including hiring affected people, developing advisory committees, and actively communicating before, during, and after the research. This approach takes advantage of the knowledge and skills of the affected community. Although often time-consuming and resource-intensive, in our view it is cost-effective in terms of the research outcome and community acceptance of the findings and their implication. However, we believe the third and deepest level of academic involvement with communities is even more effective. This is the level in which the research agenda is actually set in consultation with the affected community. Answering the questions that most concern those who are affected can be an effective shortcut to achieving environmental health goals. Although perhaps counterintuitive, we find that developing research responsive to community concerns may also lead to basic advances through research that would not have begun were it not for listening to concerns of the community. There are, of course, many pitfalls to setting the research agenda in cooperation with the community. Most important is be open, respectful, and transparent. It is also crucial to avoid promising more than can be accomplished. For example, epidemiological power calculations are an abstruse art, but it is possible to explain the basic concept that a large enough population size is needed before certain questions can be asked—just try using examples like whether a pitcher is a better home run hitter than Mark McGwire because, in one baseball game, a pitcher hit a home run and McGwire did not; or whether because it rained in Phoenix yesterday, but not in Seattle, we can conclude that Seattle is more likely to be a desert.

THE CHALLENGE

It is fair to say that many of the astounding gains in public health in the past century primarily represented advances in environmental health. It is also fair to say that the major challenges of the twenty-first century remain those that must be met by advances in environmental health. These advances include more widespread distribution to many less developed areas of our world of gains in sanitation, housing, vector control, workplace health and safety, and air and water pollution. In the developed world, among the many challenges facing environmental health is that of the poor health of so many among us due to unexplained symptoms. We need to confront with compassion and with innovation the etiology and the pathogenesis of these problems. Our most likely path of success is to continue to build upon the strengths of environmental health sciences that have been the basis for our gains to the present.

ACKNOWLEDGMENTS

EOHSI is a joint program of UMDNJ–Robert Wood Johnson Medical School and Rutgers–The State University of New Jersey

REFERENCES

1. THE PRESIDENTIAL/CONGRESSIONAL COMMISSION ON RISK ASSESSMENT AND RISK MANAGEMENT. 1997. Framework for Environmental Health Risk Management. Final Report Volume 1. Washington, D.C.
2. SPANOS, N.P. & J. GOTTLIEB. 1976. Ergotism and the Salem Village witch trials. Science **194**(4272): 1390–1394.
3. GOLDSTEIN, B.D. 1995. The need to restore the public health base for environmental control. Am. J. Public Health **85**(4): 481–483.
4. KIPEN, H.M. & N. FIEDLER. 1999. Sensitivities to chemicals—context and implications. Am. J. Epidemiol. **150**(1): 13–16.
5. FIEDLER, N., H. KIPEN, J. DELUCA *et al.* 1996. Controlled comparison of multiple chemical sensitivity and chronic fatigue syndrome. Psychosom. Med. **58**(1): 38–49.
6. NATIONAL RESEARCH COUNCIL (NRC). 1983. Risk Assessment in the Federal Government: Managing the Process. National Academy Press. Washington, D.C.
7. GOLDSTEIN, B.D., S. ERDAL, J. BURGER *et al.* 2000. Stakeholder participation for community health risk evaluation: experience from the CRESP program. Annu. Rev. Energy Environ. In press.

Sensitization, Subjective Health Complaints, and Sustained Arousal

HOLGER URSIN AND HEGE R. ERIKSEN

Department of Biological and Medical Psychology, University of Bergen, N-5009 Bergen, Norway

ABSTRACT: The purpose of this presentation is to discuss the possibility that sensitization is a psychobiological mechanism underlying not only multiple chemical sensitivity (MCS), but a much more general cluster of illness, referred to as "subjective health complaints". Sustained arousal, or sustained "stress" responses, may be an important factor for the development of these conditions. Patients with subjective complaints without objective changes are sometimes referred to as having "fashionable diagnoses" or "unexplained symptoms". They may be given diagnoses like MCS, epidemic fatigue, chronic fatigue syndrome, burnout, stress, a variety of intoxications, environmental illness, radiation, multiple chemical hypersensitivity, food intolerance, functional dyspepsia, irritable bowel, myalgic encephalitis, postviral syndrome, yuppie flu, fibromyalgia, or vital exhaustion. One issue is whether this is one general condition or separate entities. Another issue is whether sensitization may be the psychobiological mechanism for most or all of these conditions. Finally, is it likely that sustained arousal may facilitate the development of sensitization in some or many neural circuits? In this review, the main emphasis will be on musculoskeletal pain. This is the most frequent and most expensive condition for sickness compensation and disability. The comorbidity of other complaints, however, will also be taken into account.

ONE GENERAL CONDITION?

The General Condition: Subjective Health Complaints

Subjective health complaints,[1–4] or "unexplained symptoms",[5] are very common, so common that in the light stages they are almost "normal". At least 75% of a normal population has had at least one complaint during the last 30 days, from the musculoskeletal system, gastrointestinal tract, or urogenital system, or "pseudoneurological" complaints, like fatigue, tiredness, dizziness, vertigo, and headaches.[3] There is no pathophysiological explanation or the complaints are beyond what is "reasonable" from a medical point of view. The plurality of us do not seek medical assistance for these complaints—they are a part of everyday life.

The distribution of complaints (FIG. 1) reveals no cut point, which could help us decide when the complaints are turning intolerable and requiring help. There are no clear thresholds that define the border between what everyone has been bothered by and what becomes intolerable and a burden for the patient and for society.[6]

Subjective health complaints are the most frequent sources of long-term sickness compensation, of permanent inability to work, and for encounter with health services, particularly frequent in frequent attenders.[2,7] When pronounced, the com-

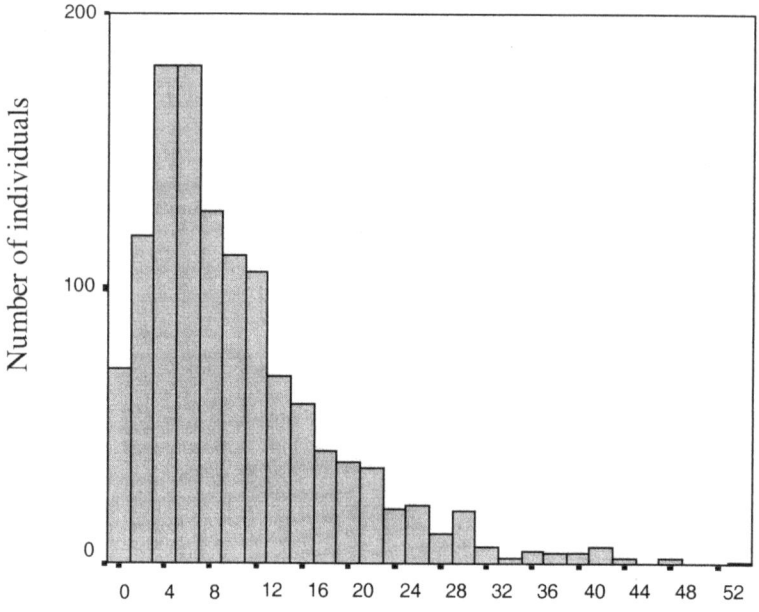

FIGURE 1. Total sum of health complaints in a cross-sectional representative sample of the Norwegian population ($n = 1000$).[6]

plaints qualify as Somatization Disorder within the DSM-IV classification system for mental disorders.[8] When less pronounced, they may qualify as Undifferentiated Somatoform Disorder. However, most patients with these complaints do not qualify for the "mental disorder" and should not be regarded as psychiatric cases, even if there is a comorbidity with psychiatric diagnostic entities.

The DSM-IV classifications seem to represent only a tip of an iceberg and it is the iceberg that is the most costly clinical and social problem. The diagnostic criteria require a certain duration, a certain number of complaints, and that the condition is causing distress and represents a clinically significant impairment. This makes practical sense, particularly for anyone located at endpoints of the referral system of medicine. However, these principles are of little help or comfort for the general practitioner that has to deal with the conditions before they may be referred to the specialist. An analysis of high utilizers of primary care in the United States confirms this picture. The clinical and behavioral features of somatization do not change dramatically at the diagnostic threshold for somatization.[9]

Present classification systems seem to invite a more dualistic approach than what is suggested by contemporary psychobiological thinking. The complaints should not be classified or treated as being either psychological or somatic. Current systems do not offer any general or common heading for subjective health complaints. Each physical complaint will have to be listed under the proper organ heading or as pain conditions, and the totality is lost. The term "subjective health complaints" should therefore be considered.[1] It comprises all the states included in the iceberg and it does not involve any assumption on etiology.

Subjective Health Complaints: One or Several Conditions?

The syndrome as it was described by Briquet[10] and by Beard[11] seems to be fairly identical to a syndrome based on subjective health complaints. In later literature, the syndrome appears sometimes as an entity, for instance, as "fashionable diagnoses" or plain DSM-IV somatization or somatoform disorders,[4] or as simply "subjective health complaints",[1] with sensitization as the common denominator.

There seems to be consensus that there is a very high degree of comorbidity, but the issue of one versus several conditions is not solved. It may be that the iceberg of subjective health complaints has many tips, but it is still one iceberg. Clauw[12] pointed out that, even if the musculoskeletal features define fibromyalgia, there is considerable overlap with chronic fatigue syndrome, migraine and tension headaches, irritable bowel syndrome, and affective disorders. Patients appearing for treatment for chronic facial pain show a high comorbidity of complaints like irritable bowel, cystitis, premenstrual syndromes, and general muscle pain.[13,14]

IS SENSITIZATION THE PSYCHONEUROBIOLOGICAL SUBSTRATE FOR SUBJECTIVE HEALTH COMPLAINTS?

Sensitization

The main position of this paper is as follows: one possible psychobiological mechanism explaining why some develop more complaints than others is that neural pathways involved in the complaints are sensitized.[1] Repeated use of synapses in the nervous system may lead to changes in synaptic efficiency for long time periods. These changes are, in principle, of two types. Sensitization is an increased efficiency in the synapse due to repeated use. Habituation is a decreased efficiency due to repeated use.[15] These two processes occur at the synaptic level, and the synaptic changes concomitant with them are known in considerable detail. The same terminology is used for complex responses, even if we do not know the neuronal network involved.

There are data suggesting that sensitization may be involved in several manifestations of subjective health complaints, when such complaints become intolerable. Patients with generalized muscle pain (fibromyalgia) have lower threshold for muscle pain than normal controls, ascribed to sensitization of neurons in the dorsal horn.[16] Pain sensitivity is a significant correlate for clinical status in patients with chronic low back pain.[17] Patients with functional gastrointestinal problems have lower sensory threshold for gut stimuli than others.[18,19] Patients with multiple chemical sensitivity respond more strongly (heart rate) to stressful tasks.[20] Subjects reporting illness from environmental chemicals also report multiple medical diagnoses, multiple subjective complaints, and psychological distress.[21] People complaining of traffic noise have higher self-reported sensitivity and annoyance to noise.[22] Sensitization has also been discussed as a model for posttraumatic stress disorder.[23]

Sensitization has also been suggested as the underlying mechanism for comorbid disorders. Major depression, panic disorder, mania, phobic disorder, irritable bowel, ovarian cysts, and anxiety may depend on "kindling" of limbic structures.[24,25] Kindling may be regarded as a time-dependent sensitization of limbic neurons.[26] The basic hypothesis is that subconvulsive kindling of limbic structures may explain why some subjects get more sensitive than others to a wide variety of stimuli. This would explain the high comorbidity of these subjective states and would offer a model for cross-sensitization from one source of stimuli to another.[24,27]

The amygdala nuclei may be the most interesting of the limbic structures for clinically relevant sensitization. Amygdala, and the ventral tegmental area, is necessary for the behavioral sensitization to cocaine.[28] The central nucleus of amygdala may be particularly important since it is involved in emotional arousal and exploration.[29] The neurons in the central nucleus produce corticotrophin-releasing hormone (CRH), but respond with increased production to increased levels of glucocorticoids rather than the expected decrease.[30] A similar alteration in this axis has been reported for patients with chronic pain and posttraumatic stress disorders.[31] Changes in receptor sensitivity and the regulation of CRH and glucocorticoids may be an interesting supplement to the kindling and sensitization hypotheses.

The kindling/sensitization hypothesis has also been offered as an explanation for the possible impact that early experiences might have on these patients. There is a high correlation between subjective health complaints (somatization) and reports of exposure to physical, verbal, or sexual abuse.[32] The problem with these data is the systematic overreporting by these patients and their unreliable histories, one of the DSM-IV characteristics of somatization patients. The sensitization hypothesis covers this eventuality. The truth value of the statement of misuse may be questioned; however, if these patients are more sensitive than the rest of the population, they are also more vulnerable.

Sensitization in Pain Pathways

There is no habituation to pain stimulation. Quite to the contrary, a common characteristic of pain, particularly for tissue damage, is hyperalgesia, an enhanced pain report to natural stimuli. Pain spreads to adjacent areas, and the injured part and surrounding areas become hypersensitive. The tissue damage releases signal molecules from injured afferents, damaged tissue, and inflammatory cells. These signal molecules spread to the surrounding tissue and depolarize primary afferent nociceptors, contributing to sensitization and hyperalgesia. Since these signal molecules interact, inflammation increases pain sensitivity.[33]

Sensitization is also affected by a feed-forward effect from the sympathetic nerves to the area (release of neuropeptide or ATP)[34] and by release of substance P from the afferent terminals.[35] An involvement of sympathetic nerves has been suggested for rheumatoid arthritis[36,37] and for fibromyalgic patients.[38]

In addition to these peripheral and feed-forward mechanisms, there is also sensitization in central pain pathways. The best known mechanisms are in the dorsal horn of the spinal cord. Activation of neurons at N-methyl-D-aspartate (NMDA) receptor sites by excitatory amino acids such as glutamate and aspartate[39] produce hyperexcitability, expansion of receptive fields, and hyperalgesia. Chronic pain may result from neuropeptides enhancing NMDA receptor excitability, possibly leading to excessive depolarization and excitotoxicity, which finally may lead to a loss of inhibitory interneurons and a loss of inhibitory mechanisms.[40] The sensitization produced by inflammation has a central factor as well, apparently by A-fibers switching to express substance P, like C-fibers do, thus contributing to the hypersensitivity.[33]

Recent data also point to long-term potentiation of nociceptive evoked responses in neurons in the dorsal horn of rats.[41,42] Similar long-term increases may also be induced by natural noxious stimulation.[41,43]

Central mechanisms also play a role in the sensitization to pain. There is a complex system of descending fibers modulating the pain transmission in the dorsal horn, both facilitating and inhibiting the transfer, involving several signal systems.[44] The dorsal reticular nucleus is involved in the facilitation of pain behavior, probably through reciprocal connections with the dorsal horn.[45] Thalamic transmission and the complex circuits involved in pain behavior are probably also modifiable by sensitization mechanisms. These circuits appear to be too complex for analyses at the neuronal level, but the kindling phenomenon suggests similar mechanisms in the limbic structures.

The neurobiological data on pain sensitization mechanisms offer an attractive model for the development of chronic muscle pain.[46] The animal models are developed based on injury of other tissues, but it is reasonable to accept these models also for muscle pain. The model implies that muscle pain depends on local mechanisms, spinal mechanisms, and interactions with central nervous mechanisms, all of which are subject to sensitization. In plain talk, psychological factors influence the synaptic mechanisms and feed-forward loops from the brain, affecting behavior and muscle tension, and these psychobiological circuits may reinforce themselves through sensitization. If this is true, it must also be possible to affect these circuits by psychological and behavioral interventions.

SUSTAINED AROUSAL, SENSITIZATION, AND SUBJECTIVE HEALTH COMPLAINTS

Cognitive Arousal Theory of Stress (CATS), Sustained Arousal, and Disease

If the stress *response* is explained within the framework of arousal or activation theory, as it is known in neurophysiology,[47,48] stress or arousal should be regarded as an essential element in the total adaptive system of the organism.[49] The stress response increases wakefulness and vigilance and affects the endocrine systems, vegetative nervous system, and immune systems as well as the biochemistry of the brain.[49]

The response occurs whenever there is a discrepancy between what the organism is expecting (set value) and what really exists (actual value of the same variable). The stress response, therefore, is simply the alarm in the homeostatic system.[49] This reformulation of stress theory may be referred to as a cognitive arousal theory of stress (CATS).[50] The response is uncomfortable and drives the organism to provide specific solutions to abolish the source of the alarm, but should not be interpreted as anything pathological or unwanted. Why would it then be so widespread in biology?

The reason to refer to the theory as "cognitive" is that the alarm depends on evaluation of expected outcomes of events and of the strategies available to the individual. Briefly, the alarm, or "stress", is dampened if the individual uses psychological defense mechanisms to deny threats and dangers or expects to be able to handle the situation with a positive result ("coping"). On the other hand, the alarm will occur if the defense mechanisms are overtaxed[51] or if the individual does not believe that his or her coping strategies are adequate.[49,52] When the expectancy is that the outcome is negative, the state is referred to as "hopelessness".[49] When the expectancy is that there are no relationships between available responses and results, the condition is referred to as "helplessness".[49,53,54] All these expectancies have a tendency to generalize. This affects mood and also health. Individuals that cope report few health problems,[55] even if they have high job demands.[52] Hopelessness and helplessness, in humans and animals, may produce a sustained alarm and sustained arousal, which again may produce pathology.

The concept is related to, but not identical with, the "allostasis" of McEwen.[56] Both positions emphasize the homeostatic principle of restoring balance—allostasis covers "stability through change". In CATS, the pathophysiological factor is the sustained arousal when there is no solution; for McEwen, it is the allostatic system itself that is overtaxed, overstimulated, or not functioning properly. He refers to that as "allostatic load", "the price for adaptation", which includes conditions like frequent activation, failure to shut the system off, or inadequate response of the allostatic systems.

Sustained Arousal Theory of Disease and Illness

Demonstrations of changes in acute stress situations do not imply pathology; it is the long-lasting arousal that may be linked to straining effects. The type of pathology and the choice of organ system depend on an interaction of genetic factors, environmental factors, and the sustained arousal. The pathophysiological mechanisms through which sustained arousal may produce disease are reasonably well defined[49,57] for the cardiovascular system, gastric mucosa, and biochemical composition of the brain in animals.[58]

For illness or subjective health complaints, the models are more hypothetical. In a comparison of chronic pain states, in particular fibromyalgia, and chronic fatigue syndromes, Clauw and Chrousos[59] concluded that such syndromes are "caused by central nervous dysfunction". This "dysfunction" should include the hypothalamic-pituitary axes, the pain processing pathways, and the autonomic nervous system. Within this context, changes in immune functions, for instance, would be secondary to the changes in the CNS and not the cause of the illnesses.

Within the CATS framework, the point is that it is not necessarily any pathology in the CNS. The illness is a consequence of a sustained arousal involving sensitization of key neuronal circuits. The kindling hypothesis for limbic structures is attractive and receives some support from the evidence of changes in the regulatory mechanisms of the hypothalamic-pituitary-adrenal (HPA) axis in depression and posttraumatic stress disorder.[31] Patients with fibromyalgia, chronic low back pain, and chronic fatigue all have signs of "dysregulation" of the HPA axis.[59–61] Sustained arousal also seems to have effects on the biochemical composition of the brain,[62] findings that may link this concept also to psychiatric morbidity. These changes in the stress response are compatible with the sustained arousal theory and sensitization of psychobiological loops. However, the relations are still speculative.

It has also been difficult to demonstrate peripheral physiological evidence of sustained arousal. In most experiments, any such change is drowned in diurnal and episodic influences and by homeostatic self-regulatory principles. The evidence from field research is indirect, but offers some support for the relevance of sustained arousal and subjective health complaints. Insufficient recovery after work-related exertion may start a vicious circle that, in the long run, will cause more severe health complaints.[63–65] Supporting this view are findings of high levels of subjective health complaints in individuals that report that they are not coping with their high job demands.[52] High levels are also found in individuals working in environments with poor learning climate, where the employees do not feel that they learn new facts and skills,[66] and in individuals that report an increased need for recovery, along with sleep problems and feelings of "burnout".[63,64] A possible psychobiological link is offered by the strong correlations between several work-related neuroendocrine recovery parameters (cortisol and adrenaline in urine) and momentary health status.[63,64]

The concept of the possibility of sustained arousal producing ill effects is not new. Both Briquet (1859)[10] and Beard (1869)[11] ascribed hysteria or asthenia to an overload of a weak ("asthenic") system. The treatment most often recommended was rest and isolation from the humdrum of daily life. These concepts are not far from present-day concerns about stress and burnout. The only new contribution that we could begin to offer is a more rational pathophysiological model for the resulting pathology or complaints.

Sustained Arousal and Therapy

Individuals with positive response outcome expectancies (coping) have no sustained arousal and, correspondingly, good health. The same principles are assumed to work in therapeutic situations. Therefore, sustained arousal may be a factor in formulating effective preventive and therapeutic programs. Predictive factors for fast recovery from low back pain include the hope of getting well and feelings of "internal control" for health—that is, the patient realizes that he or she may influence his or her condition.[67] Lifestyle factors, like physical activity, may also be related to the personal feelings of being in control of oneself. For the successful treatment of low back pain, the most important item seems to be to reduce the fear of the condition.[68] The loss of control and positive expectancies seem to aggravate common illness and may reinforce the perception of the illness, which in turn may aggravate the condition.[69] Therapy and prevention may be directed at these emotional and cognitive mechanisms.[70]

CONCLUSIONS

From Traditional Psychosomatic Medicine to Behavioral Medicine

Traditional psychosomatic models have less predictive value and less therapeutic importance than what was hoped for. The main contribution from behavioral factors on somatic disease is related to lifestyle. The effectiveness of many of the therapeutic interventions is so high that one may be tempted to disregard additional psychosocial factors. However, a very high number of patients are not served by our abilities to treat disease. These patients have illnesses, which in this context means conditions where we do not have a rational or organic explanation of their complaints, or that the complaints go beyond what is regarded as "reasonable" by the physician.

There is, therefore, more attention directed to "unexplained" or subjective health complaints. "Unexplained symptoms" have always been a challenge to medicine and to psychology. They may signal a condition that is unexplained because our diagnostic abilities and knowledge are inadequate. They may also remain unexplained simply because they do not represent any pathology in the classical sense. There is no demonstrable pathophysiological process. A better understanding of the psychobiology of our natural responses to stress and challenge may improve the situation. Sensitization in neurobiological loops maintained by sustained arousal may offer an acceptable model.

The attitude and the expectancies attached to health affect health and the prognosis for treatment of disease and illness. These factors are not psychiatric factors; they are consequences of the interaction between normal psychological factors and normal complaints. The main issue remains why some people are more sensitive than others. This may depend on early experience, genetics, or both. If we understood the rules and laws of sensitization and somatization, we could make an impact on very substantial portions of the health-care budgets in industrialized countries. This understanding may also offer a handle on changing health behavior, which may have an even greater impact on health-care budgets and life quality.

REFERENCES

1. URSIN, H. 1997. Sensitization, somatization, and subjective health complaints: a review. Int. J. Behav. Med. **4:** 105–116.
2. ERIKSEN, H.R., R. SVENDSRØD, G. URSIN & H. URSIN. 1998. Prevalence of subjective health complaints in the Nordic European countries in 1993. Eur. J. Public Health **8:** 294–298.
3. ERIKSEN, H.R., C. IHLEBÆK & H. URSIN. 1999. A scoring system for subjective health complaints (SHC). Scand. J. Soc. Med. **1:** 63–72.
4. FORD, C.V. 1997. Somatization and fashionable diagnoses: illness as a way of life. Scand. J. Work Environ. Health **238**(suppl. 3): 7–16.
5. NIMNUAN, C., M. HOTOPF & S. WESSELY. 2000. Medically unexplained symptoms: how often and why are they missed? QJM **93:** 21–28.
6. IHLEBÆK, C., H.R. ERIKSEN & H. URSIN. 2000. Prevalence of subjective health complaints (SHC) in Norway. Submitted.
7. KARLSSON, H., M. JOUKAMAA, I. LAHTI et al. 1997. Frequent attender profiles: different clinical subgroups among frequent attender patients in primary care. J. Psychosom. Res. **42:** 157–166.
8. AMERICAN PSYCHIATRIC ASSOCIATION. 1994. Diagnostic and Statistical Manual of Mental Disorders. Fourth edition. Amer. Psychiatric Assoc. Washington, D.C.
9. KATON, W., E. LIN, M. VON KORFF et al. 1991. Somatization: a spectrum of severity. Am. J. Psychiatry **148:** 34–40.
10. GUZE, S.B. 1975. The validity and significance of the clinical diagnosis of hysteria (Briquet's syndrome). Am. J. Psychiatry **132:** 138–141.
11. CHATEL, J.C. & R. PEELE. 1970. The concept of neurasthenia. Int. J. Psychiatry **9:** 36–49.
12. CLAUW, D.J. 1995. The pathogenesis of chronic pain and fatigue syndromes, with special reference to fibromyalgia. Med. Hypotheses **44:** 369–378.

13. KORSZUN, A., E. PAPADOPOULUS, M. DEMITRACK et al. 1998. The relationship between temporomandibular disorders and stress-associated syndromes. Oral Surg. Oral Med. Oral Pathol. **86:** 416–420.
14. KROGSTAD, B.S., A. JOKSTAD, B.L. DAHL & O. VASSEND. 1996. Relationships between risk factors and treatment outcome in a group of patients with temporomandibular disorders. J. Orofac. Pain **10:** 48–53.
15. THOMPSON, R.F. & W.A. SPENCER. 1966. Habituation: a model phenomenon for the study of neuronal substrates of behavior. Psychol. Rev. **73:** 16–43.
16. VÆRØY, H., R. HELLE, Ø. FØRRE et al. 1988. Elevated CSF levels of substance P and high incidence of Raynaud phenomenon in patients with fibromyalgia: new features for diagnosis. Pain **32:** 21–26.
17. CLAUW, D.J., D. WILLIAMS, W. LAUERMAN et al. 1999. Pain sensitivity as a correlate of clinical status in individuals with chronic low back pain. Spine **24:** 2035–2041.
18. MEARING, F., X. DE-RIBOT, A. BALBOA et al. 1995. Does *Helicobacter pylori* infection increase gastric sensitivity in functional dyspepsia? Gut **37:** 47–51.
19. LEMBO, T., J. MUNAKATA, H. MERTZ et al. 1994. Evidence for the hypersensitivity of lumbar splanchnic afferents in irritable bowel syndrome. Gastroenterology **107:** 1686–1696.
20. BELL, I.R., E.J. MARKLEY, D.S. KING et al. 1993. Polysymptomatic syndromes and autonomic reactivity to nonfood stressors in individuals with self-reported adverse food reactions. J. Am. Coll. Nutr. **12:** 227–238.
21. BELL, I.R., J.M. PETERSON & G.E. SCHWARTZ. 1995. Medical histories and psychological profiles of middle-aged women with and without self-reported illness from environmental chemicals. J. Clin. Psychiatry **56:** 151–160.
22. NIVISON, M.E. & I.M. ENDRESEN. 1993. An analysis of relationships among environmental noise, annoyance, and sensitivity to noise, and the consequences for health and sleep. J. Behav. Med. **16:** 257–276.
23. FRIEDMAN, M.J. 1994. Neurobiological sensitization models of post-traumatic stress disorder: their possible relevance to multiple chemical sensitivity syndrome. Toxicol. Ind. Health **10:** 449–462.
24. BELL, I.R., C.S. MILLER & G.E. SCHWARTZ. 1992. An olfactory-limbic model of multiple chemical sensitivity syndrome: possible relationships to kindling and affective spectrum disorders. Biol. Psychiatry **32:** 218–242.
25. GODDARD, G.V. 1987. Development of epileptic seizures through brain stimulation of low intensity. Nature **214:** 1020.
26. ANTELMAN, S.M., J.C. SOARES & S. GERSHON. 1997. Time-dependent sensitization—possible implications for clinical psychopharmacology. Behav. Pharmacol. **8:** 505–514.
27. BELL, I.R. 1994. White paper: neuropsychiatric aspects of sensitivity to low-level chemicals—a neural sensitization model. Toxicol. Ind. Health **10:** 277–312.
28. KALIVAS, P.W. & J.E. ALESDATTER. 1993. Involvement of N-methyl-D-aspartate receptor stimulation in the ventral tegmental area and amygdala in behavioral sensitization to cocaine. J. Pharmacol. Exp. Ther. **267:** 486–495.
29. JELLESTAD, F.K., G.S. FOLLESØ & H. URSIN. 1991. The neurobiological foundation of exploration. *In* Curiosity and Exploration, pp. 43–63. Springer. New York/Berlin.
30. SCHULKIN, J., B.S. MCEWEN & P.W. GOLD. 1994. Allostasis, amygdala, and anticipatory anxiety. Neurosci. Biobehav. Rev. **18:** 385–396.
31. YEHUDA, R., D. BOISONEAU, M.T. LOWY & E.L. GILLER. 1996. Dose-response changes in plasma cortisol and lymphocyte glucocorticoid receptors following dexamethasone administration in combat veterans with and without posttraumatic stress disorder. Arch. Gen. Psychiatry **52:** 583–593.
32. PRIBOR, E.F., S.H. YUTZY, J.T. DEAN & R.D. WETZEL. 1993. Briquet's syndrome, dissociation, and abuse. Am. J. Psychiatry **150:** 1507–1511.
33. NEUMANN, S., T.P. DOUBELL, T. LESLIE & C.J. WOOLF. 1996. Inflammatory pain hypersensitivity mediated by phenotypic switch in myelinated primary sensory neurons. Nature **384:** 360–364.
34. RAJA, S., J.N. MEYER & R.A. MEYER. 1988. Peripheral mechanisms of somatic pain. Anaesthesiology **68:** 571–590.
35. NAKAMURA-CRAIG, M. & T.W. SMITH. 1989. Substance P and peripheral inflammatory hyperalgesia. Pain **38:** 91–98.

36. LEDEN, I., A. ERIKSSON, B. LILJA *et al.* 1983. Autonomic nerve function in rheumatoid arthritis of varying severity. Scand. J. Rheumatol. **12:** 166–170.
37. LEVINE, J.D., Y.O. TAIWO, S.D. COLLINS & J.K. TAM. 1986. Noradrenaline hyperalgesia is mediated through interaction with sympathetic postganglionic neurone terminals rather than activation of primary afferent nociceptors. Nature (Lond.) **323:** 158–160.
38. VÆRØY, H., R. HELLE, Ø. FØRRE *et al.* 1988. Cerebrospinal fluid levels of beta-endorphin in patients with fibromyalgia (fibrositis syndrome). J. Rheumatol. **15:** 1804–1806.
39. WOLF, C.J. & W.N. THOMPSON. 1991. The induction and maintenance of central sensitization is dependent on N-methyl-D-aspartic acid receptor activation; implications for the treatment of post-injury pain hypersensitivity states. Pain **44:** 293–299.
40. DUBNER, R. & M.A. RUDA. 1992. Activity dependent neuronal plasticity following tissue injury and inflammation. Trends Neurosci. **15:** 96–103.
41. LIU, X. & J. SANDKUHLER. 1997. Characterization of long-term potentiation of C-fiber-evoked potentials in spinal dorsal horn of adult rat: essential role of NK1 and NK2 receptors. J. Neurophysiol. **78:** 1973–1982.
42. SVENDSEN, F., A. TJOLSEN, F. RYKKJA & K. HOLE. 1999. Behavioural effects of LTP-inducing sciatic nerve stimulation in the rat. Eur. J. Pain **3:** 355–363.
43. RYGH, L.J., F. SVENDSEN, K. HOLE & A. TJOLSEN. 1999. Natural noxious stimulation can induce long-term increase of spinal nociceptive responses. Pain **82:** 305–310.
44. MACARTHUR, L., K. REN, E. PFAFFENROTH *et al.* 1999. Descending modulation of opioid–containing nociceptive neurons in rats with peripheral inflammation and hyperalgesia. Neuroscience **88:** 499–506.
45. ALMEIDA, A., R. STORKSON, D. LIMA *et al.* 1999. The medullary dorsal reticular nucleus facilitates pain behaviour induced by formalin in the rat. Eur. J. Neurosci. **11:** 110–122.
46. URSIN, H., I.M. ENDRESEN, E. HÅLAND & N. MJELLEM. 1993. Sensitization: a neurobiological theory for muscle pain. *In* Progress in Fibromyalgia and Myofascial Pain, pp. 411–425. Elsevier. Amsterdam/New York.
47. MORUZZI, G. & H.W. MAGOUN. 1949. Brain stem reticular formation and activation of the EEG. Electroencephalogr. Clin. Neurophysiol. **1:** 455–473.
48. VANDERWOLF, C.H. & T.E. ROBINSON. 1981. Reticulo-cortical activity and behavior: a critique of the arousal theory and a new synthesis. Behav. Brain Sci. **4:** 459–514.
49. LEVINE, S. & H. URSIN. 1991. What is stress? *In* Stress: Neurobiology and Neuroendocrinology, pp. 3–21. Dekker. New York.
50. URSIN, H. & H.R. ERIKSEN. 2000. The cognitive arousal theory of stress. Behav. Brain Sci. Submitted (http://www.uib.no/ibmp/back/msCATS.html).
51. OLFF, M. 1999. Stress, depression, and immunity: the role of defense and coping styles. Psychiatry Res. **85:** 7–15.
52. ERIKSEN, H.R. & H. URSIN. 1999. Subjective health complaints: is coping more important than control? Work Stress **13:** 238–252.
53. OVERMIER, J.B. & M.E.P. SELIGMAN 1967. Effect of inescapable shock upon subsequent escape and avoidance responding. J. Comp. Physiol. Psychol. **63:** 28–33.
54. OVERMIER, J.B. 1988. Psychological determinants of when stressors stress. *In* Neurobiological Approaches to Human Disease—Neuronal Control of Bodily Function: Basic and Clinical Aspects. Vol. 2, pp. 236–259. Huber. Toronto.
55. ERIKSEN, H.R., M. OLFF & H. URSIN. 1997. The CODE: a revised battery for coping and defence and its relations to subjective health. Scand. J. Psychol. **38:** 175–182.
56. MCEWEN, B.S. 1998. Stress, adaptation, and disease: allostasis and allostatic load. Ann. N.Y. Acad. Sci. **840:** 33–44.
57. URSIN, H. 1980. Personality, activation, and somatic health: a new psychosomatic theory. *In* Coping and Health, pp. 259–279. Plenum. New York.
58. URSIN, H. & R. MURISON, Eds. 1983. Biological and Psychological Basis of Psychosomatic Disease. Pergamon. Oxford.
59. CLAUW, D.J. & G.P. CHROUSOS. 1997. Chronic pain and fatigue syndromes: overlapping clinical and neuroendocrine features and potential pathogenic mechanisms. Neuroimmunomodulation **4:** 134–153.

60. GRIEP, E.N., J.W. BOERSMA, E.G. LENTJES *et al.* 1998. Function of the hypothalamic-pituitary-adrenal axis in patients with fibromyalgia and low back pain. J. Rheumatol. **25:** 1374–1381.
61. DEMITRACK, M.A. & L.J. CROFFORD. 1998. Evidence for and pathophysiological implications of hypothalamic-pituitary-adrenal axis dysregulation in fibromyalgia and chronic fatigue syndrome. Ann. N.Y. Acad. Sci. **840:** 684–697.
62. COOVER, G., H. URSIN & R. MURISON. 1983. Sustained activation and psychiatric illness. *In* Biological and Psychological Basis of Psychosomatic Disease, pp. 249–258. Pergamon. Oxford.
63. SLUITER, J.K., A.J. VAN DER BEEK & M.H.W. FRINGS-DRESEN. 1999. The influence of work characteristics on the need for recovery and experienced health: a study on coach drivers. Ergonomics **42:** 573–583.
64. SLUITER, J.K., A.J. VAN DER BEEK & M.H.W. FRINGS-DRESEN. 1998. Work stress and recovery measured by urinary catecholamines and cortisol excretion in long distance coach drivers. Occup. Environ. Med. **55:** 407–413.
65. MEIJMAN, T.F., G. MULDER, M. VAN DORMOLEN & R. CREMER. 1992. Workload of driving examiners: a psychophysiological field study. *In* Enhancing Industrial Performance, pp. 245–258. Taylor & Francis. London.
66. MIKKELSEN, A., P.Ø. SAKSVIK, H.R. ERIKSEN & H. URSIN. 1999. The impact of learning opportunities and decision authority on occupational health. Work Stress **13:** 20–31.
67. HALDORSEN, E.M.H., K. KRONHOLM, J.S. SKOUEN & H. URSIN. 1998. Predictors for outcome of a multimodal cognitive behavioural treatment program for low back patients—a 12-month follow-up study. Eur. J. Pain **4:** 293–307.
68. INDAHL, A., L. VELUND & O. REIKERÅS. 1995. Good prognosis for low back pain when left untampered: a randomized clinical trial. Spine **20:** 473–477.
69. MOSS-MORRIS, R., K.J. PETIRE & J. WEINMAN. 1996. Functioning in chronic fatigue syndrome: do illness perceptions play a regulatory role? Br. J. Health Psychol. **1:** 15–25.
70. WILHELMSEN, I., T.T. HAUG, H. URSIN & A. BERSTAD. 1994. Effect of short-term cognitive psychotherapy on recurrence of duodenal ulcer: a prospective randomized trial. Psychosom. Med. **56:** 440–448.

Representation of Acute and Persistent Pain in the Human CNS: Potential Implications for Chemical Intolerance

PIERRE RAINVILLE,[a,b] M. CATHERINE BUSHNELL,[c] AND GARY H. DUNCAN[d]

[b]*Département de Stomatologie, Faculté de Médecine Dentaire, Université de Montréal, Montréal, Québec H3C 3J7, Canada, and Department of Neurology, University of Iowa Hospitals and Clinic, Iowa City, Iowa 52242, USA*

[c]*Department of Anesthesiology, McGill University, Montréal, Québec H3A 1A1, Canada*

[d]*Faculté de Médecine Dentaire, Université de Montréal, Montréal, Québec H3C 3J7, Canada*

ABSTRACT: The study of pain may be relevant to the study of chemical intolerance (CI) in many ways. Pain is often reported as a symptom of CI and it is defined as a subjective experience similar to many other symptoms of CI, making its objectification difficult. Furthermore, the CNS plastic changes that underlie the development of persistent pain states and abnormal pain responses may share some similarities with those involved in the sensitization to environmental chemicals. Functional brain imaging studies in humans demonstrate that acute pain evoked by nociceptive stimulation is accompanied by the activation of a widely distributed network of cerebral structures, including the thalamus and the somatosensory, insular, and anterior cingulate cortices. Abnormal activity within these regions has been associated with the experience of pain following damage to the peripheral or central nervous system (neuropathic pain) in a number of clinical populations. In normal individuals, activity within this network is correlated with subjective pain perception, is highly modifiable by cognitive interventions such as hypnosis and attention, and has been associated with emotions. Other cognitive mediators such as expectations can also produce robust changes in pain perception (e.g., in placebo analgesia). These effects likely depend on both higher-order cerebral structures and descending mechanisms modulating spinal nociceptive activity. These psychological processes can be solicited to reduce clinical pain and we speculate that they may further attenuate or promote central mechanisms involved in the transition from acute to persistent pain states. The investigation of central determinants of subjective experience is essential to assess the possibility that higher-order brain/psychological processes modulate and/or mediate the development of persistent pain states. These factors may contribute to the development of symptoms in CI.

[a]*Address for correspondence:* Département de Stomatologie, Faculté de Médecine Dentaire, Université de Montréal, CP 6128, Succursale Centre-ville, Montréal, Québec H3C 3J7, Canada. Voice: 514-343-6111, ext. 3935; fax: 514-343-5647.

pierre.rainville@umontreal.ca

INTRODUCTION

The symptoms grouped under the terms chemical intolerance (CI), multiple chemical sensitivity (MCS), and toxicity-induced loss of tolerance (TILT) have been suggested to reflect a pathological response to the exposure to environmental chemical substances.[1-3] The study of pain within this context may be relevant in many ways. First, pain is one of the multiple symptoms often reported in CI/MCS/TILT. Second, the similarities with other syndromes in which pain is a dominant feature such as fibromyalgia raise the possibility of common mechanisms. Third, CI/MCS/TILT has been hypothesized to develop in two stages, with (1) an "initiating exposure" presumed to trigger plastic changes in the CNS followed by (2) an "elicitation phase" characterized by an enhanced reaction to exposure levels below the normal threshold for the manifestation of a toxic response.[3] This temporal dynamic has been hypothesized to reflect central plastic changes potentially similar to those involved in the transition from an acute pain episode to the development of a persistent pathological pain state and abnormal increases in pain sensitivity. Fourth, diagnosis of CI/MCS/TILT relies on identification of many symptoms, which can only be gained through *subjective experiences* reported by the patient (e.g., fatigue, changes in mood). In this perspective, pain provides a model for studying central determinants of subjective experience and thereby may provide insight into the study of similar phenomena.

This article briefly reviews evidence indicating that the subjective experience of pain is accompanied by a characteristic pattern of cerebral activity in humans. Examples are described suggesting that pathological pain states and responses may arise from abnormal activity within this same network of cerebral structures. Experimental studies demonstrate that psychological factors (i.e., higher-order brain processes) can influence the experience of pain and modify brain activity within the identified network. As these psychological factors can readily influence clinical pain, it is suggested that they may modulate the CNS plastic changes involved in the transition from acute to persistent pathological pain states. This attempt to draw a parallel between CI/MCS/TILT and pathological pain states is admittedly speculative and should be understood within the context of an exploration of possible similar or overlapping mechanisms.

THE PRIVATE EXPERIENCE OF PAIN

Pain has been defined as an unpleasant sensory or emotional experience, which we primarily associate with tissue damage or describe in terms of tissue damage, or both.[4] This definition adopted by the International Association for the Study of Pain recognizes that pain is a subjective state—a private, "first-person", experience. This implies that the subjective report of pain *cannot* be validated or invalidated with certainty by an external observer. In contrast, nociception refers to the multiple "objective" physiological and behavioral responses produced when an organism is exposed to stimuli that are actually or potentially damaging to tissues (nociceptive stimuli). The notions of toxicity and chemical sensitivity have some similarities with the concepts of nociception and pain, respectively. Toxins or poisons are substances that, when ingested, inhaled, or absorbed, or applied to, injected into, or developed within the body, may damage structures or disturb functions. In contrast, the sensitivity to chemicals in the context of CI/MCS/TILT refers, at least in part, to unpleasant subjective experiences or feelings of illness attributed to the exposure to environmental chemicals.

In spite of the difficulties in assessing the subjective experience of pain, psychophysical and neurophysiological methods show that, when pain is experienced in response to clearly delineated and well-controlled nociceptive stimuli, there is a reliable correspondence between the physical properties of the stimuli, the peripheral and CNS physiological activity, and the subjective reports of pain.[5] Similarly, subjective feelings of illness normally characterize the exposure to toxic doses of chemicals. However, there are situations in which no pain is felt in the presence of extensive tissue damage and, conversely, pain may be experienced without an obvious indication of peripheral tissue damage (*nonnociceptive* pain). This latter condition can be observed in patients with a variety of nervous system dysfunctions, including neuralgias produced by herpes zoster, diabetes, or HIV; spinal cord injury; multiple sclerosis; or stroke. Nonnociceptive pain is often the result of abnormal activity within the neural systems involved in the transmission of nociceptive signals or in endogenous neural pain-modulatory circuits, and in brain areas underlying the subjective experience of pain itself. Likewise, the multiple symptoms of CI/MCS/TILT are reported at low (subtoxic) levels of environmental chemicals (chemical sensitivity without toxicity), they are not clearly associated with the stimulus (equivocal dose-response function), and they lack chemical specificity.[2,3] Pain arising from CNS abnormalities may be *attributed to* or *described in terms of* tissue damage. For example, a patient who experiences a deep aching pain in his/her leg as the result of a stroke involving the thalamus (thalamic pain syndrome) may believe that the pain was caused by a torn muscle. Similarly, symptoms of chemical sensitivity may be *attributed to* the exposure to chemical substances, a process often associated with the experience of odors or with a specific environment (e.g., in sick-building syndrome). However, the example of the thalamic pain syndrome illustrates that there is no guarantee that this attribution is indeed valid. Thus, it is necessary to distinguish between subjective experience, which cannot be invalidated with certitude, and the attribution of the experience to a specific cause. In view of those similarities, it appears reasonable to hypothesize that, like pain due to abnormal activity in the CNS, CI/MCS/TILT may reflect abnormal function in the central systems underlying the normal response to toxic substances. If those mechanisms contribute significantly to the condition, the constellation of symptoms reported may reflect the effect of the abnormal CNS activity on various organs, including the brain itself. Furthermore, the brain structures involved may be precisely those that are critically involved in the generation of the unpleasant subjective experiences themselves that normally characterize a toxic exposure. New methods in cognitive neuroscience may aid in investigating these possibilities by facilitating the examination of cerebral correlates of subjective experience.

THE REPRESENTATION OF PAIN IN THE BRAIN

Modern brain imaging techniques such as positron emission tomography (PET), single photon emission computed tomography, functional magnetic resonance imaging (fMRI), high-density EEG, and magnetoencephalography provide important tools to investigate the cerebral correlates of the subjective experience of pain in humans. Recent investigations of the cerebral responses to experimental nociceptive stimuli using those methods have led to the identification of a subset of cortical and subcortical structures activated when pain is experienced.[6,7] These structures include the thalamus as well as primary (S1) and secondary (S2) somatosensory cortices, the insular cortex (IC), and the anterior cingulate cortex (ACC). Sites activated are most often contralateral to the stimulation, but bilateral activation has been consistently observed in mainly S2 and the IC, and sometimes in the ACC and thalamus. The level of activation within those areas is correlated with the subjects' ratings of pain.[8] Anatomical and electrophysiological studies confirm that each of the cortical areas activated in imaging studies receives nociceptive input from the dorsal horn of the spinal cord through spino-thalamo-cortical pathways.[6] Activation within this network of structures has been reported in response to experimental heat and cold pain,[9–11] electric shocks to the skin and muscle,[12] cutaneous injections of capsaicin[13] or ethanol,[14] and painful mechanical stimulation of the viscera.[15] Other subcortical sites reported less consistently in those studies include the basal ganglia, the hypothalamus, the brain stem, and the cerebellum. Additional cortical activation has been reported in the supplementary motor and premotor areas and in prefrontal and lateral posterior parietal cortices. Decreases in activity have been noted sporadically in the occipital, medial parietal, and temporal lobes. The consistent pattern of activation identified in response to various noxious experimental stimuli and the positive relationship observed with pain ratings suggest that this network is critically involved in pain perception. These experimental studies provide the necessary basic observations to start the investigation of pain-related brain activity in clinical populations.

ABNORMAL BRAIN ACTIVITY IN PATHOLOGICAL PAIN STATES

Studies investigating brain activity in pathological pain states following lesions of the peripheral or central nervous system have implicated the areas activated in response to experimental pain stimuli in normal subjects. Peripheral nerve compression, nerve section, or limb amputation often leads to nonnociceptive spontaneous pain in the denervated area (neuropathic pain). PET studies performed in patients experiencing neuropathic pain have reported abnormally *low* levels of rCBF in the thalamus contralateral to the spontaneous pain.[16] The electrical stimulation of the somatosensory thalamus contralateral to the neuropathic side can provide some relief from neuropathic pain[17] and has been shown, using PET, to produce increases in rCBF in the thalamus, as well as over S1 and the IC.[18] This pattern of rCBF changes in response to thalamic stimulation suggests that activation of the somatosensory thalamus and of cortical areas involved in tactile (S1)[19,20] and thermal perception (IC)[21] may contribute to pain relief. Changes in the organization of somatotopic maps in S1 have also been shown to correlate with the experience of phantom pain in amputees[22,23] and with chronic back pain.[24] Further, changes in opioid-receptor binding have been reported in patients with trigeminal neuralgia in the thalamus, the IC, and the ACC, in addition to the basal ganglia and prefrontal and parietal cortices.[25] These effects suggest that chronic pain may be associated with abnormal activity and functional reorganization within thalamocortical pathways projecting to S1, the IC, and the ACC.

Central nervous system lesions may also lead to the development of persistent nonnociceptive pain (central pain). A recent theoretical model proposes that the development of central pain in some cases may be a consequence of reduced inhibition normally exerted by the lateral pathways on medial pathways.[26] This condition may result from the loss of afferent activity in spinothalamic pathways projecting to areas of the lateral and posterior thalamus involved in tactile (VPL/VPM) and thermal sensation (VMpo). This reduced inhibition is suggested to result in abnormal activity within the medial thalamus. Consistent with this possibility, abnormal thalamo-cortical activity has been associated with positive symptoms in various neurological and psychiatric diseases including persistent pain states.[27] Furthermore, a surgical lesion in the medial thalamus at sites showing abnormal bursting activity has been shown to provide some relief of those symptoms.[28] This aberrant activity associated with pain would likely result in abnormal activity in cortical areas that receive medial thalamic afferents such as the ACC.[29] Surgical lesions of the ACC have been shown to produce some impairment in the perception of experimental pain[30] and have been performed, albeit with equivocal results, to produce pain relief.[31,32]

An increase in pain sensitivity is observed during inflammation and may also be experienced by patients with peripheral nerve damage or a CNS lesion. Allodynia, the pain felt in response to stimuli that do not normally provoke pain, has been shown to involve central plastic changes in spinal nociceptive processes.[33] Activation of S2, the IC, and the ACC has been observed during mechanical allodynia in a patient with neuropathic pain resulting from peripheral nerve injury, while the same innocuous stimulus applied to a normal area of the skin produced a nonpainful sensation and activated only S1 and S2.[34] In patients with allodynia resulting from CNS damage, imaging studies suggest that multiple mechanisms may be involved. Whereas ACC activation was observed in response to tactile allodynia in a patient with a large cortical lesion,[35] ACC activation was not seen during allodynia in a patient with central pain due to lateral medullary lesions.[36] Although additional studies are required to demonstrate the reliability and specificity of those effects, such findings suggest that a number of pathological conditions may be associated with dysfunction in various cerebral areas involved in the processing of noxious stimulation and in pain perception.

The investigation of brain activity in pain patients is in its infancy. Although there is no simple equation between the measures used in PET or fMRI and the level of neuronal activity, these preliminary findings are consistent with the notion that persistent pathological pain states involve functional abnormalities in the thalamus and the cortical areas activated by noxious experimental stimuli in normal subjects. The mechanisms leading to the abnormal activity in those areas remain largely to be elucidated. The observed functional changes may be the consequence of local plastic changes as well as alterations of nociceptive activity at lower levels of the neuraxis.[33,37]

THE COGNITIVE MODULATION OF PAIN

The notion that pain, like many other symptoms of CI/MCS/TILT, is a subjective phenomenon raises important questions about the contribution of psychological factors to its generation and modulation. Hypnosis, attention, and placebos have all been shown to modulate pain. These interventions may act through a variety of neurophysiological processes.

In the laboratory, hypnotic analgesia has been found to modulate pain-evoked autonomic activity[38,39] and pain-evoked cerebral potentials recorded over the scalp[40] and in the ACC.[41] In a series of experimental studies using PET and tonic heat pain in normal subjects, hypnosis was also found to modulate activity in multiple brain areas. In separate experiments, suggestions were given to modulate either the affective dimension of pain or its subjective sensory intensity.[42] In the first experiment, pain-evoked activity in the ACC was modulated in correlation with reports of pain unpleasantness.[43] In contrast, the primary modulation of pain intensity produced rCBF changes mainly in S1.[44] Hypnotic suggestions also produced widespread bilateral frontal increases in rCBF that may reflect the direct or indirect influences exerted by frontal cortices on pain-related activity.[45]

Although the cortical sites of pain-related activity are hypothesized to constitute the substrate for the hypnotic modulation of the pain experience, they are only a subset of numerous potential sites for modulation. For example, hypnotic suggestions of analgesia have been shown to modulate the amplitude of the R-III reflex (a spinal nociceptive reflex).[46,47] A recent psychophysical study further indicates that hypnotic analgesia can be produced in specific body areas, suggesting that endogenous pain-modulatory mechanisms may act in a somatotopic fashion on nociceptive pathways, rather than as a generalized effect.[48] These effects imply that the physiological mechanisms underlying the hypnotic modulation of pain (1) can affect specific components of the neural network underlying the different dimensions of the experience, (2) involve both cortical processes and descending mechanisms that modulate spinal cord nociceptive activity, and (3) are somatotopically organized.

The direction of attention toward or away from pain (distraction) constitutes another powerful means to modulate pain perception. When painful heat stimuli are presented, subjects report less pain if they are concurrently performing a cognitive task[49,50] or a sensory-discrimination task in the visual[51] or auditory modality.[52] These decreases in pain are accompanied by reduction of pain-related activity in S1[44,52] and in the region of S2[50] and could be functionally dependent upon attention-related activity in the ACC.[49]

Other cognitive factors have also been shown to influence pain processes. For example, the administration of a placebo can produce a reliable decrease in pain perception when patients expect relief.[5] Although no functional brain imaging study has investigated the brain correlates of placebo analgesia yet, available psychophysical and pharmacological data suggest that central mechanisms involved in pain perception are involved in this phenomenon. In an experimental study, Amanzio and Benedetti showed that the tolerance to ischemic pain to the arm is significantly increased when subjects receive saline injections and are told that an analgesic substance is administered.[53] This placebo effect is blocked by the opioid antagonist naloxone, indicating a mediation by endorphins, as previously demonstrated.[5] This study further shows an increase in placebo analgesia when subjects are preexposed to morphine analgesia in previous days within the same experimental context, suggesting that conditioning mechanisms may contribute to the effect. The contributions of prior exposure and expectations can be further dissociated by telling the subjects that the substance injected has no analgesic effect. In this case, the effect of prior exposure is maintained (conditioning effect), but the expectation-related effect is abolished, with the result that the placebo analgesia is reduced. The residual analgesic effect associated with the prior exposure to morphine is again blocked by the administration of naloxone. Amanzio and Benedetti further demonstrated that the component of placebo analgesia associated with the preexposure (conditioning) is blocked by naloxone only if the conditioning was done with morphine and not if it was done with a nonopioid drug (ketorolac).[53] Furthermore, there is evidence that the placebo effect associated with expectations can be somatotopically specific. In a separate study, subjects were treated with a placebo cream on the left hand before the injection of capsaicin to both hands and feet.[54] In those conditions, placebo analgesia was observed specifically on the left hand where the placebo cream had been applied and this effect was again blocked by naloxone. Importantly, the mechanical allodynia measured 30 minutes after the capsaicin injection was also reduced only at the site of placebo analgesia. Taken together, these studies indicate that (1) both expectations and conditioning by prior exposure may contribute to placebo analgesia, (2) conditioning effects depend on drug-specific mechanisms, while expectation-related analgesia depends on opioid-mediated mechanisms, and (3) placebo effects can be somatotopically specific and can attenuate the development of allodynia. These effects suggest that expectations may engage somatotopically organized opioid-mediated descending modulatory mechanisms that alter spinal nociceptive activity[5] and influence the development of central sensitization and allodynia. The above-mentioned changes in opioid-binding receptors in pain-related thalamocortical sites in trigeminal neuralgia raise the possibility that opioid-mediated placebo effects may depend on a combination of actions at many levels of the CNS.

Although the effects of the psychological interventions described are produced transiently in well-controlled experimental conditions, it is likely that the mechanisms involved are recruited in natural environments. This is consistent with the notion that the CNS is not passively registering peripheral nociceptive activity and that a variety of mechanisms associated with cognitive processes are continuously modulating activity at multiple stages of nociceptive processing. Indirect evidence from clinical studies further indicates that these mechanisms may influence the development of pain in various pathological states.

POTENTIAL IMPLICATIONS FOR PERSISTENT PAIN STATES

Many psychological variables have been identified that may contribute to the development of persistent, nonnociceptive pain. In a review of the literature, Turk identified a series of predictors that received consistent support from multiple studies investigating pain of various origins.[55] These factors can be grouped into three categories: (1) subjective pain severity, (2) emotional state, and (3) cognitive processes. The severity of pain during the initiating episode may be one of the most important factors.[55–57] Pain intensity at the time of acute onset has been found to be a good predictor of chronicity for persistent back pain, postherpetic neuralgia, and postoperative pain. Preemptive pharmacological analgesia in the days preceding and following surgical amputations has been used in an attempt to reduce the incidence of phantom pain, although a rigorous evaluation of this procedure's efficacy has been difficult to achieve.[57] The emotional state of the individual at the time of the acute pain episode may also contribute to the development of persistent pain states. Emotions most consistently implicated are anxiety, depression, and lassitude/malaise/loneliness. Emotions have been associated with activity in brain areas involved in pain and in the regulation of body states, such as various nuclei of the brain stem (e.g., parabrachial nucleus, periaqueductal gray area) and the hypothalamus, S2, IC, and cingulate and orbitofrontal cortices.[58] Many additional factors are grouped under the category cognitive processes. Maladaptive coping, passive cognition, perceived stress/stressful life events, disease conviction, perception of poor health, and perceived severity of illness or disability have all been associated with the development of persistent pain in multiple studies. The respective contribution of the "objective" severity of the trauma or pathology and the subjective perception of severity and pain should be assessed more systematically to evaluate the potential specific and overlapping contribution of these factors. Furthermore, many of the cognitive factors identified reflect the individuals' subjective perception and appraisal of their own condition and are likely to interact with their emotional state, which may, in turn, affect pain.[5] In any case, these studies are consistent with the possibility that pain, emotions, and cognitive factors reflect central mechanisms that may mediate or at least modulate the transition from acute to persistent pain. The specificity of these effects and their underlying physiological mechanisms remain to be clarified.

The experimental studies performed in normal subjects on pain modulation led to the conclusion that various psychological factors can influence acute experimental pain and the corresponding pain-related CNS activity at both the spinal and cerebral levels. The beneficial effects of those interventions have been reported on both perioperative[59,60] and persistent pain.[61] A recent PET study further confirms that hypnotic interventions can produce changes in cortical activity in pain-related areas in amputees.[62] In this study, hypnotic suggestions were given to produce comfortable nonpainful or painful phantom experiences. Phantom pain was accompanied by stronger activation within the thalamus, the ACC, and the orbitofrontal cortex. Most interestingly, in this study, subjective ratings of pain were also correlated to the activity within the ACC, a result similar to the experiment on hypnotic modulation of pain unpleasantness in normal subjects.[43] Similar effects have been observed in the cingulate cortex during hypnotic analgesia in fibromyalgia patients.[63] This convergence of results provides a critical link between experimental and clinical studies and indicates that similar mechanisms may be recruited in both conditions. Given that the modulation of clinical pain may be mediated at least in part by those mechanisms, psychological interventions may help prevent the development of persistent pain states by reducing pain in the acute phase. Further advances in our understanding of the neurophysiological mechanisms involved in both the central plastic changes associated with pain and the psychological modulation of pain may help in designing psychological interventions to better prevent the initiation, or attenuate the progression, of persistent pain states. These developments are also necessary for evaluating potential mechanisms underlying the putative *psychogenic* pain states, which have been hypothesized to involve abnormal ACC and prefrontal activity.[64] Within the present context, these states may reflect a determinant influence of higher-order brain mechanisms in the initiation of central plastic changes within pain-related structures, leading to nonnociceptive persistent pain.

CONCLUSIONS

The parallel tentatively drawn between CNS mechanisms of persistent pain and CI/MCS/TILT is admittedly speculative. Abnormal activity within specific CNS structures that are involved in the normal representation of pain can lead to persistent pathological pain states. The first simple implication of this observation is that the experience of symptoms characterizing CI/MCS/TILT may reflect abnormal activity within CNS structures involved in the normal toxic response, some of which may be involved in pain and emotion as well. One of the main limitations of functional brain imaging studies is that the observation of abnormal activity in pain-related areas may only passively reflect changes taking place at lower levels of the neuraxis. However, brain processes are likely to contribute to the development of pathological pain states and they are undoubtedly more proximal to the mechanisms underlying the subjective experience of pain. Studies on the psychological modulation of pain demonstrate the multiplicity, versatility, and potential efficacy of psychological processes influencing acute and persistent pain. Although in many cases these mechanisms may only have modulating effects, the value of psychological variables in predicting the transition from acute to persistent pain states indicates that they should not be neglected. These psychological factors, conceived as higher-order brain mechanisms, may also *mediate* the development of certain forms of persistent pain states, and similar mechanisms may be at play in certain forms of CI/MCS/TILT. However, this possibility is usually considered only as a last resort and with prudence, when all alternatives have been excluded. This state of affairs reflects how little we know about CNS mechanisms that underlie psychological functions and subjective experience. Ultimately, these questions may only be resolved when we achieve an adequate understanding of the neurophysiological determinants of consciousness.

ACKNOWLEDGMENTS

This article was written with the financial support of The Human Frontier Science Program to Pierre Rainville.

REFERENCES

1. MILLER, C.S. 1997. Toxicant-induced loss of tolerance—an emerging theory of disease? Environ. Health Perspect. **105:** 445–453.
2. BELL, I.R. *et al.* 1999. Neural sensitization model for multiple chemical sensitivity: overview of theory and empirical evidence. Toxicol. Ind. Health **15:** 295–304.
3. SORG, B. 1999. Multiple chemical sensitivity: potential role for neural sensitization. Crit. Rev. Neurobiol. **13:** 283–316.
4. MERSKEY, H. & F.G. SPEAR. 1967. The concept of pain. J. Psychosom. Res. **11:** 59–67.
5. PRICE, D.D. 1999. Psychological Mechanisms of Pain and Analgesia. IASP Press. Seattle.
6. TREEDE, R.D. *et al.* 1999. The cortical representation of pain. Pain **79:** 105–111.
7. RAINVILLE, P., G.H. DUNCAN & M.C. BUSHNELL. 2000. Représentation cérébrale de l'expérience subjective de la douleur chez l'homme. Méd./Sci. **16:** 519–527.
8. COGHILL, R.C. *et al.* 1999. Pain intensity processing within the human brain: a bilateral, distributed mechanism. J. Neurophysiol. **82:** 1934–1943.

9. TALBOT, J.D. et al. 1991. Multiple representations of pain in human cerebral cortex. Science **251:** 1355–1358.
10. JONES, A.K.P. et al. 1991. Cortical and subcortical localization of response to pain in man using positron emission tomography. Proc. R. Soc. Lond. Ser. B Biol. Sci. **244:** 39–44.
11. CASEY, K.L. et al. 1994. Positron emission tomography analysis of cerebral structures activated specifically by repetitive noxious heat stimuli. J. Neurophysiol. **71:** 802–807.
12. SVENSSON, P. et al. 1997. Cerebral processing of acute skin and muscle pain in humans. J. Neurophysiol. **78:** 450–460.
13. IADAROLA, M.J. et al. 1998. Neural activation during acute capsaicin-evoked pain and allodynia assessed with PET. Brain **121:** 931–947.
14. HSIEH, J.C. et al. 1995. Traumatic nociceptive pain activates the hypothalamus and the periaqueductal gray: a positron emission tomography study. Pain **64:** 303–314.
15. AZIZ, Q. et al. 1997. Identification of human brain loci processing esophageal sensation using positron emission tomography. Gastroenterology **113:** 50–59.
16. IADAROLA, M.J. et al. 1995. Unilateral decrease in thalamic activity observed with positron emission tomography in patients with chronic neuropathic pain. Pain **63:** 55–64.
17. DUNCAN, G.H., M.C. BUSHNELL & S. MARCHAND. 1991. Deep brain stimulation: a review of basic research and clinical studies. Pain **45:** 49–59.
18. DUNCAN, G.H. et al. 1998. Stimulation of human thalamus for pain relief: possible modulatory circuits revealed by positron emission tomography. J. Neurophysiol. **80:** 3326–3330.
19. FOX, P.T., H. BURTON & M.E. RAICHLE. 1987. Mapping human somatosensory cortex with positron emission tomography. J. Neurosurg. **67:** 34–43.
20. COGHILL, R.C. et al. 1994. Distributed processing of pain and vibration by the human brain. J. Neurosci. **14:** 4095–4108.
21. CRAIG, A.D. et al. 2000. Thermosensory activation of insular cortex. Nat. Neurosci. **3:** 184–190.
22. FLOR, H. et al. 1995. Phantom-limb pain as a perceptual correlate of cortical reorganization following arm amputation. Nature **375:** 482–484.
23. BIRBAUMER, N. et al. 1997. Effects of regional anesthesia on phantom limb pain are mirrored in changes in cortical reorganization. J. Neurosci. **17:** 5503–5508.
24. FLOR, H. et al. 1997. Extensive reorganization of primary somatosensory cortex in chronic back pain patients. Neurosci. Lett. **224:** 5–8.
25. JONES, A.K. et al. 1999. Measurement of changes in opioid receptor binding *in vivo* during trigeminal neuralgic pain using [11C] diprenorphine and positron emission tomography. J. Cereb. Blood Flow Metab. **19:** 803–808.
26. CRAIG, A.D. 1998. A new version of the thalamic disinhibition hypothesis of central pain. Pain Forum **7:** 1–14.
27. LLINAS, R.R. et al. 1999. Thalamocortical dysrhythmia: a neurological and neuropsychiatric syndrome characterized by magnetoencephalography. Proc. Natl. Acad. Sci. U.S.A. **96:** 15222–15227.
28. JEANMONOD, D., M. MAGNIN & A. MOREL. 1996. Low-threshold calcium spike bursts in the human thalamus: common physiopathology for sensory, motor, and limbic positive symptoms. Brain **119:** 363–375.
29. VOGT, B.A., R.W. SIKES & L.J. VOGT. 1993. Anterior cingulate cortex and the medial pain system. *In* Neurobiology of Cingulate Cortex and Limbic Thalamus: A Comprehensive Handbook, pp. 313–344. Birkhäuser. Basel/Boston.
30. DAVIS, K.D. et al. 1994. Altered pain and temperature perception following cingulotomy and capsulotomy in a patient with schizoaffective disorder. Pain **59:** 189–199.
31. FOLTZ, E.L. & L.E. WHITE. 1968. The role of rostral cingulotomy in "pain" relief. Int. J. Neurol. **6:** 653–673.
32. HURT, R.W. & H.T. BALLANTINE. 1974. Stereotaxic anterior cingulate lesions for persistent pain: a report on 68 cases. Clin. Neurosurg. **21:** 334–351.
33. WOOLF, C.J. & M.W. SALTER. 2000. Neuronal plasticity: increasing the gain in pain. Science **288:** 1765–1768.

34. HOFBAUER, R.K. *et al.* 2000. Peripheral and central mechanisms underlying allodynia in a nerve injured patient [abstract]. Soc. Neurosci. Abstr. **26:** no. 160.7.
35. OLAUSSON, H. *et al.* 2000. Central pain in a hemispherectomized patient. In preparation.
36. PEYRON, R. *et al.* 1998. Allodynia after lateral-medullary (Wallenberg) infarct: a PET study. Brain **121:** 345–356.
37. JONES, E.G. 2000. Cortical and subcortical contributions to activity-dependent plasticity in primate somatosensory cortex. Annu. Rev. Neurosci. **23:** 1–37.
38. LENOX, J.R. 1970. Effect of hypnotic analgesia on verbal report and cardiovascular responses to ischemic pain. J. Abnorm. Psychol. **75:** 199–206.
39. HILGARD, E.R. *et al.* 1974. Heart rate changes in pain and hypnosis. Psychophysiology **11:** 692–702.
40. ARENDT-NIELSEN, L., R. ZACHARIAE & P. BJERRING. 1990. Quantitative evaluation of hypnotically suggested hyperaesthesia and analgesia by painful laser stimulation. Pain **42:** 243–251.
41. KROPOTOV, J.D., H.J. CRAWFORD & Y.I. POLYAKOV. 1997. Somatosensory event-related potential changes to painful stimuli during hypnotic analgesia: anterior cingulate cortex and anterior temporal cortex intracranial recordings. Int. J. Psychophysiol. **27:** 1–8.
42. RAINVILLE, P. *et al.* 1999. Dissociation of pain sensory and affective dimensions using hypnotic modulation. Pain **82:** 159–171.
43. RAINVILLE, P. *et al.* 1997. Pain affect encoded in human anterior cingulate, but not somatosensory cortex. Science **277:** 968–971.
44. BUSHNELL, M.C. *et al.* 1999. Pain perception: is there a role for primary somatosensory cortex? Proc. Natl. Acad. Sci. U.S.A. **96:** 7705–7709.
45. RAINVILLE, P. *et al.* 1999. Cerebral mechanisms of hypnotic induction and suggestion. J. Cogn. Neurosci. **11:** 110–125.
46. KIERNAN, B.D. *et al.* 1995. Hypnotic analgesia reduces R-III nociceptive reflex: further evidence concerning the multifactorial nature of hypnotic analgesia. Pain **60:** 39–47.
47. DANZIGER, N. *et al.* 1998. Different strategies of modulation can be operative during hypnotic analgesia: a neurophysiological study. Pain **75:** 85–92.
48. BENHAIEM, J-M. *et al.* 2001. Local and remote effects of hypnotic suggestions of analgesia. Pain. In press.
49. PEYRON, R. *et al.* 1999. Haemodynamic brain responses to acute pain in humans—sensory and attentional networks. Brain **122:** 1765–1779.
50. PETROVIC, P. *et al.* 2000. Pain-related cerebral activation is altered by a distracting cognitive task. Pain **85:** 19–30.
51. MIRON, D., G.H. DUNCAN & M.C. BUSHNELL. 1989. Effects of attention on the intensity and unpleasantness of thermal pain. Pain **39:** 345–352.
52. CARRIER, B. *et al.* 1998. Attentional modulation of pain-related activity in human cerebral cortex. Soc. Neurosci. Abstr. **24:** 1135.
53. AMANZIO, M. & F. BENEDETTI. 1999. Neuropharmacological dissection of placebo analgesia: expectation-activated opioid systems versus conditioning-activated specific subsystems. J. Neurosci. **19:** 484–494.
54. BENEDETTI, F., C. ARDUINO & M. AMANZIO. 1999. Somatotopic activation of opioid systems by target-directed expectations of analgesia. J. Neurosci. **19:** 3639–3648.
55. TURK, D.C. 1997. The role of demographic and psychosocial factors in transition from acute to chronic pain. *In* Proceedings of the Eighth World Congress on Pain, pp. 185–213. IASP Press. Seattle.
56. KALSO, E. 1997. Prevention of chronicity. *In* Proceedings of the Eighth World Congress on Pain, pp. 215–230. IASP Press. Seattle.
57. KATZ, J. 1997. Perioperative predictors of long-term pain following surgery. *In* Proceedings of the Eighth World Congress on Pain, pp. 231–240. IASP Press. Seattle.
58. DAMASIO, A.R. 1999. The Feeling of What Happens: Body and Emotion and the Making of Consciousness. Hartcourt, Brace. New York.
59. LANG, E.V. *et al.* 2000. Adjunctive non-pharmacological analgesia for invasive medical procedures: a randomized trial. Lancet **355:** 1486–1490.
60. BENEDETTI, F. *et al.* 1998. The specific effects of prior opioid exposure on placebo analgesia and placebo respiratory depression. Pain **75:** 313–319.

61. BARBER, J. 1996. Hypnosis and Suggestion in the Treatment of Pain: A Clinical Guide. Norton. New York.
62. WILLOCH, F. *et al.* 2000. Phantom limb pain in the human brain: unravelling neural circuitries of phantom limb pain sensations using positron emission tomography. Ann. Neurol. **48:** 842–849.
63. WIK, G. *et al.* 1999. Functional anatomy of hypnotic analgesia: a PET study of patients with fibromyalgia. Eur. J. Pain **3:** 7–12.
64. DERBYSHIRE, S.W. *et al.* 1994. Cerebral responses to pain in patients with atypical facial pain measured by positron emission tomography. J. Neurol. Neurosurg. Psychiatry **57:** 1166–1172.

Role of Neurotransmitters in Sensitization of Pain Responses

WILLIAM D. WILLIS, JR.[a]

Department of Anatomy and Neurosciences, University of Texas Medical Branch, Galveston, Texas 77555-1069, USA

> ABSTRACT: Injection of capsaicin into the skin results in pain, primary heat and mechanical hyperalgesia, and secondary mechanical allodynia and hyperalgesia. Sensory receptors in the area of secondary mechanical allodynia and hyperalgesia are unaffected, and so the sensory changes must be due to central actions of the initial intense nociceptive discharge that follows the capsaicin injection. Central sensitization of the responses of spinothalamic tract neurons lasts several hours, but can be prevented by spinal cord administration of non-NMDA and NMDA glutamate receptor antagonists or NK1 substance P receptor antagonists. The long-lasting increase in excitability of spinothalamic tract cells depends on the activation of several second messenger cascades (PKC, PKA, and NO/PKG signal transduction pathways). The excitability change also depends on activation of calcium/calmodulin-dependent kinase II, which is consistent with the proposal that this central sensitization response is a form of long-term potentiation.

INTRODUCTION

Chemicals that damage tissues of the body or that are released as a consequence of inflammation can activate and sensitize primary afferent nociceptors, leading to pain and primary hyperalgesia in response to later stimulation of the same receptors.[1] Parallel changes in dorsal horn neuronal activity model these events. For example, the injection of formalin[2] or bee venom[3] into the skin causes a prolonged activation of primary afferent C-nociceptors, resulting in enhanced activity of nociceptive dorsal horn neurons. Because formalin kills receptors in the vicinity of the injection and leaves a scar, the injection site becomes anesthetic. By contrast, stimulation of the skin following a bee venom injection causes greater dorsal horn neuronal activity than the same stimulus before the chemical injection.[3] Presumably, much of this activity can be attributed to the activation of sensitized primary afferent nociceptors, although sensitization of central nociceptive neurons is likely as well.

---

[a]Address for correspondence: William D. Willis, Jr., M.D., Ph.D., Department of Anatomy and Neurosciences, University of Texas Medical Branch, 301 University Boulevard, Galveston, TX 77555-1069. Voice: 409-772-2103; fax: 409-772-4687.
wdwillis@utmb.edu

CAPSAICIN MODEL OF SECONDARY MECHANICAL ALLODYNIA AND HYPERALGESIA

Following cutaneous injury in some pain models, it is possible to stimulate an area of undamaged skin adjacent to the damaged tissue and to evoke pain by either an innocuous stimulus (secondary allodynia) or more pain by a previously painful stimulus (secondary hyperalgesia).[4–7] Primary afferent fibers supplying the area of secondary allodynia and hyperalgesia are not sensitized.[6,8] However, it should be noted that the process of central sensitization is a consequence of input from primary afferent nociceptors that supply an area of damage or of inflammation. It is the input from these nociceptors to the central nervous system that leads to a transient central sensitization.[7]

An example of secondary allodynia and hyperalgesia is the response of human subjects to the intradermal injection of capsaicin.[5–7] If 100 µg of capsaicin (dissolved in 10 µL of vehicle) is injected into the hairy skin of the forearm, there is an immediate and strong sense of burning pain that lasts about 15–20 min. Following this, it is possible to demonstrate an analgesic area of skin at the injection site (presumably due to the desensitization or destruction of primary afferent nociceptors supplying the area), surrounded by a region of primary mechanical and heat hyperalgesia. In addition, an elongated region of secondary mechanical allodynia and hyperalgesia develops over 15–20 min in adjacent skin that was not directly affected by the capsaicin injection. The secondary mechanical allodynia lasts about 1–2 h.

FIGURE 1 shows a diagram of the neural mechanism that was proposed by Hardy, Woolf, and Goodell[4] to account for such sensory changes following application of a strong noxious stimulus to the skin. According to their model, pain is produced by the activation of nociceptors, which in turn evoke discharges in spinothalamic tract (STT) neurons (and presumably other nociceptive ascending tract cells as well). However, the nociceptive input also activates neural circuits in the spinal cord dorsal horn that cause the sensitization of other STT cells that receive input from mechanoreceptors and nociceptors that supply an adjacent region of skin that was unaffected by the capsaicin. The enhanced responses of these STT neurons to innocuous and noxious stimuli applied to normal skin result in secondary allodynia and hyperalgesia.

The following question can then be asked: what causes the central sensitization of STT cells?

PRIMATE MODEL OF CENTRAL SENSITIZATION

Central sensitization involves a complex sequence of chemical events that result in an enhanced responsiveness of nociceptive dorsal horn neurons that transmit signals to the brain, leading to the sensation of pain. To study the chemical mechanisms that underlie central sensitization, we have developed an animal model in which changes in the responses of primate STT neurons are used to model human sensation. Recordings can readily be made from antidromically identified STT neurons of the lumbosacral spinal cord in anesthetized monkeys.[9] If capsaicin is injected into the skin in the central region of the receptive field on the hind limb, the background

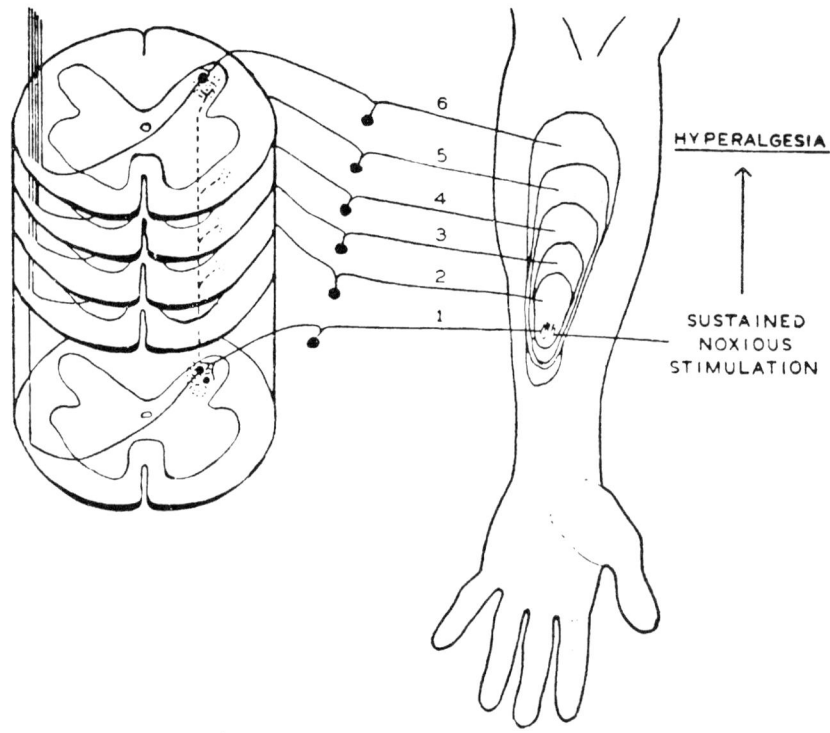

FIGURE 1. Diagram showing the possible central mechanisms underlying the pain, primary hyperalgesia, and secondary allodynia and hyperalgesia that follow application of a strong noxious stimulus to the skin. (From ref. 4, with permission.)

discharges of the STT cells typically increase substantially for about 15–20 min (FIG. 2A and B).[10,11] We believe that this response underlies the pain experienced by human subjects following capsaicin injection, although obviously the monkey can feel no pain because it is anesthetized. Stimulation in the vicinity of the injection site may produce either smaller or larger responses to mechanical stimuli, modeling areas of analgesia and primary hyperalgesia. Stimulation with heat pulses near the injection site reveals a reduced threshold and larger responses than in the control state, modeling primary heat hyperalgesia. Innocuous mechanical stimuli applied in a region of skin a few centimeters distal or proximal to the injection site evoke larger responses than before, modeling secondary mechanical allodynia (FIG. 2C and D), and noxious mechanical stimuli often produce larger responses, as would be expected in secondary mechanical hyperalgesia (FIG. 2E–H). Heat pulses that are applied in the secondary region produce smaller responses than before the injection,[12] consistent with the absence of secondary heat hyperalgesia in human subjects following intradermal injection of capsaicin.[13]

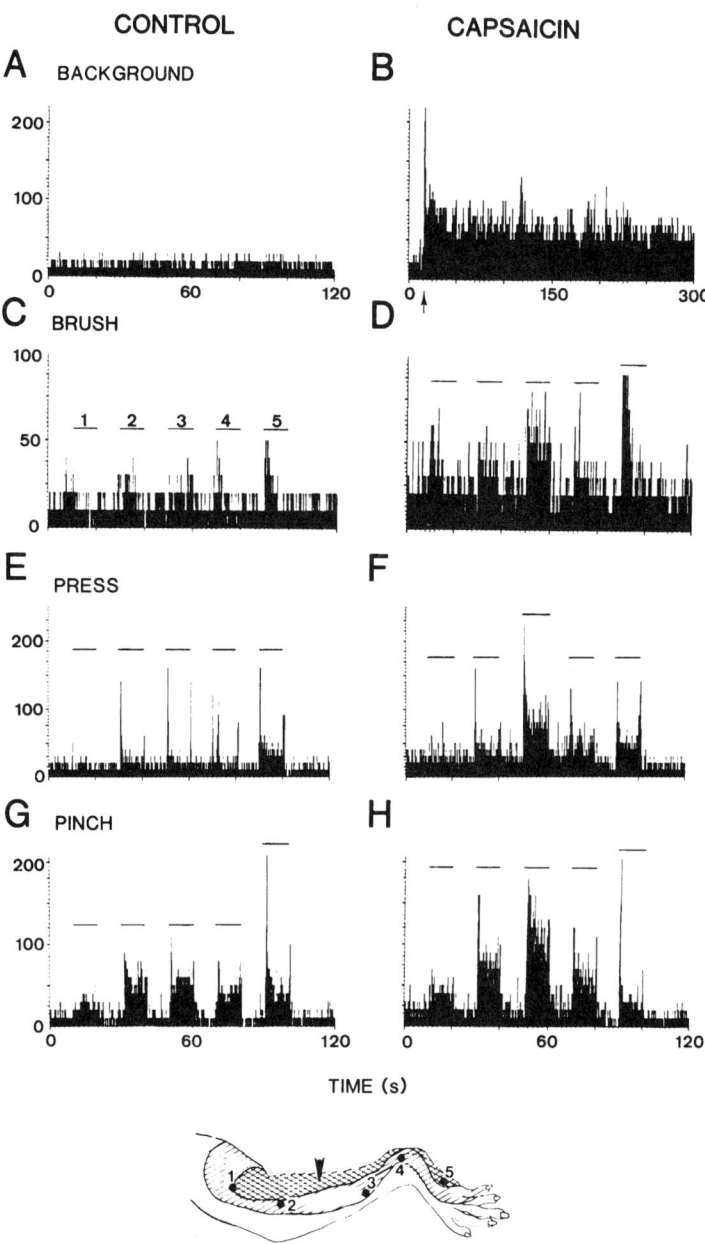

FIGURE 2. Responses of a primate spinothalamic tract (STT) cell to intradermal injection of capsaicin. The drawing at the bottom of the illustration shows the receptive field of the STT cell before (*double-hatched area*) and after (additional *single-hatched area*) capsaicin. The arrowhead indicates the injection site. The numbered dots show the sites that were

ROLE OF NEUROTRANSMITTER RECEPTORS IN DORSAL HORN ON CENTRAL SENSITIZATION

Capsaicin is known to activate nociceptors in the skin that contain VR-1 receptors.[14,15] VR-1 receptors are present on at least two classes of primary afferent nociceptors: those that contain neuropeptides, such as substance P (SP) and/or calcitonin gene-related peptide (CGRP), and those that stain positively for the lectin, IB4.[15] Capsaicin administration in adult animals causes depletion of peptides from the peptidergic nociceptors and also eliminates fluoride-resistant acid phosphatase activity,[14] which is believed to be present in nociceptors that can be labeled for IB4. In neonatal rats, the excitotoxic effects of capsaicin administration can result in the permanent loss of most C-nociceptors.[14] Peptide-containing primary afferent terminals in the dorsal horn contain colocalized glutamate.[16] Activation of these afferent fibers by capsaicin causes the synaptic release of glutamate and peptides.[17,18] Aspartate is also released following capsaicin injection,[17] but this excitatory amino acid may originate from interneurons. STT cells receive synaptic contacts that contain glutamate, SP, and CGRP,[19–21] and release of these substances from synaptic terminals would be expected to activate STT cells. The synaptic endings that contain CGRP must be made by primary afferent fibers because CGRP in the dorsal horn is found only in primary afferents.[22]

We have performed experiments using both microiontophoresis and microdialysis techniques to determine what neurotransmitter receptors and signal transduction pathways are involved in the central sensitization of STT neurons that follows intradermal injection of capsaicin. Iontophoretic release of excitatory or inhibitory amino acids or SP allowed a test of the responsiveness of excitatory and inhibitory amino acid and neurokinin receptors on STT cells. Microdialysis administration of peptides or of neurotransmitter receptor antagonists, as well as activators or inhibitors of signal transduction pathways, was used as an alternative approach when it was appropriate to apply a drug throughout much of the dorsal horn. In either case, drugs were confined to the spinal cord. An important aspect of the experimental design for this work is that the effects of intradermal injection of capsaicin largely wear off within 2 h after the injection. Two successive injections of capsaicin separated by 2 h each produce essentially the same degree and duration of central sensitization, provided that the injections are placed in separate locations within the receptive field (FIG. 3A, left).[23] This allows a drug to be administered before either the first or the second capsaicin injection, so within-neuron statistical comparisons can be employed.

FIGURE 3 shows the effects of several neurotransmitter receptor antagonists that were administered by microdialysis into the dorsal horn on the sensitization of re-

---

stimulated either by an innocuous or a noxious mechanical stimulus before and after capsaicin injection. The column of peristimulus time histograms at the left shows the activity of the STT cell before capsaicin and the column at the right the corresponding activity after capsaicin. (**A**) The initial background activity of the neuron is shown. (**B**) The greatly enhanced activity following capsaicin injection at the time indicated by the *arrow* is shown. In **C–D** the responses to brushing the skin (BRUSH) at sites 1–5 before and after capsaicin are shown. **E–F** show the responses to application of a large arterial clip (PRESS) to the skin, and **G–H** the responses to application of a small arterial clip (PINCH) before and after capsaicin. (From ref. 11, with permission.)

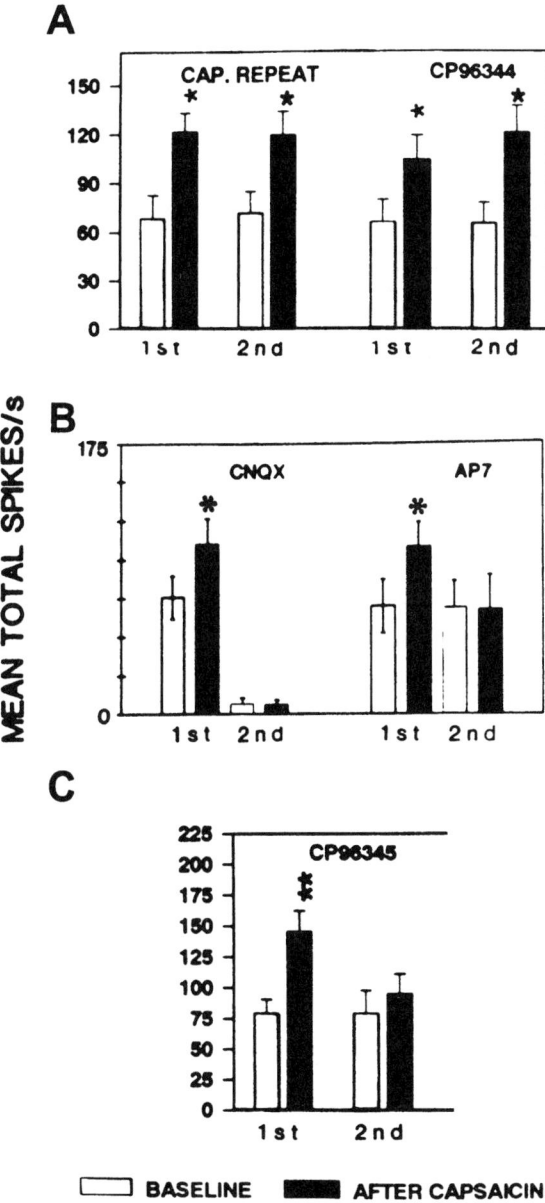

FIGURE 3. Interaction of neurotransmitter receptor antagonists administered by microdialysis into the dorsal horn with the central sensitization of responses of SDTT cells to innocuous mechanical (BRUSH) stimuli before and after intradermal injection of capsaicin. The bar graphs show the mean baseline responses (*open bars*) and the responses following capsaicin (*filled bars*). Two pairs of bars are shown for each experimental condition. The

sponses of STT cells to innocuous (brushing the skin) mechanical stimuli applied to the skin in the secondary area, several centimeters away from the capsaicin injection sites. STT neurons were isolated within about 1 mm of the dialysis fiber so that the drug effects would occur within a reasonable time (15–60 min) following the beginning of dialysis. In FIGURE 3A (left set of bars), no drug was given. The responses to innocuous mechanical stimulation of the skin before the first and the second injections of capsaicin were the same. Both injections of capsaicin caused essentially the same enhancement of the responses. FIGURE 3B (left set of bars) shows that microdialysis administration of the non-NMDA excitatory amino acid receptor antagonist, CNQX, essentially eliminated the responses of the neuron to mechanical stimulation and prevented the sensitization from occurring.[24] On the other hand, administration of the NMDA receptor antagonist, AP7, did not affect the responses to brush and press stimuli (FIGURE 3B, right set of bars), but completely prevented the central sensitization. Thus, the central sensitization of primate STT neurons is dependent on the activation of NMDA receptors. FIGURE 3C shows that microdialysis administration of the NK1 antagonist, CP96, 345,[23] also prevented central sensitization of the STT neuron (whereas the inactive isomer CP96, 344 had no effect; FIG. 3A, right set of bars). We conclude that both NMDA and NK1 receptors are crucially involved in the initiation of central sensitization.

The iontophoresis experiment in FIGURE 4 shows how the dose of AP7 used for the experiment of FIGURE 3B was determined.[24] Graded doses of several glutamate receptor agonists, including NMDA, aspartate, AMP, and glutamate, were used before administration of AP7 to test for the responsiveness of the neuron to these agents. Then, a concentration of AP7 was infused through the microdialysis fiber that was estimated to result in an effective concentration at the level of the cell, based on known concentrations used in *in vitro* experiments, the likely reduction in concentration across the dialysis membrane and the further reduction following diffusion in the tissue. Iontophoretic release of the agonists was again done, using the same graded current doses. The AP7 prevented any response to NMDA and blocked most of the responses to aspartate. However, the responses to AMPA and glutamate were essentially unchanged. It was concluded that an appropriate concentration of AP7 was used in the dialysis fluid (and that aspartate may act chiefly on NMDA re-

---

first pair of bars of each set shows the enhancement of the responses to the BRUSH stimuli that occurred following capsaicin in the absence of a neurotransmitter receptor antagonist. After a wait of 2 h to allow recovery from the first injection of capsaicin, a neurotransmitter receptor antagonist was administered by microdialysis into the dorsal horn near the STT cell under observation. After recording control responses, a second injection of capsaicin was made. In **A**, left set of bars, no antagonist was infused, but rather just artificial cerebrospinal fluid. In **A**, right set of bars, the inactive isomer of an NK1 receptor antagonist, CP96, 344, was infused. In each of these experiments, the responses were elevated to essentially the same extent following each of the two capsaicin injections.[23] In **B**, left set of bars, the administration of the non-NMDA receptor antagonist, CNQX, nearly completely blocked the BRUSH responses, and there was no increase following capsaicin.[24] In **B**, right set of bars, administration of the NMDA receptor antagonist, AP7, did not alter the BRUSH response but prevented its enhancement following capsaicin.[24] In **C**, a similar action was produced by administration of the NK1 receptor antagonist, CP96, 345. (Panels A and C, from ref. 23, with permission; panel B, from ref. 24, with permission.)

WILLIS: NEURAL PLASTICITY & CHEMICAL INTOLERANCE 149

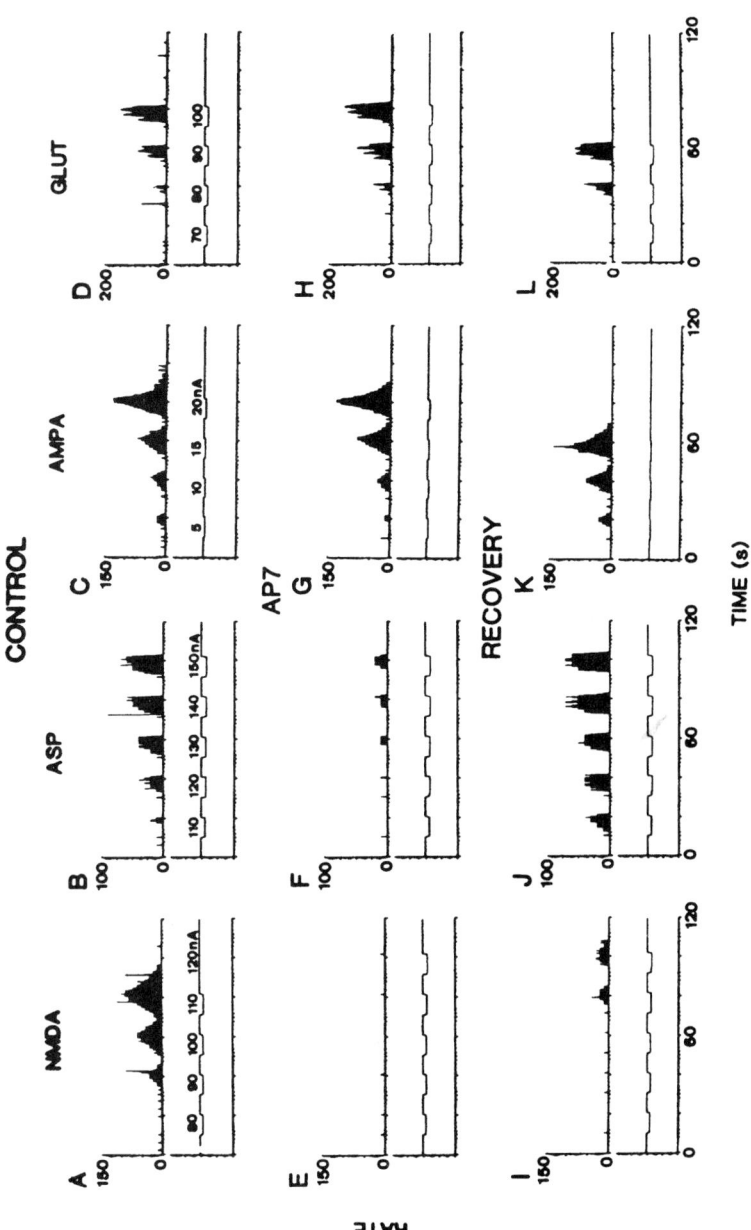

FIGURE 4. *See following page for caption.*

ceptors and glutamate on non-NMDA receptors in STT cells). SP could not be tested in this manner, because we often saw little evidence of a change in firing rate when SP was released iontophoretically near STT cells. Instead, we chose a dose that was estimated to be in the range that is used in *in vitro* experiments, based on the expected reduction in concentration that was produced by the microdialysis membrane and diffusion.

We have also been able to show that a cooperative action of NMDA and SP can sensitize individual STT neurons.[25] For example, in FIGURE 5G, graded doses of NMDA alone were applied repeatedly and it was found that the responses showed a gradual tachyphylaxis. Iontophoretic release of SP (at the dose chosen) by itself had only a slight excitatory effect on the discharges of STT neurons (not illustrated). However, corelease of NMDA and SP sensitized the STT neuron illustrated to later applications of NMDA (FIG. 5B and C–F). The responses continue to increase over a period of 20 min and they remained increased for hours.

Recently, we have also shown that groups I, II, and III metabotropic glutamate receptors can modulate central sensitization of primate STT cells.[26,27]

We have not as yet tested antagonists of the receptors for other peptides, such as CGRP. We suspect that CGRP, and perhaps fast neurotransmitters other than excitatory amino acids, may also be involved in central sensitization.

ROLE OF SIGNAL TRANSDUCTION PATHWAYS IN CENTRAL SENSITIZATION

The long duration of central sensitization argues strongly against the notion that it results simply from interactions between excitatory neurotransmitters and their receptors since such interactions last milliseconds to minutes. Thus, it is a reasonable hypothesis that the time course of central sensitization, which lasts hours, reflects the activation of one or more signal transduction pathways (perhaps coupled with inactivation of protein phosphatase activity).

To determine the possible role of signal transduction pathways in central sensitization, we administered into the dorsal horn activators or inhibitors of a number of signal transduction pathways by microdialysis and have shown that the protein kinase C, NO/protein kinase G, and protein kinase A pathways all contribute to central sensitization of STT cells.[28–31] The evidence is consistent with the coactivation of all of these signal transduction pathways, although there appear to be some dif-

---

FIGURE 4. Evidence that the dose of AP7 administered by microdialysis produced a selective block of NMDA, but not non-NMDA, glutamate receptors.[24] In **A–D** are shown the responses to graded current doses of several glutamate receptor agonists, including NMDA, aspartate (ASP), AMPA, and glutamate (GLUT) released near the STT cell by microiontophoresis. After control records were made, AP7 was administered into the adjacent dorsal horn by microdialysis. The appropriate dose to be tried was estimated based on that used for *in vitro* experiments and the predicted reduction in concentration across the dialysis membrane and after tissue diffusion. In **E–H**, it is seen that the dose of AP7 used completely blocked the responses to NMDA, most of the responses to ASP, but had little or no effect on the responses to AMPA and GLUT. **I–L** show that partial recovery occurred within 2 h. (From ref. 24, with permission.)

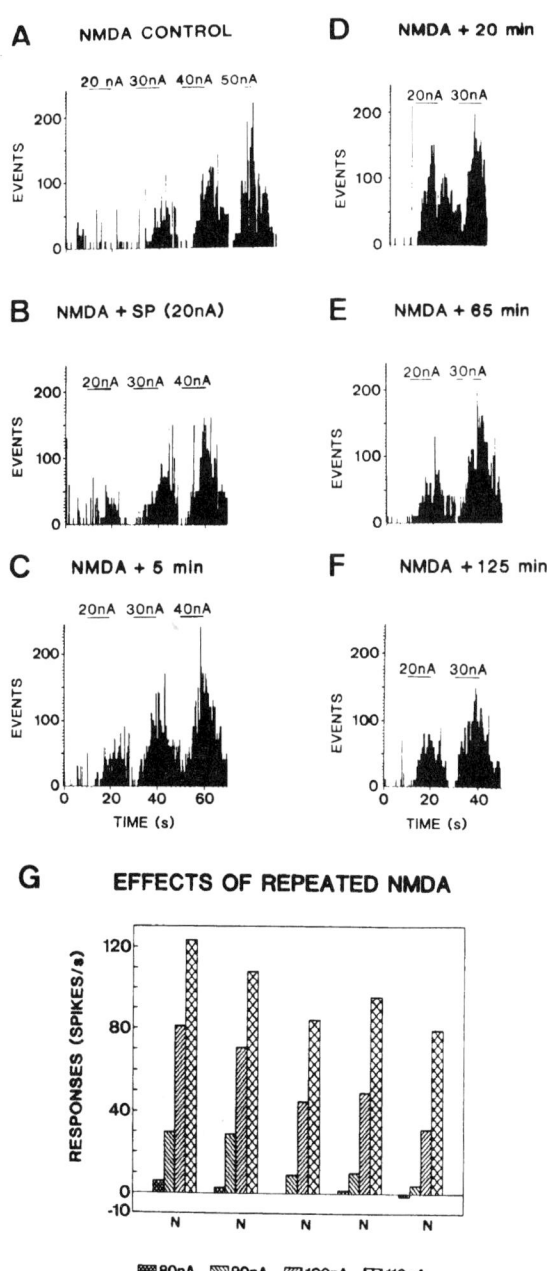

FIGURE 5. Iontophoretic coapplication of NMDA and substance P (SP) can result in central sensitization of STT cells.[25] The peristimulus time histograms in **A–F** show the responses of an STT cell to graded current doses of NMDA. In the control recording in **A**, the lowest dose (20 nA) had no effect on the activity of the cell. During the coapplication of

ferences in the actions of particular pathways. We presume that the influx of calcium ions into neurons in dorsal horn circuits that impinge on STT neurons or into STT neurons themselves, as well as actions on G-protein coupled receptors, such as NK1 and metabotropic glutamate receptors, activate the signal transduction pathways, leading to the phosphorylation of proteins in the dorsal horn neurons, including STT cells.

ALTERED RESPONSIVENESS OF EXCITATORY AND INHIBITORY AMINO ACID RECEPTORS ON SPINOTHALAMIC TRACT NEURONS DURING CENTRAL SENSITIZATION

During the central sensitization that follows intradermal injection of capsaicin, the responses of STT neurons to iontophoretic release of excitatory amino acids are generally increased,[11] whereas the responses to released inhibitory amino acids are reduced (FIG. 6).[32] It is known that protein kinase C enhances NMDA-activated currents by reducing the Mg^{2+} block and by increasing the probability of channel openings.[33] Furthermore, protein kinase action can reduce the activity of inhibitory amino acid receptors.[34,35] Thus, we hypothesize that central sensitization is produced by the phosphorylation by protein kinases of excitatory and inhibitory amino acids receptors, increasing the responsiveness of the former and reducing the responsiveness of the latter.

We have recently completed an initial experiment to test this idea.[36] STT cells in rats were retrogradely labeled by injection of fluorogold into the lateral thalamus bilaterally. Antibodies were used to label NR1 subunits of the NMDA receptor and phosphorylated NR1 subunits. Counts of STT neuron profiles showed that intradermal injection of capsaicin increased the proportion of STT neurons that contained recognizable phospho-NR1-like immunoreactivity on the side of the capsaicin injection, but not on the contralateral side. The increase in labeled STT cells lasted between 1 and 2 h. Vehicle injection had no effect. The proportion of STT cells that contained recognizable NR1-like immunoreactivity did not change. We conclude that the effect of capsaicin in enhancing the phosphorylation of NMDA receptors in STT cells is consistent with our working hypothesis. We are now examining whether capsaicin also causes an increase in the phosphorylation of AMPA receptors.

RELATIONSHIP BETWEEN CENTRAL SENSITIZATION AND LTP

It is our view that central sensitization is a spinal cord variety of long-term potentiation (LTP).[37] A number of investigators have reported LTP in the spinal cord.[38–40] To test this idea further, we have recently obtained preliminary evidence that intra-

---

SP (20 nA) (**B**), there was a small response to the lowest current dose of NMDA (20 nA). However, following cessation of the SP application, the responses to NMDA increased progressively over at least 20 min (**C–D**), and the responses to the lowest NMDA dose remained elevated at 65 and 125 min (**E–F**). In **G**, repeated sets of graded current doses of NMDA in the absence of SP resulted in a progressive tachyphylaxis. (A–F from ref. 25, with permission.)

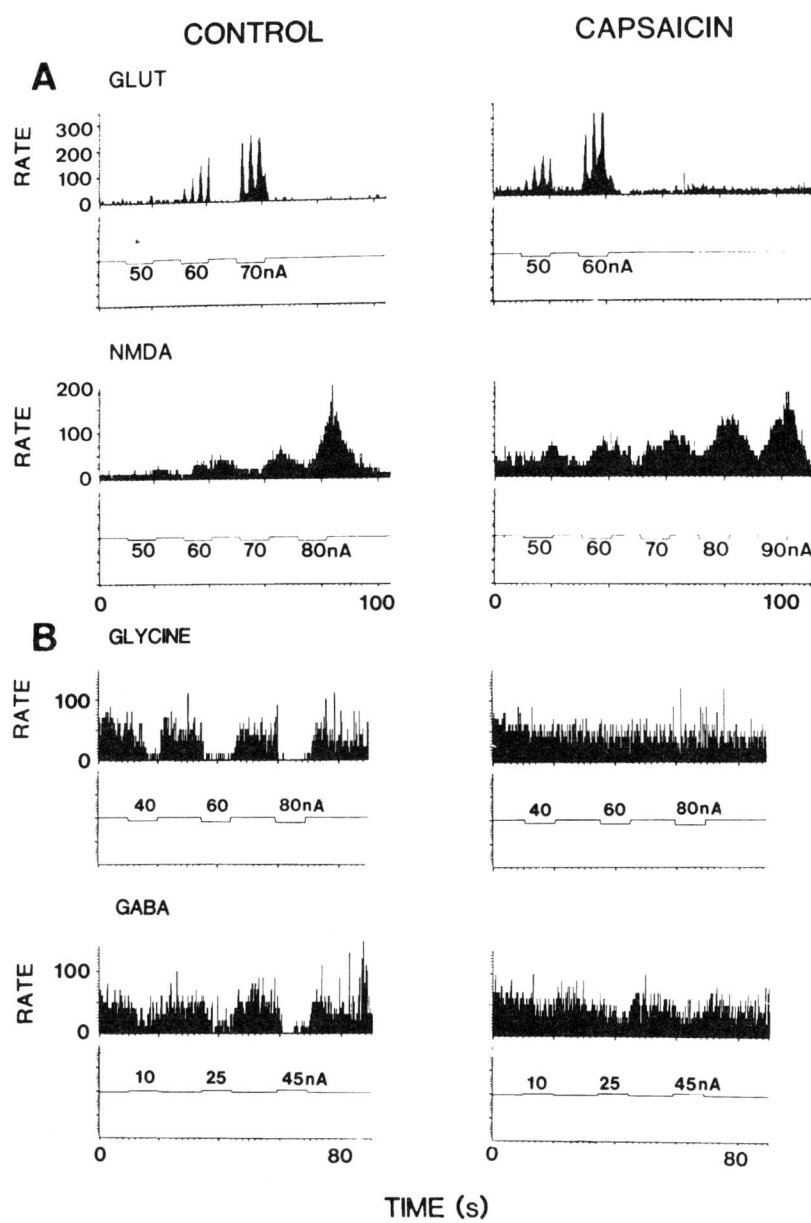

FIGURE 6. Enhancement of excitatory amino acid responses and reduction in inhibitory amino acid responses of STT cells following intradermal injection of capsaicin.[11,32] The peristimulus time histograms in **A** show the responses of an STT cell to iontophoretic application of graded current doses of GLUT and of NMDA before and after capsaicin. The histograms in **B** show the responses of another STT cell to graded current doses of glycine and GABA before and after capsaicin. (A, from ref. 11, with permission; B, from ref. 32, with permission.)

dermal capsaicin causes an increased phosphorylation of calcium/calmodulin-dependent kinase II (CamKII) in the spinal cord within 5 min of the injection and that the CaMKII inhibitor, KN-93, can block central sensitization of dorsal horn interneuronal responses. We plan to continue to test for parallels between central sensitization and LTP.

CONCLUSIONS

Intradermal injection of capsaicin in human subjects results in pain and primary mechanical and heat hyperalgesia in the area of the injection and in secondary allodynia and hyperalgesia in response to innocuous and noxious mechanical, but not heat, stimuli applied to adjacent, unaltered skin. Corresponding changes in the responses of primate spinothalamic tract (STT) neurons are observed, suggesting that these changes in neuronal responses can serve as a predictive model for human sensation, an example of an across-species comparison. Secondary allodynia and hyperalgesia following capsaicin injection are likely to be produced by sensitization of central nociceptive neurons, such as STT cells, because the capsaicin does not alter the sensitivity of sense organs that supply the skin in the secondary area. Administration of neurotransmitter receptor antagonists into the spinal cord shows that central sensitization of primate STT cells following capsaicin injection depends on the activation of non-NMDA, NMDA, and metabotropic glutamate receptors and NK1 (substance P) receptors. The short-lasting action of these neurotransmitters is succeeded by the activation of several signal transduction cascades, including those involving a number of protein kinases, such as CamKII, PKC, PKG, and PKA. Consequences of activation of protein kinases include an enhanced responsiveness of excitatory amino acid receptors and a reduced responsiveness of inhibitory amino acid receptors to their agonists. Initial experiments indicate that there is an increase in the proportion of STT cells in rats that contain phophorylated NMDA receptors for more than an hour following capsaicin injection. It is suggested that central sensitization of primate STT cells represents a spinal cord form of LTP.

REFERENCES

1. MEYER, R.A. & J.N. CAMPBELL. 1981. Myelinated nociceptive afferents account for the hyperalgesia that follows a burn to the hand. Science **213:** 1527–1529.
2. DICKENSON, A.H. & A.F. SULLIVAN. 1987. Peripheral origins and central modulation of subcutaneous formalin-induced activity of rat dorsal horn neurones. Neurosci. Lett. **83:** 207–211.
3. CHEN, J., C. LUO & H-L. LI. 1998. The contribution of spinal neuronal changes to development of prolonged, tonic nociceptive responses of the cat induced by subcutaneous bee venom injection. Eur. J. Pain **2:** 359–376.
4. HARDY, J.D., H.G. WOOLF & H. GOODELL. 1967. Pain Sensations and Reactions. Hafner Pub. New York.
5. LAMOTTE, R.H., D. SHAIN, D.A. SIMONE et al. 1991. Neurogenic hyperalgesia: psychophysical studies of underlying mechanisms. J. Neurophysiol. **66:** 190–211.
6. LAMOTTE, R.H., L.E.R. LUNDBERG & H.E. TOREBJÖRK. 1992. Pain, hyperalgesia, and activity in nociceptive C units in humans after intradermal injection of capsaicin. J. Physiol. (Lond.) **448:** 749–764.

7. TOREBJÖRK, H.E., L.E.R. LUNDBERG & R.H. LAMOTTE. 1992. Central changes in processing of mechanorceptive input in capsaicin-induced secondary hyperalgesia in humans. J. Physiol. (Lond.) **448:** 765–780.
8. BAUMANN, T.K., D.A. SIMONE, C. SHAIN *et al.* 1991. Neurogenic hyperalgesia: the search for the primary cutaneous afferent fibers that contribute to capsaicin-induced pain and hyperalgesia. J. Neurophysiol. **66:** 212–227.
9. TREVINO, D.L., J.D. COULTER & W.D. WILLIS. 1973. Location of cells of origin of spinothalamic tract in lumbar enlargement of the monkey. J. Neurophysiol. **36:** 750–761.
10. SIMONE, D.A., L.S. SORKIN, U. OH *et al.* 1991. Neurogenic hyperalgesia: central neural correlates in responses of spinothalamic tract neurons. J. Neurophysiol. **66:** 228–246.
11. DOUGHERTY, P.M. & W.D. WILLIS. 1992. Enhanced responses of spinothalamic tract neurons to excitatory amino acids accompany capsaicin-induced sensitization in the monkey. J. Neurosci. **12:** 883–894.
12. SLUKA, K.A., H. REES, P.S. CHEN *et al.* 1997. Inhibitors of G-proteins and protein kinases reduce the sensitization to mechanical stimulation and the desensitization to heat of spinothalamic tract neurons induced by intradermal injection of capsaicin in the primate. Exp. Brain Res. **115:** 15–24.
13. ALI, Z., R.A. MEYER & J.N. CAMPBELL. 1996. Secondary hyperalgesia to mechanical but not heat stimuli following a capsaicin injection in hairy skin. Pain **68:** 401–411.
14. HOLZER, P. 1991. Capsaicin: cellular targets, mechanisms of action, and selectivity for thin sensory neurons. Pharmacol. Rev. **43:** 143–201.
15. TOMINAGA, M., M.J. CATERINA, A.B. MALMBERG *et al.* 1998. The cloned capsaicin receptor integrates multiple pain-producing stimuli. Neuron **21:** 531–543.
16. DE BIASI, S. & A. RUSTIONI. 1988. Glutamate and substance P coexist in primary afferent terminals in the superficial laminae of spinal cord. Proc. Natl. Acad. Sci. U.S.A. **85:** 7820–7824.
17. GAMSE, R., A. MOLNAR & F. LEMBECK. 1979. Substance P release from spinal cord slices by capsaicin. Life Sci. **25:** 629–636.
18. SORKIN, L.S. & D.J. MCADOO. 1993. Amino acids and serotonin are released into the lumbar spinal cord of the anesthetized cat following intradermal capsaicin injections. Brain Res. **607:** 89–98.
19. WESTLUND, K.N., S.M. CARLTON, D. ZHANG *et al.* 1992. Glutamate-immunoreactive terminals synapse on primate spinothalamic tract cells. J. Comp. Neurol. **322:** 519–527.
20. CARLTON, S.M., C.C. LAMOTTE, C.N. HONDA *et al.* 1985. Ultrastructural analysis of substance P and other synaptic profiles innervating an identified primate spinothalamic tract neuron. Neurosci. Abstr. **11:** 578.
21. CARLTON, S.M., K.N. WESTLUND, D. ZHANG *et al.* 1990. Calcitonin gene-related peptide containing primary afferent fibers synapse on primate spinothalamic tract cells. Neurosci. Lett. **109:** 76–81.
22. CHUNG, K., W.T. LEE & S.M. CARLTON. 1988. The effects of dorsal rhizotomy and spinal cord isolation on calcitonin gene-related peptide containing terminals in the rat lumbar dorsal horn. Neurosci. Lett. **90:** 27–32.
23. DOUGHERTY, P.M., J. PALECEK, V. PALECKOVA *et al.* 1994. Neurokinin 1 and 2 antagonists attenuate the responses and NK1 antagonists prevent the sensitization of primate spinothalamic tract neurons after intradermal capsaicin. J. Neurophysiol. **72:** 1464–1475.
24. DOUGHERTY, P.M., J. PALECEK, V. PALECKOVA *et al.* 1992. The role of NMDA and non-NMDA excitatory amino acid receptors in the excitation of primate spinothalamic tract neurons by mechanical, chemical, thermal, and electrical stimuli. J. Neurosci. **12:** 3025–3041.
25. DOUGHERTY, P.M. & W.D. WILLIS. 1991. Enhancement of spinothalamic neuron responses to chemical and mechanical stimuli following combined micro-iontophoretic application of N-methyl-D-aspartic acid and substance P. Pain **47:** 85–93.
26. NEUGEBAUER, V., P-S. CHEN & W.D. WILLIS. 1999. Role of metabotropic glutamate receptor subtype mGluR1 in brief nociception and central sensitization of primate STT cells. J. Neurophysiol. **82:** 272–282.
27. NEUGEBAUER, V., P-S. CHEN & W.D. WILLIS. 2000. Groups II and III metabotropic glutamate receptors differentially modulate brief and prolonged nociception in primate STT cells. J. Neurophysiol. **84:** 2998–3009.

28. LIN, Q., Y.B. PENG & W.D. WILLIS. 1996. Possible role of protein kinase C in the sensitization of primate spinothalamic tract neurons. J. Neurosci. **16:** 3026–3034.
29. LIN, Q., Y.B. PENG, J. WU *et al.* 1997. Involvement of cGMP in nociceptive processing by and sensitization of spinothalamic neurons in primates. J. Neurosci. **17:** 3293–3302.
30. LIN, Q., J. WU & W.D. WILLIS. 1997. The effects of protein kinase A activation on the responses of primate spinothalamic neurons to mechanical and thermal stimuli. Neurosci. Abstr. **23:** 2357.
31. LIN, Q., J. PALECEK, V. PALECKOVA *et al.* 1999. Nitric oxide mediates the central sensitization of primate spinothalamic tract neurons. J. Neurophysiol. **81:** 1075–1089.
32. LIN, Q., Y.B. PENG & W.D. WILLIS. 1996. Inhibition of primate spinothalamic tract neurons by spinal glycine and GABA is reduced during central sensitization. J. Neurophysiol. **76:** 1005–1014.
33. CHEN, L. & L-Y.M. HUANG. 1992. Protein kinase C reduces Mg^{2+} block of NMDA-receptor channels as a mechanism of modulation. Nature **356:** 521–523.
34. LEIDENHEIMER, N.J., S.J. MCQUILKIN, L.D. HAHNER *et al.* 1992. Activation of protein kinase C selectively inhibits the γ-aminobutryic acid$_A$ receptor: role of desensitization. Mol. Pharmacol. **41:** 1116–1123.
35. VAELLO, M.L., A. RUIZ-GÓMEZ, J. LERMA *et al.* 1994. Modulation of inhibitory glycine receptors by phosphorylation by protein kinase C and cAMP-dependent protein kinase. J. Biol. Chem. **269:** 2002–2008.
36. ZOU, X., Q. LIN & W.D. WILLIS. 2000. Enhanced phosphorylation of NMDA receptor NR1 subunits in spinal cord dorsal horn and spinothalamic tract neurons after intradermal injection of capsaicin in rats. J. Neurosci. **20:** 6989–6997.
37. WILLIS, W.D. 1997. Is central sensitization of nociceptive transmission in the spinal cord a variety of long-term potentiation? A commentary on the article by Svendsen, Tjolsen, and Hole. NeuroReport **8:** iii.
38. RANDIC, M., M.C. JIANG & R. CERNE. 1993. Long-term potentiation and long-term depression of primary afferent neurotransmission in the rat spinal cord. J. Neurosci. **13:** 5228–5241.
39. LIU, X-G. & J. SANDKÜHLER. 1997. Characterization of long-term potentiation of C-fiber-evoked potentials in spinal dorsal horn of adult rat: essential role of NK1 and NK2 receptors. J. Neurophysiol. **78:** 1973–1982.
40. SVENDSEN, F., A. TJOLSEN & K. HOLE. 1997. LTP of spinal Aβ and C-fibre evoked responses after electrical sciatic nerve stimulation. NeuroReport **8:** 3427–3430.

Central Neuroplasticity and Pathological Pain

RONALD MELZACK, TERENCE J. CODERRE,[a] JOEL KATZ,[b]
AND ANTHONY L. VACCARINO[c]

Department of Psychology, McGill University, Montreal, Quebec H3A 1B1, Canada

ABSTRACT: The traditional specificity theory of pain perception holds that pain involves a direct transmission system from somatic receptors to the brain. The amount of pain perceived, moreover, is assumed to be directly proportional to the extent of injury. Recent research, however, indicates far more complex mechanisms. Clinical and experimental evidence shows that noxious stimuli may sensitize central neural structures involved in pain perception. Salient clinical examples of these effects include amputees with pains in a phantom limb that are similar or identical to those felt in the limb before it was amputated, and patients after surgery who have benefited from preemptive analgesia which blocks the surgery-induced afferent barrage and/or its central consequences. Experimental evidence of these changes is illustrated by the development of sensitization, wind-up, or expansion of receptive fields of CNS neurons, as well as by the enhancement of flexion reflexes and the persistence of pain or hyperalgesia after inputs from injured tissues are blocked. It is clear from the material presented that the perception of pain does not simply involve a moment-to-moment analysis of afferent noxious input, but rather involves a dynamic process that is influenced by the effects of past experiences. Sensory stimuli act on neural systems that have been modified by past inputs, and the behavioral output is significantly influenced by the "memory" of these prior events. An increased understanding of the central changes induced by peripheral injury or noxious stimulation should lead to new and improved clinical treatment for the relief and prevention of pathological pain.

INTRODUCTION

The relationship between central neuroplasticity and chronic, pathological pain is not a simple one. Phantom limbs, for example, reveal the complexities of the relationship. It is well known that, after a hand is amputated, punctate stimulation of the skin of the forearm produces sensations not only at the stimulated sites, but also in specific parts of the phantom hand.[1-3] An excellent somatotopic map of the phantom hand is revealed on the forearm which is reasonably assumed to reflect neuroplastic changes in representations of the hand and forearm in the central nervous system from spinal cord to cerebral cortex. These changes in somatotopic maps at both the forearm and brain are found within hours after amputation, suggesting that they are due to the removal of inhibition of existing neurons (rather than growth of

[a]Current address: Department of Anesthesia, McGill University, Montreal, Quebec H3A 1B1, Canada.
[b]Current address: Department of Anesthesia, Toronto General Hospital, Toronto, Ontario M5G 2C4, Canada.
[c]Current address: Department of Psychology, University of New Orleans, New Orleans, LA 70148.

new neurons) in the hand area, which now respond to stimulation of the forearm. The dynamic changes over time are further revealed as the somatotopic-referred map at the forearm expands greatly to cover almost the whole lower arm, then contracts and undergoes further changes over a period of a year or more.

After these remarkable changes, we would expect that the target cells in the brain must also undergo fundamental changes in the functions they subserve. Several months after amputation of a hand or fingers, the denervated areas of the thalamus and cortex respond exclusively to stimulation of adjacent body areas. However, astonishingly, it seems that stimulation of the denervated brain areas does not produce sensations in the body areas that have "taken over". Despite the neuroplasticity, stimulation of the cortex[4] or thalamus[5] in human paraplegics with major spinal cord injuries produces sensations in anesthetic body areas *below* the spinal transection. This suggests that there is a change in the *input* pattern to these cells, but their *output* pattern retains essential components that produce the perception of the originally innervating part of the body. That is, the neural network—or neuromatrix—of the body-self is partly built-in and partly modified by sensory inputs. The built-in part may explain why the output pattern continues to produce the perception of the genetically determined body part. The marked plasticity in brain representation after amputation may explain telescoping of the phantom and probably some portion of the characteristics of the pain and other abnormal, hyperesthetic experiences reported by amputees. However, we have just seen that the neuroplastic changes in sensory brain areas may hide a built-in, immutable core that continues to send signals for perception and response related to the body area for which it was genetically designated.

Another example of neuronal plasticity that must be examined with caution is the body of evidence that prolonged epidural blocks of sensory input prior to amputation of a limb may prevent or diminish the probability that the patient will suffer phantom limb pain.[6–8] However, the early evidence indicating a marked "preemptive" effect by the presurgical and intrasurgical anesthetic blocks has been challenged by a few failures to replicate the earlier studies.[9] Although the results are contentious,[10–12] this is an exciting, important area for research that has potentially valuable implications for both understanding neuroplasticity and putting that knowledge to use by preventing pathological pain.

These observations teach us that neuroplasticity certainly occurs, but within limits. It is physiologically evident in brain structures, but it does not completely change their functional role in the total activity of the brain. So too, preemptive analgesia does not produce huge clinical effects, but it has been repeatedly demonstrated in well-designed experiments. Clearly, we must keep a balanced perspective on plasticity and genetic determination.

NEURAL PLASTICITY IN HISTORICAL PERSPECTIVE

Pain research and therapy, at any period in history, are determined by the dominant theory of brain function at the time. Until the last half of this century, pain was thought to be produced by a passive, direct-transmission system from peripheral receptors to cortex. There was no place in this concept of the nervous system for plasticity, in which neuronal and synaptic functions are capable of being molded or shaped so that they influence subsequent perceptual experiences. Plasticity related to pain represents persistent functional changes, or somatic memories,[13] produced in the nervous system by injuries or other pathological events. The recognition that such changes can occur is essential to understanding the chronic pain syndromes, such as low back pain and phantom limb pain, that persist and often destroy the lives of the people who suffer them.

The theory of pain that we inherited in the twentieth century was proposed by Descartes three centuries earlier.[14] It holds that injury activates specific pain receptors and fibers that, in turn, project pain impulses through a spinal pain pathway to a pain center in the brain. The psychological experience of pain, therefore, was virtually equated with physical injury. In the 1950s, there was no room for psychological contributions to pain, such as attention, past experience, and the meaning of the situation. Instead, pain experience was held to be proportional to peripheral injury or pathology. Patients who suffered chronic pain without presenting signs of organic disease were often sent to psychiatrists.

In 1965, Melzack and Wall[15] proposed the gate control theory of pain. The emphasis of the theory on the modulation of inputs in the spinal dorsal horns and the dynamic role of the brain in pain processes had a clinical as well as a scientific impact. Psychological factors, which were previously dismissed as reactions to pain, were now seen to be an integral part of pain processing, and new avenues for pain control were opened. Similarly, cutting nerves and pathways was gradually replaced by a host of methods to modulate the input. Physical therapists and other health care professionals who use a multitude of modulation techniques (including acupuncture) were brought into the picture, and transcutaneous electrical nerve stimulation (TENS) became an important modality for the treatment of chronic and acute pain.[14]

The gate control theory's most important contribution to biological and medical science was its emphasis on central nervous system (CNS) mechanisms. The theory forced the medical and biological sciences to accept the brain as an active system that filters, selects, and modulates inputs. The dorsal horns, too, were not merely passive transmission stations but sites at which dynamic activities—inhibition, excitation, and modulation—occurred. The theory highlighted the CNS as an essential component in pain processes.

Even though the Cartesian concept of direct transmission has dominated our ideas about pain for the past 200 years, descriptions of plasticity related to pain—that is, the idea that injury can produce alterations in CNS function affecting subsequent pain sensitivity—have been proposed by a few courageous clinical observers. MacKenzie[16] suggested that increased pain sensitivity and referred pain could be the result of increased sensitivity of CNS structures. He proposed that sensory impulses arising from injured tissues create an "irritable focus" in spinal cord segments onto which they impinge. In relation to perioperative anesthesia, Crile[17] wrote that patients given inhalational anesthesia still need to be protected by regional anesthesia; otherwise they might incur persistent CNS changes and enhanced postoperative pain. According to Hardy et al.,[18] secondary hyperalgesia and referred cutaneous hyperalgesia occur because an injury produces a state of hyperexcitability in the spinal cord. This hyperexcitability is sustained following the activation of a network of internuncial neurons, which produces a spreading facilitation of adjacent neurons in the spinal cord, allowing for the spread of hyperalgesia to uninjured regions of the body. Similarly, Livingston[19] suggested that the afferent activity generated by injured peripheral nerves elicits an abnormal firing pattern within the spinal cord. He proposed that a disturbance occurs in an internuncial pool of dorsal horn interneurons and results in reverberatory activity which eventually spreads to other parts of the spinal cord, including areas that affect the sympathetic chain. Increased activity in sympathetic efferents would disrupt vasoregulation and induce further hypersensitivity of peripheral tissue, leading to increased afferent input and a vicious circle of peripheral-central activity.

Aside from descriptive references to irritable foci, reverberatory activity, and vicious circles, the above theories do not provide empiral evidence for, or details of, the nature of the CNS changes that occur following noxious stimulation. Only recently has there been specific empirical evidence indicating noxious stimulus-induced changes in CNS function. Kenshalo et al.[20] demonstrated that noxious peripheral stimuli produce changes in the sensitivity of dorsal horn neurons to further stimulation, and Woolf and Wall[21,22] provided empirical evidence for a primary afferent input triggering sustained increases in central excitability. Woolf[21] demonstrated that injury-induced increases in spinal cord excitability could be maintained even after local anesthesia of the injured site, providing empirical evidence that acute injury could produce lasting spinal changes. Woolf and Wall[22] showed that the amount of morphine required to prevent the development of this spinal hyperexcitability was 10-fold less than the amount required to reverse it after it was established, and provided the experimental basis for subsequent clinical investigations of the use of preemptive analgesia for the prevention or alleviation of postoperative pain.

These studies indicate that noxious stimulation or injury can produce dramatic alterations in spinal cord function, including sensitization, wind-up, or the expansion of the receptive fields of spinal neurons. Recently, several investigators have proposed detailed theories of how noxious stimuli produce these changes in CNS function. Unlike previous theories of central sensitization, recent theories propose that, in addition to a contribution of neuronal hyperactivity to pathological pain, there are specific cellular and molecular changes that affect membrane excitability and induce new gene expression, thereby allowing for enhanced responses to future stimulation. These studies have recently been reviewed by Coderre et al.[23,24] The effect of these changes includes an expansion of dorsal horn receptive fields and hyperexcitability which, if allowed to persist, would presumably produce prolonged changes in excitability that could be maintained without further noxious peripheral input.

PAIN IN PHANTOM LIMBS AND DEAFFERENTATED STRUCTURES

A striking property of phantom limb pain is the persistence of a pain that existed in a limb prior to its amputation. This type of phantom limb pain, characterized by the persistence or recurrence of a previous pain, has the same qualities and is experienced in the same area of the limb as the preamputation pain. Case studies of amputees[13] have demonstrated pain "memories" of painful diabetic and decubitus ulcers, gangrene, corns, blisters, ingrown toenails, cuts, and deep tissue injury. In addition, the phantom limb may assume the same painful posture as that of the real limb prior to amputation, especially if the arm or leg had been immobilized for a prolonged period.[13]

The literature indicates that the proportion of amputees who report that their phantom pains are similar to those felt in the limb before amputation may be as high as 79%.[13] Reports of pain memories in phantom limbs appear to be less common when there has been a discontinuity, or a pain-free interval, between the experience of pain and the amputation. This is consistent with the observation that relief of preamputation pain by continuous epidural block for 3 days prior to amputation decreases the incidence of phantom limb pain 6 months later.[6] Furthermore, if pain is experienced at or near the time of amputation, there is a higher probability that it will persist in the phantom limb.[13,25]

Pain also persists in patients with deafferentation that does not involve amputation. Patients with brachial plexus avulsion[26] or spinal cord injuries[27] often experience pain in the anesthetic, deafferentated region. For example, Nathan[28] described a patient who continued to feel the pain of an ingrown toenail after a complete spinal cord break. In addition, patients undergoing spinal anesthesia[29] and those with injuries of the brachial plexus[26] or spinal cord[27] sometimes report that a limb is in the same uncomfortable, often painful, posture it was in prior to the injury or block. These postural phantom sensations do not usually persist beyond several days, and in most cases are at least temporarily reversed by competing visual inputs which reveal a dissociation between the real and perceived limb.

A literature also exists on the persistence of painful and nonpainful sensations associated with removal or deafferentation of body structures other than the limbs, including breasts,[30] teeth,[31,32] and internal and special sense organs. Ulcer pain has been reported to persist after vagotomy[33] or subtotal gastrectomy with removal of the ulcer.[34] Similarly, patients have reported labor pain and menstrual cramps following total hysterectomy,[35] rectal and hemorrhoid pain following removal of the rectum,[36] the burning pain of cystitis after complete removal of the bladder,[37] and the pain of a severely ulcerated cornea after enucleation of an eye.[38]

When a missing or completely anesthetic limb continues to be the source of pain which resembles an old injury, it is reasonable to assume that the pain is centrally represented, but it is not clear whether deafferentation per se is necessary for pain memories to develop. The interruption of afferent input associated with deafferentation may facilitate the central neural changes that contribute to the formation of pain memories by removing normal inhibitory control mechanisms. In addition, because amputation also results in the loss of visual and tactile information related to the limb, the central influences that normally inhibit the established pain "traces" may be reduced further by the absence of information from external sources that could confirm or disconfirm the percept arising from the peripheral injury.

There is evidence that in some instances the reactivation of pain memories requires a peripheral trigger. Leriche[39] described a patient who did not experience phantom limb pain until six years after amputation, when an injection into the stump instantly, and permanently, revived the pain of a former painful ulceration of the Achilles tendon. Nathan[28,40] reported a similar phenomenon when applying noxious stimulation to the stump of an amputee who later reexperienced the pain of an ice-skating injury he had sustained five years earlier when the leg was intact. Noordenbos and Wall[41] also described seven patients with partial peripheral nerve injury, and subsequent pain, who underwent complete nerve resection and graft or ligation. Following regeneration and a pain-free period, all redeveloped pain of the same quality and in the same location as the pain they had experienced prior to nerve resection, although in some patients the recurrence of pain was restricted to a smaller area within the originally painful region. These studies and case reports indicate that past pains may be reactivated months or even years after the original injury, in some cases by a peripheral trigger that provides the input required to activate the central neural structures subserving the memory trace.

Deafferentation by peripheral neurectomy or dorsal rhizotomy in rodents is followed by self-mutilation (autotomy) in which the animals bite and scratch the insensate paw to the point of amputation.[42] There is evidence that autotomy behavior is produced by ongoing pain or dysesthesia, associated with increased neuronal activity, which is referred to the anesthetic region.[43] Autotomy behavior is dramatically affected by alterations in the level of noxious input present at the time of, or prior to, nerve section. Thus, noxious chemical,[44,45] thermal,[46,47] and electrical[47,48] stimulation prior to nerve sections significantly increases the severity of autotomy following neurectomy or rhizotomy. These findings suggest that the prior injury produces central changes that influence nociceptive behavior, after nerve sections, at a time when inputs from the injured region are no longer capable of transmitting their message centrally.

The above findings are similar to clinical reports that phantom limb pain is more likely to occur in amputees who had pain in their limb prior to amputation, and strongly suggest that central neuroplasticity is crucial to the development of phantom limb pain. The clinical relevance of these findings is indicated by the observation that in human amputees the incidence of phantom limb pain at 7 days and 6 months after amputation is significantly greater in patients whose pain is not treated by epidural block with bupivacaine and morphine prior to amputation surgery.[6] In contrast to the effect of increasing noxious inputs at the time of nerve injury, reducing or eliminating the afferent barrage induced by nerve section produces a dramatic reduction in autotomy. When the afferent barrage induced by nerve cuts in rats is blocked by treating the sciatic and saphenous nerves with local anesthetics prior to sectioning them, a significant reduction is found in the incidence and severity of autotomy.[48]

An animal model has recently been developed[47] that parallels the observation that human amputees report similar pains in a limb before and after amputation. In this animal model, rats selectively initiated autotomy in either the lateral or medial half of a hind paw if that particular half had been given a thermal injury prior to sciatic and saphenous nerve sections. The selective attack on the previously injured region, despite the fact that the entire foot was deafferented, suggests that the rats were responding to pain referred to the injured area, which was produced by the prior injury and the central trace it created. Rats injured after neurectomy did not show a similar preference indicating that the rats were not responding simply to peripheral cues associated with the injury.

DENERVATION HYPERSENSITIVITY AND NEURONAL HYPERACTIVITY

Sensory disturbances associated with nerve injury have been closely linked to alterations in CNS function. Markus *et al.*[49] have demonstrated that the development of hypersensitivity in a rat's hind paw following sciatic nerve section occurs concurrently with the expansion of the saphenous nerve's somatotopic projection in the spinal cord. Nerve injury may also lead to the development of increased neuronal activity at various levels of the somatosensory system. In addition to spontaneous activity generated from the neuroma,[50] peripheral neurectomy also leads to increased spontaneous activity in the dorsal root ganglion[51] and spinal cord.[52] Furthermore, after dorsal rhizotomy, increases in spontaneous neural activity occur in the dorsal horn,[53] the spinal trigeminal nucleus,[54] and the thalamus.[55]

Clinical neurosurgery studies reveal a similar relationship between denervation and CNS hyperactivity. Neurons in the somatosensory thalamus of patients with neuropathic pain display high spontaneous firing rates, abnormal bursting activity, and evoked responses to stimulation of body areas that normally do not activate these neurons.[56,57] The site of abnormality in thalamic function appears to be somatotopically related to the painful region. In patients with complete spinal cord transection and dysesthesias referred below the level of the break, neuronal hyperactivity was observed in thalamic regions that had lost their normal sensory input, but not in regions with apparently normal afferent input.[58] Furthermore, in patients with neuropathic pain, electrical stimulation of subthalamic, thalamic, and capsular regions may evoke pain and in some instances even reproduce the patient's pain.[40,59] Direct electrical stimulation of spontaneously hyperactive cells evokes pain in some, but not all pain patients, raising the possibility that in certain patients the observed changes in neuronal activity may contribute to the perception of pain.[58] Studies of patients undergoing electrical brain stimulation during brain surgery reveal that pain is rarely elicited by test stimuli unless the patient suffers from a chronic pain problem. However, brain stimulation can elicit pain responses in patients with chronic pain that does not involve extensive nerve injury or deafferentation. Nathan[40] describes a patient who underwent thalamic stimulation for a movement disorder. The patient had been suffering from a toothache for 10 days prior to the operation. Electrical stimulation of the thalamus reproduced the toothache.

It is possible that receptive field expansions and spontaneous activity generated in the CNS following peripheral nerve injury are, in part, mediated by alterations in normal inhibitory processes in the dorsal horn. Within four days of a peripheral nerve section, a reduction occurs in the dorsal root potential, and therefore in the presynaptic inhibition it represents.[60] Nerve section also induces a reduction in the inhibitory effect of A-fiber stimulation on activity in dorsal horn neurons.[61] Furthermore, nerve injury affects descending inhibitory controls from brain stem nuclei. In the intact nervous system, stimulation of the locus coeruleus[62] or the nucleus raphe magnus[63] produces an inhibition of dorsal horn neurons. Following dorsal rhizotomy, however, stimulation of these areas produces excitation, rather than inhibition, in half the cells studied.[64]

EFFECTS OF ANESTHETIC OR ANALGESIC PRETREATMENT ON POSTINJURY PAIN

As noted above, deafferentation pain in rats is significantly reduced if the injured nerves are locally anesthetized prior to nerve injury. Thus, autotomy after nerve sections,[48] or hyperalgesia following nerve ligation,[65] is significantly reduced if the sciatic and saphenous nerves are locally anesthetized prior to the nerve injury. Recent evidence indicates that persistent pain induced by tissue injury is also reduced by pretreatment with local anesthetics or opioids prior to the injury, suggesting a contribution of central plasticity to nociceptive pain. A subcutaneous injection of dilute formalin produces a biphasic nociceptive response with an early phase of intense pain that occurs in the first few minutes and a later tonic phase of moderate pain occurring about 20–60 min after formalin injection.[66] The nociceptive response to subcutaneous formalin is matched by a corresponding biphasic increase in the activity of dorsal horn neurons after formalin injection.[67] Dickenson and Sullivan[68] have demonstrated that intrathecal administration of a μ-opiate agonist significantly inhibits the prolonged increase in dorsal horn activity produced by subcutaneous formalin injection. However, this inhibition occurs only if the drug is given before the formalin injection, and not if it is given 2 min after the injection. These results imply that the dorsal horn activity associated with the late phase of the formalin test depends upon spinal activation during the early phase immediately after formalin injection.

Behavioral studies support the electrophysiological finding that the late phase response to formalin is, in part, dependent on spinal changes generated during the early phase. Tonic nociceptive responses in the late phase of the formalin test (30–60 min after formalin) are not eliminated by complete anesthetic blockade of the formalin-injected area at the time of testing during the late phase, but are virtually abolished if the area was also blocked by local anesthetics at the time of formalin injection.[69] Furthermore, late-phase nociceptive responses are significantly reduced by spinal anesthesia induced immediately prior to formalin injection, but not by spinal anesthesia administered 5 min after formalin injection—that is, after the early phase had already occurred.[69] These results suggest that central neural changes, which occur during the early phase of the formalin test, are essential for the development of the later tonic phase of the formalin test.

Evidence suggests that peripheral tissue injury also induces plasticity in supraspinal structures, which affects persistent pain behavior. This evidence comes from assessing the effects of preinjury treatment with local anesthetics (in this case injected into discrete brain regions) on postinjury pain responses. Nociceptive responses to subcutaneous formalin injection into the rat hind paw are suppressed after focal injection of lidocaine into specific limbic system sites such as the cingulum bundle and the fornix pathway. The lidocaine injection produces analgesia during the late phase of the formalin test (30–70 min after formalin injection) when injected into these areas 10 min before, but not 10 min after, the formalin injection.[70] These results suggest that activity in the cingulum bundle and fornix during the early-phase response to formalin is critical to the development of the late-phase response to formalin. The cingulum bundle and fornix are part of a neural loop that projects from the anterior thalamic nuclei to the cingulate cortex, hippocampus, and mammillary bodies, and returns to the anterior thalamic nuclei.[71] It is proposed that activation of this "closed" circuit during the early phase of the formalin response induces a sensitized state within the limbic system, enhancing responses to subsequent stimulation. Recent physiological evidence supports this concept. Brain stem stimulation has been found to enhance the responsiveness of the anterior thalamic nuclei to stimulation of the mammillary bodies and cingulate cortex.[72] Furthermore, noxious peripheral stimulation produces bursting activity in CA1 neurons of the hippocampus.[73] The selective blocking of neural activity in the cingulum bundle or fornix during the early phase of formalin may reduce nociceptive responses by preventing the development of long-term changes in these structures.

POSTOPERATIVE PAIN

The idea that CNS changes produced by tissue damage and noxious inputs associated with surgery could contribute to postoperative pain has existed for several decades.[17] However, it was only after the research by Woolf and Wall[22] provided a sound justification for preemptive treatment that this idea began to receive the clinical attention it deserves. Woolf and Wall[22] demonstrated in experimental animals that opioids are much more effective at reducing stimulus-induced increases in the excitability of the dorsal horn if they are administered prior to, rather than following, C-fiber electrical nerve stimulation. Recent clinical evidence supports the hypothesis that the administration of analgesic agents prior to surgery may prevent the central sensitizing effects of the surgical procedure. In this manner it may be possible to reduce postoperative pain intensity or lower postoperative analgesic requirements for periods much longer than the duration of action of the preoperatively administered agents.

McQuay et al.[74] examined the possible prophylactic effect of opiate premedication and/or local anesthetic nerve blocks on postoperative pain. They provided data showing that the time to first request for postoperative analgesics was longest among patients who had received a presurgical treatment with opiates and nerve blocks, and shortest among patients who had received neither. Similar findings have recently been reported by Kiss and Kilian,[75] who showed that opiate pretreatment increased the length of time until request for first analgesic, reduced the percentage of patients requesting analgesics, and decreased analgesic consumption in the first 48 h for patients undergoing lumbar disc surgery. Over the past few years, additional evidence has accumulated to support the hypothesis that preemptive analgesia using a variety of agents (e.g., opiates, local anesthetics, NSAIDs) prolongs the time to first request for analgesics, reduces postoperative pain intensity, or decreases postoperative analgesic requirements among patients undergoing inguinal herniography,[76] oral surgery,[77–79] tonsillectomy,[80] abdominal surgery,[81] orthopedic surgery,[82,83] lower-limb amputation,[6,84] and thoracotomy.[85]

Tverskoy et al.[76] clearly demonstrated the benefits of preincisional blockade on postoperative pain. Patients who were undergoing inguinal hemiorraphy received general anesthesia alone, general anesthesia plus subcutaneous and intramuscular injections of bupivacaine prior to surgical incision, or spinal bupivacaine administered preoperatively. All patients received the same regimen of postoperative analgesics. Twenty-four and 48 h after surgery, postoperative incisional pain, movement-associated pain, and pain induced by pressure applied to the surgical wound were all significantly lower in the two groups that had received bupivacaine prior to surgical incision compared to patients who received general anesthesia alone.

Recently, a number of well-controlled, double-blind studies have also shown that preoperative administration of NSAIDs by a variety of routes reduces postoperative pain long after the clinical duration of action of the NSAIDs. Campbell et al.[79] found that intravenous diclofenac administered before tooth extraction resulted in less postoperative pain the day after surgery when compared with pretreatment using intravenous fentanyl or a placebo. Similarly, Hutchison et al.[78] reported that, compared to patients pretreated with a placebo, significantly fewer patients who received orally administered piroxicam before tooth extraction required supplemental postoperative analgesics and their time to first postoperative analgesic request was longer.

McGlew et al.[83] demonstrated that, on days 1 to 3 after spinal surgery, postoperative pain scores and opiate consumption were significantly lower among patients who had received indomethacin suppositories compared with placebo suppositories one hour before surgery.

Taken together, these studies demonstrate that opiate premedication, regional local anesthesia, spinal anesthesia, or systemic NSAIDs administered before incision are more effective than placebo or no treatment controls. The implication of these studies for clinical pathological pain is that changes in central neural function that are induced by surgery alter subsequent perception in such a way that nociceptive inputs from the surgical wound may be perceived as more painful (hyperalgesia) than they would otherwise have been, and innocuous inputs may give rise to frank pain (allodynia).

However, these early studies on the prevention of postoperative pain with preoperative analgesics did not compare the pretreatment with the effects of the same treatments administered after surgery.[86] Demonstrating that pretreatment with analgesics, but not a placebo, lessens pain and decreases postoperative analgesic requirements at a time when the agents are no longer clinically active indicates that the central component of postoperative pain can be prevented or preempted. In the absence of a postincisional or postoperative treatment condition, it is not possible to determine the separate contributions of factors associated with the intraoperative versus the postoperative period to the enhanced postoperative pain experience. It may be that analgesic pretreatments reduce the development of local inflammation, a potential peripheral factor that could contribute to postoperative pain, rather than inhibiting central sensitization induced by noxious inputs during surgery. This may be particularly important in the case of NSAIDs,[78,79,83] which act primarily to reduce peripheral inflammation, but may also be important in the case of infiltration with local anesthetics[76] because local anesthesia would also reduce peripheral inflammation that is dependent on the efferent functions of peripheral nerves (i.e., neurogenic inflammation). Altering the timing of administration of analgesic agents (i.e., before or after incision vs. before or after surgery) may provide clues to the specific intraoperative (e.g., incision, wound retraction) or postoperative (e.g., inflammation) factors that contribute to the central neural changes underlying the enhanced pain.

Recently, studies have been directed at identifying specific intra- and postoperative factors that may contribute to surgically induced postoperative pain and hyperalgesia by comparing the effects on postoperative pain of opiates or local anesthetic agents administered either before or after surgery.[85,87–90] Rice et al.[87] found that the timing of a caudal block with bupivacaine relative to the start of surgery had no effect on postoperative pain in a pediatric population undergoing brief (30 min) ambulatory surgical procedures. Dierking et al.[89] evaluated the effects of a local anesthetic inguinal field block administered before or after inguinal hemiorraphy on postoperative pain and analgesic consumption. They also found that the timing of the block relative to surgical trauma did not produce differences in postoperative pain or analgesic use. Similarly, Dahl et al.[88] reported that postoperative pain and analgesic consumption did not depend on whether a 72-h continuous infusion of epidural bupivacaine and morphine was started before incision or immediately after surgery, approximately 2.5 h later.

In contrast, Ejlersen et al.[90] reported that even though preincisional blockade was not associated with significantly less postoperative pain, fewer patients in the preincisional group, as opposed to a postincisional group, required supplemental postoperative analgesics, and their demand for analgesics was delayed. In addition, Katz et al.[85] demonstrated that preincisional treatment with epidural fentanyl in patients undergoing thoracotomy resulted in significantly lower VAS pain scores 6 h after treatment when compared with a postincisional treatment. The significant difference in pain intensity could not be explained by lingering plasma concentrations of fentanyl, which at the time of pain assessment were equally subtherapeutic in both groups, or by PCA morphine consumption, which until this point was virtually identical in both groups. Also, between 12 and 24 h after surgery, the control group self-administered more than twice the amount of PCA morphine than the experimental group, a finding that parallels the studies by Woolf and Wall.[22,91] Recent studies by Katz and his colleagues[92,93] continue to find small, but consistent effects of pre-emptive analgesia on several types of postsurgical pain.

EXPERIMENTAL EVIDENCE OF CNS PLASTICITY

Damage of peripheral tissue and injury to nerves typically produce persistent pain and hyperalgesia. Recent evidence indicates that hyperalgesia depends, in part, on central sensitization. Hyperalgesia to punctate mechanical stimuli, which develops after intradermal injection of capsaicin, is maintained even after anesthetizing the region where capsaicin was injected.[94] However, if the skin region is anesthetized prior to capsaicin injection, cutaneous hyperalgesia does not develop. Furthermore, hyperalgesic responses to capsaicin can be prevented if the area of skin where the injection is made is rendered anesthetic by a proximal anesthetic block of the peripheral nerve which innervates it. Thus, for hyperalgesia to develop, it is critical that initial inputs from the injury reach the CNS. However, once hyperalgesia is established, it does not need to be maintained by inputs from the injured peripheral tissue.

Further evidence for a central mechanism of hyperalgesia is suggested by clinical and experimental cases of referred pain and hyperalgesia. Referred pain appears to depend on neural mechanisms because local anesthesia of the injured region blocks its expression.[95] Furthermore, the role of central neural mechanisms is supported by the observation that phrenic nerve stimulation causes referred shoulder pain even after the sectioning of all cutaneous nerves from the painful region of the shoulder[96] and by the finding that the injection of hypertonic saline into intraspinous ligaments resulted in pain referred to a phantom arm.[97] It is possible that referred pain depends on the misinterpretation of inputs from an injured region whose axons also branch to the uninjured referred area, or alternatively that axons from the injured and referred regions converge on the same cells in the sensory pathway. If referred pain could be explained exclusively by convergence, then such pains would not provide clear evidence of central sensitization. However, evidence that referred pain is also in part dependent on CNS changes is provided by findings that referred pain and hyperalgesia spread to areas that do not share the same dermatome.[19] For example, it has been shown that pain of cardiac origin is referred to sites as distant as the patient's ear.[98] The fact that pain and hyperalgesia can spread to areas far removed from the injured region implies that central changes, as opposed to convergence, are involved in the spread of hyperalgesia.

Furthermore, referred pain has often been found to spread specifically to sites of a previous injury. Henry and Montuschi[99] describe a case where the pain of an angina attack was referred to the site of an old vertebral fracture. Similarly, Hutchins and Reynolds[31] discovered that alterations in barometric pressure during high-altitude flights caused many of their patients to complain of pain localized to teeth that had been the site of previous painful stimulation (e.g., fillings, canes, and extractions), in many cases years earlier. Reynolds and Hutchins[32] were able to replicate this finding under controlled conditions. One week after damaged teeth were filled or extracted, pinprick of the nasal mucosa produced pain referred to the previously treated teeth. This phenomenon occurred among patients who had been treated under general anesthesia, but not under the influence of a local anesthetic block. Furthermore, in patients who had received bilateral dental treatment without a local anesthetic, subsequent blocks applied to one side permanently abolished the referred pain ipsilateral, but not contralateral, to the anesthetized side.

Behavioral and physiological studies in animals also demonstrate hyperalgesia or sensitization in response to stimulation of body regions that are at a distance from a cutaneous or deep tissue injury. Cutaneous[21] and deep[100] tissue injury, as well as noxious electrical stimulation of cutaneous and muscle afferent nerves,[101] also produces an increase in the excitability of the ipsilateral and contralateral flexor efferent nerves in response to noxious mechanical stimulation of the hind paw. Since the increased excitability in the contralateral flexor efferent nerve is maintained even after inputs from the injured paw are blocked by local anesthesia, the results suggest that central, not peripheral, changes underlie this effect. In this way, cutaneous hyperalgesia after injury may depend on central hypersensitivity which is produced by inputs from a peripheral injury, but does not need to be maintained by them. Behavioral studies indicate that the spread of hyperalgesia to the hind paw contralateral to the paw that received a thermal injury is unaffected by either deafferentation or anesthetic blocks of the injured hind paw following the injury, but is prevented if deafferentation or anesthetic block precedes the injury.[46] These data provide further evidence that peripheral injury can produce central changes that are maintained even after the inputs from the injury are removed.

Prolonged sensory disturbances associated with tissue injury (secondary hyperalgesia and referred pain, as well as allodynia and persistent spontaneous pain) are believed to result from either a reduction in the threshold of nociceptors or an increase in the excitability of CNS neurons involved in pain transmission. Because there is a large body of evidence documenting the sensitization of peripheral receptors following noxious stimulation, a peripheral mechanism is usually held to be responsible for the hyperalgesia that develops after injury. However, recent experimental studies suggest that sensitization within the CNS also contributes significantly to this phenomenon. Specifically, following injury, noxious stimulation, or C-fiber afferent electrical stimulation, there is a sensitization of neurons in the dorsal horn of the spinal cord and other areas in the somatosensory pathway. This sensitization is reflected by increased spontaneous activity, reduced thresholds or increased responsivity to afferent inputs, and prolonged afterdischarges to repeated stimulation.

In addition to the sensitization and prolonged excitation of dorsal horn cells, noxious stimulation associated with tissue injury also produces an expansion of the receptive fields of dorsal horn neurons. Neurons in the dorsal horn of the spinal cord with receptive fields adjacent to a cutaneous heat injury expand their receptive fields to incorporate the site of injury.[102] Similar receptive field expansions have been observed in spinal cord following mechanical, chemical, inflammatory, and nerve injuries, as well as following the induction of polyarthritis and in response to electrical nerve stimulation.[23] Receptive field expansions have also been observed in brain stem and thalamic neurons.

IMPLICATIONS FOR TREATMENT OF ACUTE AND CHRONIC PAIN

Recent advances in our understanding of the mechanisms that underlie pathological pain have important implications for the treatment of both acute and chronic pain. Since it has been established that intense noxious stimulation produces a sensitization of CNS neurons, it is possible to direct treatments not only at the site of peripheral tissue damage, but also at the site of central changes. Furthermore, it may be possible in some instances to prevent the development of central changes which contribute to pathological pain states. The fact that amputees are more likely to develop phantom limb pain if there is pain in the limb prior to amputation,[13] combined with the finding that the incidence of phantom limb pain is reduced if patients are rendered pain-free by epidural blockade with bupivacaine and morphine prior to amputation,[6] suggests that the development of neuropathic pain can be prevented by reducing the potential for central sensitization at the time of amputation. Although the latter finding is contentious,[9,10] the conclusions by Bach *et al.* remain valid.[11,12] The evidence that postoperative pain is also reduced by premedication with regional and/or spinal anesthetic blocks and/or opiates[74,76,85] suggests that acute postoperative pain can also benefit from the blocking of the afferent barrage arriving within the CNS and the central sensitization it may induce.

Whether chronic postoperative problems such as painful scars, postthoracotomy chest-wall pain, and phantom limb and stump pain can be reduced by blocking nociceptive inputs during surgery remains to be determined. Furthermore, additional research is required to determine whether multiple-treatment approaches (involving local and epidural anesthesia, as well as pretreatment with opiates and antiinflammatory drugs) that produce an effective blockade of afferent input may also prevent or relieve other forms of severe chronic pain such as postherpetic neuralgia and reflex sympathetic dystrophy. It is hoped that a combination of new pharmacological developments, careful clinical trials, and an increased understanding of the contribution and mechanisms of noxious stimulus-induced neuroplasticity will lead to improved clinical treatment and prevention of pathological pain. In particular, these improvements in the treatment and prevention of pain may lead to more effective strategies to treat the distressing pains reported by patients with chemical intolerance and multiple chemical sensitivity. Many of these pains may be due, in part at least, to prolonged pathological changes in the nervous system produced by severe trauma and stress. Therapeutic advances in pain relief due to a better understanding of neuroplasticity may lead to improvements in treating this population of patients.

ACKNOWLEDGMENTS

This work was supported by Grant A7891 from the Natural Sciences and Engineering Research Council of Canada to R.M.; Grant MT-11045 from the Medical Research Council (MRC) of Canada and Grant 900051 from Fonds de la Recherche en Santé du Québec to T.J.C.; MRC Scientist Award and Grants MCT-78169 (MRC) and NS 35480 (National Institutes of Health) to J.K.; and Grant DA11839 from the U.S. National Institute on Drug Abuse to A.L.V.

REFERENCES

1. CRONHOLM, B. 1951. Phantom limbs in amputees. Acta Psychiatr. Neurol. Scand. Suppl. **72:** 1–310.
2. DOETSCH, G.S. 1997. Progressive changes in cutaneous trigger zones for sensation referred to a phantom hand: a case report and review with implications for cortical reorganization. Somatosens. Mot. Res. **14:** 6–16.
3. DOETSCH, G.S. 1998. Perceptual significance of somatosensory cortical reorganization following peripheral denervation. NeuroReport **9:** R29–R35.
4. COHEN, L.G., H. TOPKA, R.A. COLE & M. HALLETT. 1991. Leg paresthesias induced by magnetic brain stimulation in patients with thoracic spinal cord injury. Neurology **41:** 1283–1288.
5. LENZ, F.A., H.C. KWAN, R. MARTIN et al. 1994. Characteristics of somatotopic organization and spontaneous neuronal activity in the region of the thalamic principal sensory nucleus in patients with spinal cord transection. J. Neurophysiol. **72:** 1570–1587.
6. BACH, S., M.F. NORENG & N.U. TJELLDEN. 1988. Phantom limb pain in amputees during the first 12 months following limb amputation, after preoperative lumbar epidural blockade. Pain **33:** 297–301.
7. JAHANGIRI, M., J.W.P. BRADLEY, A.P. JAYATUNGA & C.H. DARK. 1994. Prevention of phantom limb pain after major lower limb amputation by epidural infusion of diamorphine, clonidine and bupivacaine. Ann. R. Coll. Surg. **76:** 324–326.
8. SCHUG, S.A., R. BURRELL, J. PAYNE & P. TESTER. 1995. Pre-emptive epidural analgesia may prevent phantom limb pain. Reg. Anesth. **20:** 256.
9. NIKOLAJSEN, L., S. IIKJAER, J.H. CHRISTENSEN et al. 1997. Randomised trial of epidural bupivacaine and morphine in prevention of stump and phantom pain in lower-limb amputation. Lancet **350:** 1353–1357.
10. MCQUAY, H.J., R.A. MOORE & E. KALSO. 1998. Phantom limb pain (correspondence). Lancet **351:** 595.
11. KATZ, J. 1997. Phantom limb pain (commentary). Lancet **350:** 1338–1339.
12. KATZ, J. 1998. Phantom limb pain (correspondence). Lancet **359:** 595.
13. KATZ, J. & R. MELZACK. 1990. Pain "memories" in phantom limbs: review and clinical observations. Pain **43:** 319–336.
14. MELZACK, R. & P.D. WALL. 1996. The Challenge of Pain. Penguin. London.
15. MELZACK, R. & P.D. WALL. 1965. Pain mechanisms: a new theory. Science **150:** 971–979.
16. MACKENZIE, J. 1893. Some points bearing on the association of sensory disorders and visceral diseases. Brain **16:** 321–354.
17. CRILE, G.W. 1913. The kinetic theory of shock and its prevention through anociassociation (shockless operation). Lancet **ii:** 7–16.
18. HARDY, J.D., H.G. WOLFF & H. GOODELL. 1950. Experimental evidence on the nature of cutaneous hyperalgesia. J. Clin. Invest. **29:** 115–140.

19. LIVINGSTON, W.K. 1943. Pain Mechanisms. Macmillan. New York.
20. KENSHALO, D.R., R.B. LEONARD, J.M. CHUNG & W.D. WILLIS. 1982. Facilitation of the responses of primate spinothalamic cells to cold and mechanical stimuli by noxious heating of the skin. Pain **12:** 141–152.
21. WOOLF, C.J. 1983. Evidence for a central component of post-injury pain hypersensitivity. Nature **306:** 686–688.
22. WOOLF, C.J. & P.D. WALL. 1986. Morphine-sensitive and morphine-insensitive actions of C-fibre input on the rat spinal cord. Neurosci. Lett. **64:** 221–225.
23. CODERRE, T.J., J. KATZ, A.L. VACCARINO & R. MELZACK. 1993. Contribution of central neuroplasticity to pathological pain: review of clinical and experimental evidence. Pain **52:** 259–285.
24. CODERRE, T.J., K. FISHER & M.E. FUNDYTUS. 1997. The role of ionotropic and metabotropic glutamate receptors in persistent nociception. In Proceedings of the Eighth World Congress of Pain. IASP Press. Seattle, WA.
25. JENSEN, T.S., B. KREBS, J. NIELSEN & P. RASMUSSEN. 1985. Immediate and long-term phantom pain in amputees: incidence, clinical characteristics and relationship to preamputation pain. Pain **21:** 267–278.
26. JENSEN, T.S. & P. RASMUSSEN. 1994. Phantom pain and related phenomena after amputation. In Textbook of Pain, pp. 508–521. Livingstone/Churchill. Edinburgh.
27. BERGER, M. & F. GERSTENBRAND. 1981. Phantom illusions in spinal cord lesions. In Phantom and Stump Pain, pp. 66–73. Springer. Berlin.
28. NATHAN, P.W. 1985. Pain and nociception in the clinical contex. Philos. Trans. R. Soc. Lond. **308:** 219–226.
29. WALLGREN, G.R. 1954. Phantom experience at spinal anaesthesia. Ann. Chir. Gynaecol. Fenniae **43**(suppl.): 486–500.
30. KRONER, K., B. KREBS, J. SKOV & H.S. JORGENSEN. 1989. Immediate and long-term breast syndrome after mastectomy: incidence, clinical characteristics and relationship to pre-mastectomy breast pain. Pain **36:** 327–337.
31. HUTCHINS, H.C. & O.E. REYNOLDS. 1947. Experimental investigation of the referred pain of aerodontalgia. J. Dent. Res. **26:** 3–8.
32. REYNOLDS, O.E. & H.C. HUTCHINS. 1948. Reduction of central hyper-irritability following block anesthesia of peripheral nerve. Am. J. Physiol. **152:** 658–662.
33. SZASZ, T.S. 1949. Psychiatric aspects of vagotomy: IV. Phantom ulcer pain. Arch. Neurol. Psychiatry **62:** 728–733.
34. GLOYNE, H.F. 1954. Psychosomatic aspects of pain. Psychoanal. Rev. **41:** 135–159.
35. DORPAT, T.L. 1971. Phantom sensations of internal organs. Comp. Psychiatry **12:** 7–35.
36. OVESEN, P., K. KRONER, J. OMSHOLT & K. BACH. 1991. Phantom-related phenomena after rectal amputation: prevalence and clinical characteristics. Pain **44:** 289–291.
37. BRENA, S.F. & E.E. SAMMONS. 1979. Phantom urinary bladder pain—case report. Pain **7:** 197–201.
38. MINSKI, L. 1943. Psychological reactions to injury. In Rehabilitation of the War Injured, pp. 115–122. Philosophical Library. New York.
39. LERICHE, R. 1947. A propos des algies des amputees. Mem. Acad. Chir. **73:** 280–284.
40. NATHAN, P.W. 1962. Pain traces left in the central nervous system. In The Assessment of Pain in Man and Animals, pp. 129–134. Livingstone. Edinburgh.
41. NOORDENBOS, W. & P.D. WALL. 1981. Implications of the failure of nerve resection and graft to cure chronic pain produced by nerve lesions. J. Neurol. Neurosurg. Psychiatry **44:** 1068–1073.
42. WALL, P.D., J.W. SCADDING & M.M. TORNKIEWICZ. 1979. The production and prevention of experimental anesthesia dolorosa. Pain **6:** 179–182.
43. BLUMENKOPF, B. & J.J. LIPMAN. 1991. Studies in autotomy: its pathophysiology and usefulness as a model of chronic pain. Pain **45:** 203–210.
44. DENNIS, S.G. & R. MELZACK. 1979. Self-mutilation after dorsal rhizotomy in rats: effects of prior pain and pattern of root lesions. Exp. Neurol. **65:** 412–421.
45. CODERRE, T.J., R.W. GRIMES & R. MELZACK. 1986. Autotomy after nerve sections in the rat is influenced by tonic descending inhibition from locus coeruleus. Neurosci. Lett. **67:** 82–85.

46. CODERRE, T.J. & R. MELZACK. 1987. Cutaneous hyperalgesia: contributions of the peripheral and central nervous systems to the increase in pain sensitivity after injury. Brain Res. **404:** 95–106.
47. KATZ, J., A.L. VACCARINO, T.J. CODERRE & R. MELZACK. 1991. Injury prior to neurectomy alters the pattern of autonomy in rats: behavioral evidence of central neural plasticity. Anesthesiology **75:** 876–883.
48. SELTZER, Z., B.Z. BEILIN, R. GINZBURG et al. 1991. The role of injury discharge in the induction of neuropathic pain behavior in rats. Pain **46:** 327–336.
49. MARKUS, H., B. POMERANZ & D. KRUSHELNYCKY. 1984. Spread of saphaneous somatotopic projection map in spinal cord and hypersensitivity of the foot after chronic sciatic denervation in adult rat. Brain Res. **296:** 27–39.
50. WALL, P.D. & M. GUTNIK. 1974. Properties of afferent nerve impulses originating from a neuroma. Nature **248:** 740–743.
51. WALL, P.D. & M. DEVOR. 1983. Sensory afferent impulses originate from the dorsal root ganglia as well as from the periphery in normal and nerve injured rats. Pain **17:** 321–339.
52. ASADA, H., W. YASURNO & Y. YAMAGUCHI. 1990. Properties of hyperactive cells in rat spinal cord after peripheral nerve section. Pain Suppl. **5:** S22.
53. BASBAUM, A.I. & P.D. WALL. 1976. Chronic changes in the response of cells in adult cat dorsal horn following partial de-afferentation: the appearance of responding cells in a previously non-responsive region. Brain Res. **116:** 181–204.
54. MACON, J.B. 1979. Deafferentation hyperactivity in the monkey spinal trigeminal nucleus: neuronal responses to amino acid iontophoresis. Brain Res. **161:** 549–554.
55. ALBE–FESSARD, D. & M.C. LOMBARD. 1983. Use of an animal model to evaluate the origin of and protection against deafferentation pain. In Advances in Pain Research and Therapy. Vol. 5, pp. 691–700. Raven Press. New York.
56. LENZ, F.A., H.C. KWAN, J.O. DOSTROVSKY & R.R. TASKER. 1989. Characteristics of the bursting pattern of action potential that occurs in the thalamus of patients with central pain. Brain Res. **496:** 357–360.
57. RINALDI, P.C., R.F. YOUNG, D. ALBE-FESSARD & J. CHODAKIEWITZ. 1991. Spontaneous neuronal hyperactivity in the medial and intralaminar thalamic nuclei of patients with deafferentation pain. J. Neurosurg. **74:** 415–421.
58. LENZ, F.A., R.R. TASKER, J.O. DOSTROVSKY, et al. 1987. Abnormal single-unit activity recorded in the somatosensory thalamus of a quadriplegic patient with central pain. Pain **31:** 225–236.
59. TASKER, R.R. 1989. Stereotactic surgery. In Textbook of Pain, pp. 840–855. Livingstone/Churchill. Edinburgh.
60. WALL, P.D. & M. DEVOR. 1981. The effect of peripheral nerve injury on dorsal root potentials and on transmission of afferent signals into the spinal cord. Brain Res. **209:** 95–111.
61. WOOLF, C.J. & P.D. WALL. 1982. Chronic peripheral nerve section diminishes the primary afferent A–fibre mediated inhibition of rat dorsal horn neurons. Brain Res. **242:** 77–85.
62. SEGAL, M. & D. SANDBERG. 1977. Analgesia produced by electrical stimulation of catecholamine nuclei in the rat brain. Brain Res. **123:** 369–372.
63. OLIVERAS, J.L., G. GUILBAUD & J.M. BESSON. 1979. A map of serotonergic structures involved in stimulation produced analgesia in unrestrained freely moving cats. Brain Res. **164:** 317–322.
64. HODGE, C.J., A.V. APKARIAN, M.P. OWEN & B.S. HANSON. 1983. Changes in the effects of stimulation of locus coeruleus and nucleus raphe magnus following dorsal rhizotomy. Brain Res. **288:** 325–329.
65. DOUGHERTY, P.M., C.J. GARRISON & S.M. CARLTON. 1992. Differential influence of local anesthesia upon two models of experimentally induced peripheral mononeuropathy in rat. Brain Res. **570:** 109–115.
66. DUBUISSON, D. & S.G. DENNIS. 1977. The formalin test: a quantitative study of the analgesic effects of morphine, meperidine, and brain stimulation in rats and cats. Pain **4:** 161–174.

67. DICKENSON, A.H. & A.F. SULLIVAN. 1987. Evidence for a role of the NMDA receptor in the frequency dependent potentiation of deep rat dorsal horn nociceptive neurones following C fibre stimulation. Neuropharmacology **26**: 1235–1238.
68. DICKENSON, A.H. & A.F. SULLIVAN. 1987. Subcutaneous formalin-induced activity of dorsal horn neurons in the rat: differential response to an intrathecal opiate administration pre or post formalin. Pain **30**: 349–360.
69. CODERRE, T.J., A.L. VACCARINO & R. MELZACK. 1990. Central nervous system plasticity in the tonic pain response to subcutaneous formalin injection. Brain Res. **535**: 155–158.
70. VACCARINO, A.L. & R. MELZACK. 1992. Temporal processes of formalin pain: differential role of the cingulum bundle, fornix pathway and medial bulboreticular formation. Pain **44**: 257–271.
71. VINOGRADOVA, S. 1975. Functional organization of the limbic system in the process of registration of information: facts and hypothesis. *In* The Hippocampus. Vol. 2, pp. 3–69. Plenum. New York.
72. PARE, D., M. STERIADE, M. DESCHENES & D. BOUHASSIRA. 1990. Prolonged enhancement of anterior thalamic synaptic responsiveness by stimulation of a brain-stem cholinergic group. J. Neurosci. **10**: 20–33.
73. SINCLAIR, J.G. & G.F. LO. 1986. Morphine, but not atropine, blocks nociceptor-driven activity in rat dorsal hippocampal neurones. Neurosci. Lett. **68**: 47–50.
74. McQUAY, H.J., D. CARROLL & R.A. MOORE. 1988. Post-operative orthopaedic pain—the effect of opiate premedication and local anaesthetic blocks. Pain **33**: 291–295.
75. KISS, I.E. & M. KILIAN. 1992. Does opiate premedication influence postoperative analgesia? A prospective study. Pain **48**: 157–158.
76. TVERSKOY, M., C. COZACOV, M. AYACHE *et al*. 1990. Postoperative pain after inguinal hemiorraphy with different types of anesthesia. Anesth. Analg. **70**: 29–35.
77. TUFFIN, J.R., D.R. CUNLIFFE & S.R. SHAW. 1989. Do local analgesics injected at the time of third molar removal under general anesthesia reduce significantly postoperative analgesic requirements? A double-blind controlled trial. Br. J. Oral Max. Surg. **27**: 27–32.
78. HUTCHISON, G.L., S.L. CROFTS & I.G. GRAY. 1990. Preoperative piroxicam for postoperative analgesia in dental surgery. Br. J. Anaesth. **65**: 500–503.
79. CAMPBELL, W.L., R. KENDRICK & C. PATTERSON. 1990. Intravenous diclofenac sodium: does its administration before operation suppress postoperative pain? Anaesthesia **45**: 763–766.
80. JEBELES, J.A., J.S. REILLY, J.F. GUITIERREZ, E.L. BRADLEY & I. KISSIN. 1991. The effect of pre-incisional infiltration of tonsils with bupivacaine on the pain following tonsilectomy under general anesthesia. Pain **47**: 305–308.
81. MOGENSEN, T., J. BARTHOLDY, K. SPERLING *et al*. 1992. Preoperative infiltration of the incisional area enhances postoperative analgesia to a combined low-dose epidural bupivacaine and morphine regime after upper abdominal surgery. Reg. Anesth. **17**(suppl.): 74.
82. RINGROSE, N.H. & M.J. CROSS. 1984. Femoral nerve block in knee joint surgery. Am. J. Sports Med. **12**: 398–402.
83. McGLEW, I.C., D.B. ANGLISS, G.J. GEE *et al*. 1991. A comparison of rectal indomethacin with placebo for pain relief following spinal surgery. Anaesth. Int. Care **19**: 40–45.
84. MANN, R.A.M. & W.I.K. BISSET. 1983. Anaesthesia for lower limb amputation: a comparison of spinal analgesia and general anaesthesia in the elderly. Anaesthesia **38**: 1185–1191.
85. KATZ, J., B.P. KAVANAGH, A.N. SANDLER *et al*. 1992. Pre-emptive analgesia: clinical evidence of neuroplasticity contributing to postoperative pain. Anesthesiology **77**: 439–446.
86. McQUAY, H.J. 1992. Pre-emptive analgesia. Br. J. Anaesth. **69**: 1–3.
87. RICE, L.J., M.A. PUDIMAT & R.S. HANNALLAH. 1990. Timing of caudal block placement in relation to surgery does not affect duration of postoperative analgesia in paediatric ambulatory patients. Can. J. Anaesth. **37**: 429–431.

88. DAHL, J.B., B.L. HANSEN, N.C. HJORTSO *et al.* 1992. Influence of timing on the effect of continuous extradural analgesia with bupivacaine and morphine after major abdominal surgery. Br. J. Anaesth. **69:** 4–8.
89. DIERKING, G.W., J.B. DAHL, J. KANSTRUP *et al.* 1992. Effect of pre- vs. postoperative inguinal field block on postoperative pain after hemiorraphy. Br. J. Anaesth. **68:** 344–348.
90. EJLERSEN, E., H. BRYDE-ANDERSON, K. ELIASEN & T. MOGENSEN. 1992. A comparison between preincisional and postincisional lidocaine infiltration and postoperative pain. Anesth. Analg. **74:** 495–498.
91. WOOLF, C.J. & P.D. WALL. 1986. Relative effectiveness of C primary afferent fibers of different origins in evoking a prolonged facilitation of the flexion reflex in the rat. J. Neurosci. **6:** 1433–1442.
92. KATZ, J., M. CLAIREUX, B.P. KAVANAGH *et al.* 1994. Pre-emptive lumbar epidural anaesthesia reduces postoperative pain and patient-controlled morphine consumption after lower abdominal surgery. Pain **59:** 395–403.
93. KATZ, J., M. JACKSON, B.P. KAVANAUGH & A.N. SANDLER. 1996. Acute pain after thoracic surgery predicts long-term post-thoractomy pain. Clin. J. Pain **12:** 50–55.
94. LAMOTTE, R.H., C.N. SHAIN, D.A. SIMONE & E.F.P. TSAI. 1991. Neurogenic hyperalgesia: psychophysical studies of underlying mechanisms. J. Neurophysiol. **66:** 190–211.
95. ROBERTSON, S., H. GOODELL & H.G. WOLFF. 1947. Headache: the teeth as a source of headache and other head pain. Arch. Neurol. Psychiatry **57:** 277–291.
96. DORAN, F.S.A. & A.H. RATCLIFFE. 1954. The physiological mechanism of referred shoulder-tip pain. Brain **77:** 427–434.
97. HARMAN, J.B. 1984. The localization of deep pain. Br. Med. J. **1:** 188.
98. BRYLIN, M. & B. HINDFELT. 1984. Ear pain due to myocardial ischemia. Am. Heart J. **107:** 186–187.
99. HENRY, J.A. & E. MONTUSCHI. 1978. Cardiac pain referred to site of previously experienced somatic pain. Br. Med. J. **2:** 1605–1606.
100. WOOLF, C.J. & S.B. MCMAHON. 1985. Injury-induced plasticity of the flexor reflex in chronic decerebrate rats. Neuroscience **16:** 395–404.
101. WALL, P.D. & C.J. WOOLF. 1984. Muscle but not cutaneous C-afferent input produces prolonged increases in the excitability of the flexion reflex in the rat. J. Physiol. (Lond.) **356:** 443–458.
102. MCMAHON, S.B. & P.D. WALL. 1984. Receptive fields of rat lamina I projection cells move to incorporate a nearby region of injury. Pain **19:** 235–247.

Spinal Cord Neuroplasticity following Repeated Opioid Exposure and Its Relation to Pathological Pain

JIANREN MAO[a,b] AND DAVID J. MAYER[c]

[b]MGH Pain Center, Department of Anesthesia and Critical Care, Massachusetts General Hospital, Harvard Medical School, Boston, Massachusetts 02114, USA

[c]Department of Anesthesiology, Medical College of Virginia, Virginia Commonwealth University, Richmond, Virginia 23298, USA

> ABSTRACT: Convincing evidence has accumulated that indicates neuroplastic changes within the spinal cord in response to repeated exposure to opioids. Such neuroplastic changes occur at both cellular and intracellular levels. It has been generally acknowledged that the activation of N-methyl-D-aspartate (NMDA) receptors plays a pivotal role in the development of neuroplastic changes following repeated opioid exposure. Intracellular cascades can also be activated subsequent to NMDA receptor activation. In particular, protein kinase C has been shown to be a key intracellular element that contributes to the behavioral manifestation of neuroplastic changes. Moreover, interactions between NMDA and opioid receptors can lead to potentially irreversible degenerative neuronal changes in the spinal cord in association with the development of opioid tolerance. Interestingly, similar cellular and intracellular changes occur in the spinal cord following peripheral nerve injury. These findings indicate that interactions exist in the spinal cord neural structures between two seemingly unrelated conditions—chronic opioid exposure and a pathological pain state. These observations may help understand mechanisms of chemical intolerance and multiple chemical sensitivity as well as have significant clinical implications in pain management with opioid analgesics.

Over the last several years, studies from both our laboratory and others have shown a critical role of the N-methyl-D-aspartate (NMDA) receptor in the development of neuronal plastic changes within the spinal cord following repeated exposure to opioids. We have recently shown that repeated exposure to opioids can also initiate intracellular cascades including protein kinase C (PKC) translocation and activation and nitric oxide (NO)–activated poly(ADP-ribose) synthetase (PARS) activation. Similar cellular mechanisms have been implicated in neuropathic pain resulting from chronic constriction injury (CCI) of the rat's common sciatic nerve. Of particular interest is that morphological changes in the spinal cord dorsal horn, the development of so-called dark neurons, are associated with both repeated morphine

---

[a]Address for correspondence: Jianren Mao, MGH Pain Center, Department of Anesthesia and Critical Care, Massachusetts General Hospital, Harvard Medical School, 15 Parkman Street, Suite WACC 324, Boston, MA 02114.

exposure and CCI. In this article, we will summarize these recent observations from our laboratory to indicate that spinal cord neuroplastic changes are the basis for the interactions between repeated opioid exposure and CCI. Clinical implications of such interactions and their possible relation to chemical intolerance and multiple chemical sensitivity also will be discussed.

SPINAL CORD NEUROPLASTIC CHANGES FOLLOWING REPEATED EXPOSURE TO MORPHINE

Convincing evidence indicates that NMDA receptors can be activated after repeated exposure to morphine. The activation of NMDA receptors, in turn, leads to the initiation of intracellular cascades including translocation and activation of PKC. Activation of both NMDA receptors and PKC has been shown to underlie behavioral manifestations (e.g., the development of tolerance) of interactions between NMDA and opioid receptors. In addition, morphological changes of spinal cord dorsal horn neurons, in the form of so-called dark neurons, occur as a consequence of interactions between NMDA and opioid receptors. Importantly, the formation of dark neurons can be reduced by the inhibition of NO-activated PARS.

Role of NMDA Receptors

Activation of NMDA receptors within the spinal cord has been shown to play a crucial role in the development of tolerance to the analgesic effects of morphine. Tolerance is pharmacologically defined as reduced potency of the analgesic effects of morphine following its repeated administration. Coadministration of morphine with MK-801, a noncompetitive NMDA receptor antagonist, effectively prevents the development of morphine tolerance in several animal models including rats, mice, and guinea pigs.[1–5] In addition to its preventive effects on the development of morphine tolerance, the use of LY274614, a competitive NMDA receptor antagonist, also gradually (over several days) reverses tolerance to the antinociceptive effects of morphine when repeatedly given to mice rendered tolerant to morphine.[6] However, it is important to note that, unlike the reversal of hyperalgesia by a single dose of MK-801,[7] a single treatment with either MK-801[1] or LY274614[6] is ineffective in reestablishing antinociceptive effects of morphine in morphine-tolerant animals.

The spinal cord has been suggested to be a site of this NMDA receptor action since spinalization (anatomic disconnection between the spinal cord and supraspinal regions) does not stop systemic MK-801 from preventing the development of morphine tolerance.[8] Additional evidence for a spinal site of action of NMDA receptor antagonists is that intrathecal MK-801 reduces the development of tolerance induced by repeated intrathecal morphine administration in a manner similar to that seen with systemic MK-801 treatment.[9] Furthermore, MK-801 is effective for preventing antinociceptive tolerance to the highly selective μ-opioid antagonist DAMGO.[10] Thus, it is clear that NMDA receptor activation within the spinal cord plays an important role in the development of morphine tolerance.

It is of interest to note that dextromethorphan, an antitussive drug and NMDA receptor antagonist, also has been shown to be effective in preventing the development of opioid tolerance.[11,12] In a rat model of morphine tolerance, dextromethorphan prevented or diminished the development of tolerance to the antinociceptive effects of morphine (15, 24, or 32 mg/kg) when dextromethorphan was coadministered orally with morphine (ratios from 4:1 to 1:2). This combined oral treatment regimen also reduced at least one sign (teeth chattering, wet-dog shaking, or jumping) of naloxone-precipitated physical dependence on morphine in the same rats. The data reveal a constant ratio range of the morphine/dextromethorphan combination effective for preventing the development of morphine tolerance and dependence.[12] These results indicate that combined treatment with clinically available NMDA receptor antagonists and morphine may be a useful approach for preventing morphine tolerance and dependence in humans.

Role of PKC

A growing body of evidence indicates an important role of protein kinases, particularly PKC, in the development of antinociceptive tolerance.[13–17] It has been shown that intrathecal administration of GM1 ganglioside, a reported inhibitor for PKC translocation from cytoplasm to cell membrane, attenuates the development of tolerance to the antinociceptive effects of morphine in rats.[15] In addition, spinal cord levels of membrane-bound PKC increase reliably as morphine tolerance develops.[15] This increase in membrane-bound PKC occurs mainly within laminae I–II of the spinal cord dorsal horn, a region similar to the one showing increased levels of PKC translocation in nerve-injured animals with demonstrable thermal hyperalgesia.[18,19] In addition, this tolerance-associated increase in membrane-bound PKC can be reduced by intrathecal treatment with GM1 ganglioside.[15]

Independent verification of these results was provided by a recent study utilizing an immunocytochemical method. In this study, the development of morphine tolerance was shown to be associated with increases in immunoreactivity of a specific PKC isoform (PKCγ) in laminae I–II dorsal horn neurons.[20] Such increases in PKCγ immunoreactivity along with behavioral manifestations of morphine tolerance could be prevented by intrathecal administration of the noncompetitive NMDA receptor antagonist MK-801.[20] Increases in PKCγ immunoreactivity in similar spinal cord dorsal horn regions also were seen in rats with nerve injury–induced thermal hyperalgesia (see below), further suggesting the involvement of common regions of the spinal cord dorsal horn in mechanisms of hyperalgesia and morphine tolerance. These results indicate clear associations of PKC translocation/activation and behavioral manifestations of morphine tolerance. It is important to point out that activation of NMDA receptors and subsequent intracellular PKC within the spinal cord, as discussed above, reflects spinal cord neuroplastic changes following repeated exposure to opioids since spinal cord PKC levels do not differ from saline controls following a single injection of morphine.[20] Moreover, such neuroplastic changes occur as a result of interactions between spinal cord opioid and NMDA receptors because, thus far, there is no evidence that NMDA receptors can be activated directly by opioid receptor antagonists.[21]

Evidence for Spinal Cord Neuronal Degenerative Changes

A serious consequence of opioid and NMDA receptor interactions is the formation of so-called dark neurons, a form of degenerative neuronal changes that are observed in the spinal cord dorsal horn following peripheral nerve injury.[22,23] In a rat model of morphine tolerance,[24] rats that were made tolerant to morphine exhibited a reliable increase in the number of dark neurons in the dorsal horn of the lumbar spinal cord. Several features characterized this increase in dark neurons. Dark neurons were primarily located in laminae I–II and to a much lesser degree in laminae III–IV. Also, there was no statistical difference in the number of dark neurons observed on the left and right sides of the spinal cord. Importantly, the development of dark neurons following repeated exposure to opioids was reliably reduced by the selective PARS inhibitor benzamide in the same experiment. The specificity of PARS inhibition was confirmed by utilizing other PARS inhibitors, including 3-aminobenzamide and niacinamide (nicotinamide). Moreover, the development of tolerance and dark neurons in morphine-treated rats is associated with the activation of opioid receptors because the coadministration of the opioid receptor antagonist, naltrexone, and morphine reliably prevented both the development of the antinociceptive tolerance as well as the increase in dark neurons as compared to the morphine plus saline controls.[24]

The major findings of this series of studies are as follows: (a) the incidence of dark neurons increased significantly within the spinal cord dorsal horn, particularly the superficial laminae I–II, of rats injected daily for 8 days with intrathecal morphine; (b) benzamide and other PARS inhibitors reduced or prevented the development of analgesic tolerance and dark neurons; and (c) the development of dark neurons after repeated morphine injection is opioid receptor–mediated because concurrent administration of naltrexone with morphine prevents the development of dark neurons. These studies demonstrate that *in vivo* administration of morphine for 8 days produces dark neurons similar in morphology and location to transsynaptic alterations resulting from CCI of the sciatic nerve.[25] Importantly, the morphological characteristics of these cells are consistent with those of cells undergoing programmed cell death (apoptosis). Thus, opioid and NMDA receptor interactions could lead to potentially irreversible neuronal changes within the spinal cord dorsal horn.

SPINAL CORD NEUROPLASTIC CHANGES FOLLOWING PATHOLOGICAL PAIN

It has been generally acknowledged that nerve injury–induced sensitization of primary afferent nociceptive neurons accompanies and is a contributing cause of pathological pain states. Recently, it has become evident that tissue injury and inflammation are also followed by increased responsiveness of nociceptive neurons within the spinal cord and other regions of the central nervous system (CNS). Studies on the neural basis of such central changes have also indicated a crucial role of NMDA receptors and related intracellular neurochemical consequences in the development and maintenance of injury-induced central hyperactive states, a form of CNS neuronal plasticity that may well underlie behavioral manifestations of hyperalgesia, allodynia, and spontaneous pain.[19,26,27] Interestingly, recent investigations have indicated that synaptic and intracellular events similar to those that follow repeated opioid exposure occur during the development of injury-induced hyperalgesia. Moreover, the same spinal cord locus has been shown to be involved in neuroplasticity associated with repeated opioid exposure and hyperalgesia (a pathological pain state).

Role of NMDA Receptors

Compelling evidence indicates that activation of spinal cord NMDA receptors contributes to the hyperalgesia that occurs following peripheral nerve injury or inflammation. Systemic (intraperitoneal) or spinal cord (intrathecal) administration of either competitive (e.g., AP-5) or noncompetitive (e.g., MK-801) NMDA receptor antagonists reduces thermal hyperalgesia in CCI rats.[7,28–31] In addition, systemic treatment with MK-801 at 1 hour prior to and continuously (once daily for 3 days) after nerve injury also *prevents* the development and expression of thermal hyperalgesia, an effect that lasts up to 12 days after the discontinuation of MK-801 treatment in CCI rats.[7] On the other hand, intrathecal administration of NMDA (an NMDA receptor agonist) in rats produces thermal hyperalgesia similar to that induced by peripheral heat injury.[32,33] Studies using electrophysiological techniques have also demonstrated the NMDA-mediated enhancement of spinothalamic neuron responses to mechanical, thermal, and electrical stimuli.[34] These data strongly indicate that spinal cord activation of the NMDA receptor in response to peripheral tissue injury and inflammation is critical for both the development and maintenance of a pathological pain state.

Role of PKC

Similar to PKC changes following repeated exposure to opioids, PKC has been implicated in spinal cord mechanisms of pathological pain states. GM1 ganglioside, a reported intracellular inhibitor of PKC translocation and activation in both *in vivo* and *in vitro* studies, attenuates thermal hyperalgesia induced by CCI.[19,35–37] More direct evidence for a role of PKC translocation in thermal hyperalgesia is derived from a series of experiments utilizing the CCI model.[19,36] In these experiments, changes in membrane-bound PKC (translocated PKC) were assessed by employing the [^{3}H]-phorbol-12,13-dibutyrate ([^{3}H]PDBu) autoradiographic assay that measures primarily membrane-bound PKC. Concurrent with thermal hyperalgesia and spontaneous pain-related behaviors (such as lifting of the nerve-ligated hind paw) induced by CCI, CCI rats with sciatica displayed a pattern of increased membrane-bound PKC in the lumbar spinal cord in comparison to that of sham-operated rats. Reliable increases in membrane-bound PKC occurred in spinal cord dorsal horn laminae I–VI, with the greatest increase in the superficial laminae I–II. The level of this increase in spinal cord membrane-bound PKC was positively correlated with the degree of thermal hyperalgesia and spontaneous pain-related behaviors in CCI rats. Furthermore, both increases in spinal cord membrane-bound PKC and the development of nociceptive behaviors following nerve injury were prevented by once daily intrathecal treatment with GM1 ganglioside for 3 days.[19] In addition, the spinal cord PKCγ level also increases following CCI.[38] These results suggest a close relationship between PKC translocation and a pathological pain state resulting from CCI.

Evidence for Spinal Cord Neuronal Degenerative Changes

Transsynaptic alteration of spinal cord dorsal horn neurons characterized by hyperchromatosis of cytoplasm and nucleoplasm (dark neurons) occurs following CCI.[25] The incidence of dark neurons in CCI rats has been proposed to be mediated by NMDA receptor-mediated neurotoxicity. In CCI rats, dark neurons were observed bilaterally (with ipsilateral predominance) within the spinal cord dorsal horn, particularly in laminae I–II, of rats at 8 days after unilateral sciatic nerve ligation as compared to sham-operated rats. The number of dark neurons in the dorsal horn was dose-dependently reduced in CCI rats receiving once daily intrathecal treatment with the PARS inhibitor benzamide for 7 days. Consistent with the histological improvement, thermal hyperalgesia, mechanical hyperalgesia, and low threshold mechano-allodynia also were reliably reduced in CCI rats treated with benzamide. Neither dark neurons nor neuropathic pain behaviors were reliably affected by intrathecal administration of either novobiocin [a mono(ADP-ribose) synthetase] or benzoic acid (the backbone structure of benzamide), indicating a selective effect of benzamide. Intrathecal treatment with an NO synthase inhibitor N^G-nitro-L-arginine methyl ester (40 nmol, but not its inactive D-isomer) utilizing the same benzamide treatment regimen resulted in similar reductions of both dark neurons and neuropathic pain behaviors in CCI rats.[25] These results provide *in vivo* evidence indicating that benzamide is neuroprotective and that the PARS-mediated transsynaptic alteration of spinal cord dorsal horn neurons contributes to behavioral manifestations of neuropathic pain in CCI rats.

INTERACTIONS BETWEEN NEUROPLASTIC CHANGES FOLLOWING REPEATED OPIOID EXPOSURE AND PATHOLOGICAL PAIN

As discussed above, cellular and intracellular changes occur within the rat's spinal cord following repeated exposure to opioids and pathological pain. Under both circumstances, the NMDA receptor can be activated with a subsequent activation of intracellular PKC and PARS. The PARS activation is likely to contribute to degenerative neuronal changes (dark neurons) within the spinal cord. Several lines of evidence summarized above suggest that these cellular and intracellular changes are the neural basis of spinal cord neuronal plasticity responsible for the behavioral manifestation of opioid tolerance and hyperalgesia. Since these changes occur at the same spinal cord loci, it is possible that interaction may occur between changes following repeated opioid exposure and a pathological pain state. Thus, these studies suggest that opioids may exacerbate the excitotoxicity underlying at least certain types of neuropathic pain. A corollary of this is that the excitotoxicity from neuropathic pain may, under some circumstances, reduce the response to opioids. Indeed, evidence from animal studies exists that supports such a hypothesis.[39]

First, since NMDA receptors are critical for the development of both hyperalgesia and μ-opioid tolerance, conditions such as nerve injury leading to the development of hyperalgesia have been shown to decrease the antinociceptive effectiveness of opioids in the absence of repeated exposure to opioids.[40–42] The reduced opioid analgesia mimics pharmacological tolerance, thereby significantly hampering the ability of opioids to treat pathophysiological pains. Second, since repeated exposure to opioids, a process leading to the development of pharmacological tolerance, involves activation of NMDA receptors, NMDA receptor-mediated hyperalgesia does indeed occur in association with the development of μ-opioid tolerance,[9] further reducing the effectiveness of opioid analgesics. Thus, interactions between opioid and NMDA receptors play a significant role in neuroplastic changes following repeated opioid exposure and pathological pain. Mechanisms of such interactions remain poorly understood. A working hypothesis has been discussed in our previous articles.[9,39,40]

The interactions between neuroplastic changes following repeated opioid exposure and pathological pain clearly have clinical implications. For example, it is a common clinical experience that opioids are less effective and often unreliable for treating pathological pain such as neuropathic pain from peripheral nerve injury. It is conceivable that the diversity of clinical response patterns to opiate treatment in neuropathic pain patients may result from varying degrees of CNS neuronal plastic changes initiated by peripheral nerve injury. Such neuronal plastic changes may underlie the development of neuropathic pain syndromes and also may result in a reduction of the antinociceptive effects of opiates.

RELATION TO MECHANISMS OF CHEMICAL INTOLERANCE AND MULTIPLE CHEMICAL SENSITIVITY

Multiple chemical sensitivity (MCS) is a polysymptomatic phenomenon in which subjects with MCS present with multiple symptoms in response to often low levels of different chemical agents (chemical intolerance, CI).[43,44] A characteristic feature of MCS is that these subjects can be sensitive not only to those preexposed chemical agents, but also to chemical agents without preexposure. This would suggest that central neural plasticity may have occurred following a previous exposure to certain agents. More importantly, such neuroplastic changes could become the neurobiological basis for cross-reaction to other unrelated chemical agents. Current theories of MCS and CI have been discussed in several comprehensive reviews.[43,44] The data summarized in this article may provide further insights into mechanisms of MCS and CI. Our studies, as well as others, suggest that interactions of spinal cord neuroplasticity can occur between two seemingly unrelated conditions—repeated opioid exposure and a pathological pain state. In this regard, the spinal cord neural plasticity resulting from a pathological pain state could affect the response to a chemical agent such as morphine via cellular and intracellular interactions. Importantly, such neuroplastic changes may persist for a long time if the initial impact leads to potentially irreversible changes (e.g., dark neurons) in neural structures within the spinal cord.

Future studies may be directed to investigate the time course of interactions between neural plastic changes resulting from different impacts (chemical versus nonchemical). Further, it would be of particular interest to elucidate cellular and intracellular mechanisms of MCS and CI in order to prevent the development of neural plastic changes under different circumstances. For instance, our studies indicate that long-term neural plastic changes from either repeated opioid exposure or a pathological pain state may be prevented by blocking key elements of cellular (NMDA receptors) and intracellular (PKC, PARS) responses. Such studies should provide insights into clinical management of individuals with MCS and CI.

ACKNOWLEDGMENTS

This work was partially supported by NIH Grant No. DA08835.

REFERENCES

1. TRUJILLO, K.A. & H. AKIL. 1991. Inhibition of morphine tolerance and dependence by the NMDA receptor antagonist MK-801. Science **251:** 85–87.
2. TANGANELLI, S., T. ANTONELLI, M. MORARI et al. 1991. Glutamate antagonists prevent morphine withdrawal in mice and guinea pigs. Neurosci. Lett. **122:** 270–272.
3. MAREK, P., S. BEN ELIYAHU, A.L. VACCARINO & J.C. LIEBESKIND. 1991. Delayed application of MK-801 attenuates development of morphine tolerance in rats. Brain Res. **558:** 163–165.
4. MAREK, P., S. BEN ELIYAHU, M. GOLD & J.C. LIEBESKIND. 1991. Excitatory amino acid antagonists (kynurenic acid and MK-801) attenuate the development of morphine tolerance in the rat. Brain Res. **547:** 77–81.
5. BEN ELIYAHU, S., P. MAREK, A.L. VACCARINO et al. 1992. The NMDA receptor antagonist MK-801 prevents long-lasting non-associative morphine tolerance in the rat. Brain Res. **575:** 304–308.
6. TISEO, P.J. & C.E. INTURRISI. 1993. Attenuation and reversal of morphine tolerance by the competitive N-methyl-D-aspartate receptor antagonist, LY274614. J. Pharmacol. Exp. Ther. **264:** 1090–1096.
7. MAO, J., D.D. PRICE, D.J. MAYER et al. 1992. Intrathecal MK-801 and local nerve anesthesia synergistically reduce nociceptive behaviors in rats with experimental peripheral mononeuropathy. Brain Res. **576:** 254–262.
8. GUTSTEIN, H.B., K.A. TRUJILLO & H. AKIL. 1992. MK 801 inhibits the development of morphine tolerance in the rat at spinal sites (abstract). Brain Res. **626:** 332–334.
9. MAO, J., D.D. PRICE & D.J. MAYER. 1994. Thermal hyperalgesia in association with the development of morphine tolerance in rats: roles of excitatory amino acid receptors and protein kinase C. J. Neurosci. **14:** 2301–2312.
10. MAO, J., D.D. PRICE, J. LU & D.J. MAYER. 1998. Antinociceptive tolerance to the mu-opioid agonist DAMGO is dose-dependently reduced by MK-801 in rats. Neurosci. Lett. **250:** 193–196.
11. ELLIOTT, K., A. HYNANSKY & C.E. INTURRISI. 1994. Dextromethorphan attenuates and reverses analgesic tolerance to morphine. Pain **59:** 361–368.
12. MAO, J., D.D. PRICE, F.S. CARUSO & D.J. MAYER. 1996. Oral administration of dextromethorphan prevents the development of morphine tolerance and dependence in rats. Pain **67:** 361–368.
13. NARITA, M., Y. FENG, M. MAKIMURA et al. 1994. A protein kinase inhibitor, H-7, inhibits the development of tolerance to opioid antinociception. Eur. J. Pharmacol. **271:** 543–545.
14. NARITA, M., M. MAKIMURA, Y. FENG et al. 1994. Influence of chronic morphine treatment on protein kinase C activity: comparison with butorphanol and implication for opioid tolerance. Brain Res. **650:** 175–179.
15. MAYER, D.J., J. MAO & D.D. PRICE. 1995. The development of morphine tolerance and dependence is associated with translocation of protein kinase C. Pain **61:** 365–374.
16. NARITA, M., H. MIZOGUCHI & L.F. TSENG. 1995. Inhibition of protein kinase C, but not of protein kinase A, blocks the development of acute antinociceptive tolerance to an intrathecally administered mu-opioid receptor agonist in the mouse. Eur. J. Pharmacol. **280:** R1–R3.
17. NARITA, M., H. MIZOGUCHI, J.P. KAMPINE & L.F. TSENG. 1996. Role of protein kinase C in desensitization of spinal delta-opioid-mediated antinociception in the mouse. Br. J. Pharmacol. **118:** 1829–1835.
18. MAO, J., D.D. PRICE, D.J. MAYER & R.L. HAYES. 1992. Pain-related increases in spinal cord membrane-bound protein kinase C following peripheral nerve injury. Brain Res. **588:** 144–149.
19. MAO, J., D.J. MAYER, R.L. HAYES & D.D. PRICE. 1993. Spatial patterns of increased spinal cord membrane-bound protein kinase C and their relation to increases in 14C-2-deoxyglucose metabolic activity in rats with painful peripheral mononeuropathy. J. Neurophysiol. **70:** 470–481.
20. MAO, J., D.D. PRICE, L.L. PHILLIPS et al. 1995. Increases in protein kinase C gamma immunoreactivity in the spinal cord of rats associated with tolerance to the analgesic effects of morphine. Brain Res. **677:** 257–267.

21. MAO, J. 1999. NMDA and opioid receptors: their interactions in antinociception, tolerance, and neuroplasticity. Brain Res. Rev. **30:** 289–304.
22. SUGIMOTO, T., G.J. BENNETT & K.C. KAJANDER. 1989. Strychnine-enhanced transsynaptic degeneration of dorsal horn neurons in rats with an experimental painful peripheral neuropathy. Neurosci. Lett. **98:** 139–143.
23. SUGIMOTO, T., G.J. BENNETT & K.C. KAJANDER. 1990. Trans-synaptic degeneration in the superficial dorsal horn after sciatic nerve injury: effects of a chronic constriction injury, transection, and strychnine. Pain **42:** 205–213.
24. MAYER, D.J., J. MAO, J. HOLT & D.D. PRICE. 1999. Cellular mechanisms of neuropathic pain, morphine tolerance, and their interactions. Proc. Natl. Acad. Sci. U.S.A. **96:** 7731–7736.
25. MAO, J., D.D. PRICE, J. ZHU et al. 1997. The inhibition of nitric oxide–activated poly(ADP-ribose) synthetase attenuates transsynaptic alteration of spinal cord dorsal horn neurons and neuropathic pain in the rat. Pain **72:** 355–366.
26. DUBNER, R. 1991. Neuronal plasticity and pain following peripheral tissue inflammation or nerve injury. In Proceedings of the Fifth World Congress on Pain: Pain Research and Clinical Management. Vol. 5, pp. 263–276. Elsevier. Amsterdam/New York.
27. CODERRE, T.J., J. KATZ, A.L. VACCARINO & R. MELZACK. 1993. Contribution of central neuroplasticity to pathological pain: review of clinical and experimental evidence. Pain **52:** 259–285.
28. DAVAR, G., A. HAMA, A. DEYKIN et al. 1991. MK-801 blocks the development of thermal hyperalgesia in a rat model of experimental painful neuropathy (abstract). Brain Res. **553:** 327–330.
29. MAO, J., D.J. MAYER, R.L. HAYES et al. 1992. Differential roles of NMDA and non-NMDA receptor activation in induction and maintenance of thermal hyperalgesia in rats with painful peripheral mononeuropathy. Brain Res. **598:** 271–278.
30. MAO, J., D.D. PRICE, R.L. HAYES et al. 1993. Intrathecal treatment with dextrorphan or ketamine potently reduces pain-related behaviors in a rat model of peripheral mononeuropathy. Brain Res. **605:** 164–168.
31. TAL, M. & G.J. BENNETT. 1993. Dextrorphan relieves neuropathic heat-evoked hyperalgesia in the rat. Neurosci. Lett. **151:** 107–110.
32. AANONSEN, L.M. & G.L. WILCOX. 1987. Nociceptive action of excitatory amino acids in the mouse: effects of spinally administered opioids, phencyclidine, and sigma agonists. J. Pharmacol. Exp. Ther. **243:** 9–19.
33. CODERRE, T.J. & R. MELZACK. 1991. Central neural mediators of secondary hyperalgesia following heat injury in rats: neuropeptides and excitatory amino acids. Neurosci. Lett. **131:** 71–74.
34. DOUGHERTY, P.M., J. PALECEK, V. PALECKOVA et al. 1992. The role of NMDA and non-NMDA excitatory amino acid receptors in the excitation of primate spinothalamic tract neurons by mechanical, chemical, thermal, and electrical stimuli. J. Neurosci. **12:** 3025–3041.
35. HAYES, R.L., J. MAO, D.D. PRICE et al. 1992. Pretreatment with gangliosides reduces nociceptive responses associated with a rodent peripheral mononeuropathy. Pain **48:** 391–396.
36. MAO, J., R.L. HAYES, D.D. PRICE et al. 1992. Post-injury treatment with GM1 ganglioside reduces nociceptive behaviors and spinal cord metabolic activity in rats with experimental peripheral mononeuropathy. Brain Res. **584:** 18–27.
37. MAO, J., D.D. PRICE, R.L. HAYES et al. 1992. Intrathecal GM1 ganglioside and local nerve anesthesia reduce nociceptive behaviors in rats with experimental peripheral mononeuropathy. Brain Res. **584:** 28–35.
38. MAO, J., D.D. PRICE, L.L. PHILLIPS et al. 1995. Increases in protein kinase C gamma immunoreactivity in the spinal cord dorsal horn of rats with painful peripheral mononeuropathy. Neurosci. Lett. **198:** 75–78.
39. MAO, J., D.D. PRICE & D.J. MAYER. 1995. Mechanisms of hyperalgesia and opiate tolerance: a current view of their possible interactions. Pain **62:** 259–274.
40. MAO, J., D.D. PRICE & D.J. MAYER. 1995. Experimental mononeuropathy reduces the antinociceptive effects of morphine: implications for common intracellular mechanisms involved in morphine tolerance and neuropathic pain. Pain **61:** 353–364.

41. OSSIPOV, M.H., Y. LOPEZ, M.L. NICHOLS et al. 1995. The loss of antinociceptive efficacy of spinal morphine in rats with nerve ligation injury is prevented by reducing spinal afferent drive. Neurosci. Lett. **199:** 87–90.
42. WEGERT, S., M.H. OSSIPOV, M.L. NICHOLS et al. 1997. Differential activities of intrathecal MK-801 or morphine to alter responses to thermal and mechanical stimuli in normal and nerve-injured rats. Pain **71:** 57–64.
43. SORG, B.A. 1999. Multiple chemical sensitivity: potential role for neural sensitization. Crit. Rev. Neurobiol. **13:** 283–316.
44. BELL, I.R., C.M. BALDWIN, M. FERNANDEZ & G.E.R. SCHWARTZ. 1999. Neural sensitization model for multiple chemical sensitivity: overview of theory and empirical evidence. Toxicol. Ind. Health **15:** 295–304.

Cytokines and Chronic Fatigue Syndrome

ROBERTO PATARCA[a]

E. M. Papper Laboratory of Clinical Immunology, Department of Medicine,
University of Miami School of Medicine, Miami, Florida 33101, USA

> ABSTRACT: Chronic fatigue syndrome (CFS) patients show evidence of immune activation, as demonstrated by increased numbers of activated T lymphocytes, including cytotoxic T cells, as well as elevated levels of circulating cytokines. Nevertheless, immune cell function of CFS patients is poor, with low natural killer cell cytotoxicity (NKCC), poor lymphocyte response to mitogens in culture, and frequent immunoglobulin deficiencies, most often IgG1 and IgG3. Immune dysfunction in CFS, with predominance of so-called T-helper type 2 and proinflammatory cytokines, can be episodic and associated with either cause or effect of the physiological and psychological function derangement and/or activation of latent viruses or other pathogens. The interplay of these factors can account for the perpetuation of disease with remission/exacerbation cycles. A T-helper type 2 predominance has been seen among Gulf War syndrome patients and this feature may also be present in other related disorders, such as multiple chemical sensitivity. Therapeutic intervention aimed at induction of a more favorable cytokine expression pattern and immune status appears promising.

INTRODUCTION

Chronic fatigue syndrome (CFS) is a severely debilitating condition that is characterized by changes in the immunological, endocrinological, and neurological systems. The cause and effect relationships and the relative contribution of these changes to symptomatology and disease progression are areas of intense study. This review concentrates on the immunological correlates of CFS symptomatology, in particular, the role of cytokines.

The nervous and immune systems respond to internal and external challenges and communicate and regulate each other by means of shared or system-unique hormones, growth factors, neurotransmitters, and neuromodulators. For example, a decreased norepinephrine turnover in the hypothalamus and brain stem of rats occurs at the peak of the immune response to sheep red blood cells.[1–3] Increased serotonin metabolism is associated with depressed Arthus reaction and plaque-forming cell response in rats stressed either by overcrowding lasting two weeks or more or by repeated immobilization for four days.[4,5] The long-term effects of the latter acute changes are evidenced by chronic variable stress that facilitates tumor growth[6] and is associated with immune dysregulation in multiple sclerosis.[7] The hypothalamic-pituitary-adrenal (HPA) axis plays a pivotal role in stress-mediated changes, and

---

[a]Address for correspondence: E. M. Papper Laboratory of Clinical Immunology, Department of Medicine (R-42), University of Miami School of Medicine, P.O. Box 016960, Miami, FL 33101. Voice: 305-940-9047.
rpatarca@pol.net

stimulation of corticotropin-releasing factor in the central nervous system (CNS)[8,9] rapidly suppresses a variety of immune responses, an effect that can be blocked by infusion into the brain of α-melanocyte-stimulating hormone, a tridecapeptide derived from pro-opiomelanocortin.[10]

Besides external stimuli, intrinsic imbalances in neurotransmitter levels affect the immune system either directly by acting on immunocompetent cells or indirectly via induction of hormonal secretions. For instance, depression is associated with neurotransmitter imbalances and with decreased natural killer cell cytotoxic activity.[11–14] Moreover, several studies have documented the existence of striking physiologic, neuroendocrine, metabolic, and pharmacologic differences between depressed and normal subjects and between depressed and severely ill subjects.[15–20]

The examples mentioned above illustrate the fact that disorders, or persistent noxious stimulation, of the neuroimmunological circuitry can lead to, or result from, neurological, immunological, psychiatric, or multiorgan pathology. The latter link has encouraged a search for neuroimmunological markers with functional or pathological correlates.

Although the cause of CFS remains to be elucidated, many studies summarized herein have provided evidence for abnormalities in immunological markers among individuals diagnosed with CFS. A clear picture has not been achieved because of the noticeable variability in the nature and magnitude of the findings reported by different groups.[21,22] Moreover, little support has been garnered for an association between the latter abnormalities and the diverse physical and health status changes in the CFS population. For instance, Buchwald and coworkers[23] concluded that, although a subset of CFS patients with immune system activation can be identified, serum markers of inflammation and immune activation are of limited diagnostic usefulness in the evaluation of patients with CFS or in those with only chronic fatigue because changes in their values may reflect an intercurrent, transient, common condition, such as an upper respiratory infection, or may be the result of an ongoing illness-associated process. On the other hand, Patarca and colleagues[24,25] have found that CFS patients can be categorized based on immunological findings. In addition, although the degree of overlap between distributions of soluble immune mediators in CFS and controls has fueled criticism on the validity or clinical significance of immune abnormalities in CFS, the degree of overlap in the latter is not unique to CFS and is also present, for instance, in sepsis syndrome and HIV-1-associated disease, clinical entities where studies of immune abnormalities are providing insight into pathophysiology.[26]

The aim of this report is to comprehensively review the literature on the changes in the levels of cytokines in CFS, to formulate consensus by majority conclusions when possible, and to discuss how this knowledge may contribute to the understanding of the physiological and psychological function changes seen in CFS.

CYTOKINES IN CFS

Stimulated lymphoid cells either express or induce the expression in other cells of a heterogeneous group of soluble mediators that exhibit either effector or regulatory functions. These soluble mediators include cytokines, hormones, and neurotransmitters, which in turn affect immune function and may underlie many of the pathological manifestations seen in CFS.[27] In mouse models, production of cytokines by stimulated T cells has been grouped into two major patterns, T-helper 1 and T-helper 2 types, depending on whether the cytokines favor the function of macrophages and natural killer cells or of B cells, respectively. Th1-type cytokines include interleukin-2 and interferon-γ, while IL-4, IL-5, and IL-10 are examples of Th2-type cytokines. The studies of cytokines in CFS have been done in the peripheral blood compartment and a recent review by Vollmer-Conna and coworkers[28] on the immunopathogenesis of CFS concludes that neuropsychiatric symptoms in CFS patients may be more closely related to disordered cytokine production by glial cells within the CNS than to circulating cytokines. The hypothesis that expression of proinflammatory cytokines within the CNS plays a role in the pathogenesis of immunologically mediated fatigue is underscored by the study by Sheng and coworkers[29] who, using two strains of mice with differential patterns of cytokine expression in response to an injection challenge with *Corynebacterium parvum*, demonstrated that elevated interleukin-1 (IL-1) and tumor necrosis factor (TNF) cytokine messenger (m)RNA expression in the CNS corresponded to development of fatigue. Injection of antibodies specific to either IL-1 or TNF did not alter immunologically induced fatigue, an observation that suggests a lack of involvement of these cytokines produced outside of the CNS.

Despite the limitations in interpretation, the finding of cytokine imbalances in the peripheral blood compartment has implications for physiological and psychological function changes. In this respect, the decreased natural killer (NK) cell cytotoxic and lymphoproliferative activities and increased allergic and autoimmune manifestations in CFS would be compatible with the hypothesis that the immune system of affected individuals is biased towards a T-helper (Th) 2 type, or humoral immunity-oriented cytokine pattern.[30] The factors that could lead to a Th2 shift and to mood and immunoendocrine changes among CFS patients are unknown. Vaccines and stressful stimuli have been shown to lead to long-term, nonspecific shifts in cytokine balance. Therapeutic regimens that induce a systemic Th1 bias are being tested, including repeated stimulation with bacterial antigens or poly (I)–poly (C12U)[31] and *ex vivo* activation of lymph node cells.[32]

Interleukin-1 (IL-1) and Soluble IL-1 Receptors

IL-1 is the term for two distinct cytokines—IL-1α and IL-1β—that share the same cell-surface receptors (IL-1R1 and IL-1R2) and biological activities.[33,34] One study of CFS patients[35] found elevated levels of serum IL-1α, but not of plasma IL-1β, in 17% of patients studied. When the cohort was examined as to severity of symptoms, it was noted that the top quartile in terms of disability had the highest level of IL-1. Curiously, use of reverse transcriptase-coupled polymerase chain reaction (RT-PCR) revealed IL-1β, but not IL-1α mRNA, in peripheral blood mononuclear cells (PBMCs) of several CFS patients with highly elevated levels of IL-1α. RT-PCR of fractionated cell populations showed that lymphocytes accounted for the IL-1β mRNA detected in PBMCs. No IL-1 mRNA was apparent in control subjects. That IL-1α mRNA was not detectable by RT-PCR in either PBMCs or granulocytes suggests that serum IL-1α in CFS patients is probably derived from a source other than peripheral blood cells. Other potential sources are tissue macrophages, endothelial cells, lymph node cells, fibroblasts, CNS microglia, astrocytes, and dermal dendritic cells.[33]

Linde and coworkers[36] found significantly higher levels of IL-1α in CFS and mononucleosis patients, but Lloyd,[37] Peakman,[38] and Rasmussen[39] and their coworkers found no difference. Five studies, in addition to one described above by Patarca and colleagues,[35] found no difference in the levels of IL-1β in CFS patients.[36,38–41]

The signs and symptoms of CFS, which include fatigue, myalgia, and low-grade fever, are similar to those experienced by patients infused with cytokines such as interleukin-1. Elevated serum levels of IL-1α found in a significant number of CFS patients could underlie several of the clinical symptoms. IL-1 can gain access to the brain through the preoptic nucleus of the hypothalamus, where it induces fever and the release of adrenocorticotropin hormone (ACTH)–releasing factor,[42–45] which in turn would lead to release of ACTH and cortisol. The observation that cortisol levels tend to be low in CFS patients regardless of IL-1α levels suggests a role of a defective hypothalamic feedback loop in the pathogenesis of CFS. The presence of such a defect has been documented in Lewis rats, which are particularly susceptible to the induction of a variety of inflammatory and autoimmune diseases and exhibit reduced levels of ACTH-releasing hormone, ACTH, and cortisol in response to IL-1.

Besides its effects on the HPA axis, IL-1 has other effects on the pituitary; it has been shown to augment release of prolactin and growth hormone and to inhibit release of thyrotropin and luteinizing hormone.[46,47] The growth hormone deficiency state associated with CFS[48] may also be a reflection of the defect in hypothalamic feedback loop that renders it inadequately responsive to IL-1.

IL-1 and tumor necrosis factor (TNF) provoke slow-wave sleep when placed in the lateral ventricles of experimental animals.[49] The inordinate fatigue, lassitude, and excessive sleepiness associated with CFS[50,51] could well be a consequence of the direct action of these cytokines on neurons. Neurotoxic effects due to chronic overexpression of IL-1α and/or IL-1β of S100—a small (10 kDa), soluble calcium-binding protein that is synthesized and released by astroglia[52]—have been proposed to underlie progressive neurological degeneration in Alzheimer's disease.[53]

IL-1 induces prostaglandin (PGE_2, PGI_2) synthesis by endothelial and smooth muscle cells.[54] Although the levels of these substances have not been measured in CFS patients, they are potent vasodilators, and IL-1 administration in animals and humans produces significant hypotension, a feature seen in some CFS patients. IL-1 has a natriuretic effect[55] and may affect plasma volume.

Gulick and colleagues[56] showed that IL-1 and TNF inhibit β-adrenergic agonist-mediated cardiac myocyte contractility in cultures and intracellular accumulation of cyclic adenosine monophosphate. Cytokine imbalances may, therefore, also underlie the cardiovascular manifestations of CFS.

Chronic fatigue syndrome is a condition that affects women in disproportionate numbers and is often exacerbated in the premenstrual period and following physical exertion. Cannon and coworkers[57] found that isolated peripheral blood mononuclear cells from healthy women, but not CFS patients, exhibited significant menstrual cycle-related differences in IL-1β secretion that were related to estradiol and progesterone levels. IL-1 receptor antagonist (Ra) secretion for CFS patients was twofold higher than controls during the follicular phase, but luteal-phase levels were similar between groups. In both phases of the menstrual cycle, IL-1 soluble receptor (sR) II release was significantly higher for CFS patients compared to controls. The only changes that might be attributable to exertion occurred in the control subjects during the follicular phase, who exhibited an increase in IL-1β secretion at 48 h after the stress. These results suggest that an abnormality exists in IL-1β secretion in CFS patients that may be related to altered sensitivity to estradiol and progesterone. Furthermore, the increased release of IL-1Ra and sIL-1RII by cells from CFS patients is consistent with the hypothesis that CFS is associated with chronic, low-level activation of the immune system.

In contrast to the studies described above, Swanink and coworkers[58] found no obvious difference in the levels of circulating cytokines and *ex vivo* production of IL-1α and IL-1Ra. Although endotoxin-stimulated *ex vivo* production of TNF-α and IL-1β was significantly lower in CFS, none of the immunologic test results correlated with fatigue severity or psychologic well-being scores. Swanink and coworkers[58] concluded that these immunologic tests cannot be used as diagnostic tools in individual CFS patients.

Tumor Necrosis Factors (TNFs) and Soluble TNF Receptors

TNF-α and TNF-β are cytokines produced on lymphoid cell activation.[59] Twenty-eight percent of CFS patients studied by Patarca and colleagues[35] had elevations in serum levels of TNF-α and TNF-β usually with elevation in serum levels of IL-1 or sIL-2R. TNF-α expression in CFS patients is also evident at the mRNA level, which suggests *de novo* synthesis rather than release of a preformed inducible surface TNF-α protein upon activation of monocytes and CD4+ T cells.[60] The levels of spontaneously (unstimulated) produced TNF-α by nonadherent lymphocytes were also significantly increased as compared to simultaneously studied matched controls by Gupta and colleagues.[61] TNF-α may be associated with CNS pathology because it has been associated with demyelination and may also lead to loss of appetite.[59,62] A study by Dreisbach and coworkers[63] suggests that TNF-α may be involved in the pathogenesis of postdialysis fatigue. In contrast to the studies discussed above, Lloyd *et al.*[37] found no difference in the levels of TNF-α or -β in CFS patients, and Rasmussen *et al.*[39] and Peakman *et al.*[38] found no differences in the levels of TNF-α and -β, respectively. The latter discrepancies are likely due to the fact that TNF levels decrease precipitously if the serum or plasma is not frozen within 30 min from collection.[64]

Proinflammatory effects of TNF-α may be mediated by induction of gene expression for neutrophil-activating protein-1 and macrophage inflammatory proteins, resulting in neutrophil migration and degranulation.[65] Thus, it is reasonable that TNF elevations may also be associated with markers of macrophage activation such as serum neopterin (see below).

CFS patients have higher levels of sTNF-RI or sCD120a and sTNF-RII or sCD120b.[24,25] Levels of sTNF-Rs are negatively correlated with NK cell cytotoxic and lymphoproliferative activities in CFS, an observation that is consistent with the activities of these soluble mediators. The role of TNFs and their receptors in CFS needs further elucidation.

Interleukin-2 (IL-2) and Soluble IL-2 Receptor

IL-2, formerly termed T-cell growth factor, is a glycosylated protein produced by T lymphocytes after mitogenic or antigenic stimulation.[66] IL-2 acts as a growth factor[67] and promotes proliferation of T cells[68] and, under particular conditions, of B cells and macrophages.[69,70]

Although serum IL-2 levels were found to be elevated in CFS patients compared with control individuals in one study,[71] decreased levels were reported in two other studies[72,73] and no difference was reported in three studies.[35,36,41] Rasmussen and coworkers[39] reported a higher production of IL-2 by stimulated peripheral blood cells from CFS patients as compared to controls. Cheney and coworkers[71] found no obvious relation between IL-2 serum levels and severity/duration of illness in CFS.

Elevated levels of sIL-2R, a marker of lymphoid cell activation, have been found in a number of pathological conditions, including viral infections, autoimmune diseases, and lymphoproliferative and hematological malignancies.[74,75] Twelve percent of CFS patients studied by Patarca and coworkers[35] had elevated levels of sIL-2R. Since sIL-2R antagonizes the action of IL-2 and decreases the levels of functionally available IL-2, the observation of increased levels of sIL-2R in some CFS patients may be consistent with the increased proportion of activated T cells and the reduced levels of IL-2 or decreased NK cell cytotoxic activity found in several studies of CFS patients discussed above. Linde and coworkers[36] found no elevation in sIL-2R levels in CFS patients.

Interleukin-4 (IL-4)

Visser and colleagues[76] reported that, although CD4 T cells from CFS patients produce less interferon-γ than do cells from controls, IL-4 production and cell proliferation are comparable. Because interferon-γ is a Th1-type cytokine, whereas IL-4 is a Th2-type cytokine, a decreased production of the former with no change in the latter would favor a Th2-type predominance. With CD4 T cells from CFS patients (compared with cells from controls), a 10- to 20-fold lower dexamethasone (DEX) concentration was needed to achieve 50% inhibition of IL-4 production and proliferation, indicating an increased sensitivity to DEX in CFS patients. In contrast to IL-4, interferon-γ production in patients and controls was equally sensitive to DEX. A differential sensitivity of cytokines or CD4 T cell subsets to glucocorticoids might explain an altered immunologic function in CFS patients.

IL-4 acts as a growth factor for various types of lymphoid cells, including B, T, and cytotoxic T cells,[77] and has been shown to be involved in immunoglobulin isotype selection *in vivo*.[78] Activated T cells are the major source of IL-4 production, but mast cells can also produce it, and IL-4 has been associated with allergic and autoimmune reactions.[77] It is also noteworthy that many of the effects of IL-4 are antagonized by IFN-γ, and the decreased production of the latter may underlie a predominance of IL-4 over IFN-γ effects.

Interleukin-6 (IL-6) and Soluble IL-6 Receptor

CFS patients have higher levels of sIL-6R[24] and sIL-6R enhances the effects of IL-6. The levels of spontaneously produced IL-6 by both adherent monocytes and nonadherent lymphocytes were significantly increased in CFS patients as compared to controls.[61] The abnormality of IL-6 was also observed at the mRNA level. In terms of circulating IL-6, Buchwald and coworkers[23] found that IL-6 was elevated among febrile CFS patients compared to those without this finding and therefore considered it an epiphenomenon possibly secondary to infection. Chao and coworkers[79,80] also found elevated levels of IL-6 in CFS patients, but five other groups found no difference.[23,36–38,81]

Most of the cell types that produce IL-6 do so in response to stimuli such as IL-1 and TNF, among others.[82] Excessive IL-6 production has been associated with polyclonal B-cell activation, resulting in hypergammaglobulinemia and autoantibody production.[83] As is the case with IL-4, IL-6 may contribute to activation of CD5-bearing B cells, leading to autoimmune manifestations. IL-6 also synergizes with IL-1 in inflammatory reactions and may exacerbate many of the features described previously for IL-1.

A study of cytokine production by stimulated peripheral blood mononuclear cells from patients with a closely related syndrome to CFS, the post-Q-fever fatigue syndrome (QFS) (inappropriate fatigue, myalgia and arthralgia, night sweats, changes in mood and sleep patterns following about 20% of laboratory-proven, acute primary Q-fever cases), showed an accentuated release of IL-6 that was significantly in excess of medians for all four control groups (resolving QFS, acute primary Q-fever without subsequent QFS, healthy Q-fever vaccinees, and healthy controls). Levels of induced IL-6 significantly correlated with total symptom scores and scores for other key symptoms.[84]

Interleukin-10 (IL-10)

A study by Gupta and coworkers[61] revealed that spontaneously produced IL-10 by both adherent monocytes and nonadherent lymphocytes and by PHA-activated nonadherent monocytes were decreased. IL-10 is part of the Th2-type response.

Interferons (IFNs)

The IFNs comprise a multigenic family with pleiotropic properties and diverse cellular origin. Data from six studies indicate that circulating IFNs are present in 3% or less of patients studied,[85–91] which is similar to the percentage among controls.

Peripheral blood cells from children affected by postviral fatigue syndrome produced more IFN-α than did those from controls. In line with the latter observation, Vojdani and colleagues[92] found elevated IFN-α levels in CFS patients, but Linde[36] and Straus[41] and their coworkers found no difference. Fatigue occurs in more than 70% of patients treated with IFN-α and it may be associated with the development of immune-mediated endocrine diseases, in particular, hypothryoidism and HPA axis–related hormonal deficiencies, in these patients.[93,94] IFN-α therapy–associated fatigue is often the dominant dose-limiting side effect, worsening with continued therapy and accompanied by significant depression. Decreases in mental information processing speeds, verbal memory, and executive functions have also been reported at therapeutic doses of IFN-α.[95] Although the direct cause of IFN-α-induced fatigue is unknown, it is possible that neuromuscular fatigue, similar to that observed in patients with postpolio syndrome, may also be one component of this syndrome. The induction of proinflammatory cytokines observed in patients treated with IFN-α is consistent with a possible mechanism of neuromuscular pathology that could manifest as fatigue. A study by Davis and colleagues[96] also revealed that IFN-α/β is at least partially responsible for the early fatigue induced by polyI:C during prolonged treadmill running in mice.

IFN-γ is an immunoregulatory substance, enhancing both cellular antigen presentation to lymphocytes[97] and NK cell cytotoxicity[98] and causing inhibition of suppressor T-lymphocyte activity.[99] Two groups have found impaired IFN-γ production on mitogenic stimulation of peripheral blood mononuclear cells from CFS patients,[76,100] and one group[37] found increased production. In contrast with the findings on lymphocyte activation, four groups reported no difference in the levels of circulating IFN-γ.[36,38,41,76] These results are in favor of the Th2 shift described previously.

Tumor Growth Factor-β (TGF-β)

A study by Bennett and coworkers[101] found that patients with CFS had significantly higher levels of bioactive TGF-β levels compared to healthy controls and to patients with various diseases known to be associated with immunologic abnormalities and/or pathologic fatigue: major depression, systemic lupus erythematosis (SLE), and multiple sclerosis (MS) of both the relapsing/remitting (R/R) and the chronic progressive (CP) types. A total of three studies supports the finding of elevated levels of TGF-β among CFS patients.

β-2 Microglobulin

Three studies found elevated levels of β-2 microglobulin in patients with CFS,[23–25] and one study found no difference.[79] β-2 microglobulin is a marker of immune activation.

Neopterin

Neopterin is a metabolite produced during the utilization of guanosine triphosphate, and increased production of neopterin is associated with macrophage activation by IFN-γ.[102,103] Neopterin is a presumed primate homologue of nitric oxide, which activates guanylate cyclase and is involved in neurotransmission, vasodilation, neurotoxicity, inhibition of platelet aggregation, the antiproliferative action of cytokines, and reduction of oxidative stress.[104,105] Neopterin derivatives belong to the cytotoxic arsenal of the activated human macrophage and, in high doses, enhance oxidative stress through enhancement of radical-mediated effector functions and programmed cell death by TNF-α, while having an opposite effect at low doses.[104,106] Buchwald[23] and Chao[79,80] and their coworkers found elevated levels of neopterin in CFS patients, whereas Linde[36] and Patarca[35] and their coworkers found no difference. A report of nine CFS cases showed significantly elevated serum neopterin levels in association with high cognitive difficulty scale (CDS) scores,[107,108] and neopterin levels have been shown to correlate with levels of many other mediators that have been found to be dysregulated in CFS, including members of the TNF family.[23,27,35] In terms of neurotoxicity, serum neopterin and tryptophan concentrations correlate among cancer and AIDS patients, an observation that can be accounted for by activity of indoleamine 2,3-dioxygenase, a tryptophan-degrading enzyme.[109,110] The latter enzyme also converts L-tryptophan to L-kynurenine, kynurenic acid, and quinolinic acid (QUIN). QUIN is a neurotoxic metabolite that accumulates within the CNS following immune activation and is also a sensitive marker for the presence of immune activation within the CNS.[111–113] Direct conversion of L-tryptophan into QUIN by brain tissue occurs in conditions of CNS inflammation, but not by normal brain tissue. Macrophage infiltrates, and perhaps microglia, are important sources of QUIN, an observation that is consistent with the results of inoculation of poliovirus directly into the spinal cord of rhesus macaques, resulting in increased CSF levels of both QUIN and neopterin.[111,114] Elevated serum levels of neopterin correlate with the presence of brain lesions and with neurologic and psychiatric symptoms in patients with AIDS dementia complex.[108,115] It is worth noting in this context that Buchwald and colleagues[116] found subcortical lesions consistent with edema and demyelination by magnetic resonance scans in 78% of CFS patients as compared to 20% of controls.

Soluble CD8 (sCD8)

Linde and coworkers[36] found no elevation of sCD8 in CFS patients. Elevations in the levels of sCD8 have been associated with disease progression in HIV-associated disease, but this does not appear to be the case in CFS.

Soluble ICAM-1 (sICAM-1)

Patarca and coworkers[24] found higher levels of soluble intercellular adhesion molecule-1 (sICAM-1) in CFS patients, an observation that is consistent with the higher expression of ICAM-1 in monocytes of CFS patients reported by Gupta and Vayuvegula.[117]

EXPERIMENTAL THERAPY RESULTS IN AN APPARENT SHIFT FROM THE TYPE 2 TO TYPE 1 CYTOKINE PATTERN IN CFS PATIENTS

Our group completed a safety and feasibility study using lymph node extraction, *ex vivo* cell culture, followed by autologous cell reinfusion as a treatment strategy in CFS patients.[32] Lymph nodes were obtained from patients who met the current case definition for CFS and the following inclusion criteria—a history of acute onset; a Karnofsky score < 80; evidence of immune dysfunction in three or more of the following: >1 SD above controls for elevated sTNF-RI in serum; elevated sTNF-RI in PHA-stimulated blood culture; elevated IL-5 in PHA-stimulated blood culture; lymphocyte activation (CD2+CD26+ cells > 50%); or low NK cytotoxic activity (<20%). The lymph node cells were cultured for 10 to 12 days with anti-CD3 and IL-2. IL-2 is a Th1-type cytokine and a Th1-type response inducer. Both IL-2 and anti-CD3 help activate T cells. These cells were then reinfused into the donor, who was monitored for safety and possible clinical benefit. There were no adverse events noted in this phase 1 clinical trial. Of 13 subjects, 2 had palpable lymph nodes that proved fibrotic with no viable cells. Of the remaining 11 subjects, all successfully underwent expansion and reinfusion. In some of the patients, there was an elevation in the expression of IL-2 receptor on CD4 T cells in the weeks following the reinfusion. A significant decrease in IL-5 production by PHA-stimulated blood cultures was observed at 1 week, which persisted for several weeks postinfusion.

Levels of PHA-induced IFN-γ did not change. A trend toward a decrease in the ratio of IFN-γ/IL-5 was found starting at week 1 and persisting at least 12 weeks. Of the 11 subjects, 9 had significant cognitive improvement; other measures of severity of illness also trended toward improvement. The lack of adverse effects from this experimental approach to immunomodulation in CFS and the favorable clinical and immunologic results observed in the small number of patients studied suggest that further clinical trials are warranted.

STRESSORS, CYTOKINES, AND SYMPTOMS

One of our models of CFS holds that the interaction of psychological factors (distress associated with either CFS-related symptoms or other stressful life events) and immunologic dysfunction (indicated in signs of chronic overactivation with cytokine abnormalities) contribute to (a) CFS-related physical symptoms (e.g., fatigue, joint pain, cognitive difficulties, fever) and increases in illness burden, and (b) dysfunction in the immune system's ability to survey viruses, including latent herpesviruses (indicated in impaired NKCC). As discussed above, there is a decrease in the ratio of type 1/type 2 cytokines produced by lymphocytes *in vitro* following mitogen stimulation in CFS patients. This type of dysfunction should be expected to result in impaired immune surveillance associated with cytotoxic lymphocytes. For example, Cohen *et al.*[118] found an association between psychosocial stressors, immunomodulation, and the incidence and progression of rhinovirus infections in healthy normals. Here, the rates of respiratory infections and clinical colds increased in a dose-response fashion with increases in psychological stress across all five of the cold viruses studied. If viruses related to upper respiratory tract infections (URIs) are not well controlled by immune surveillance mechanisms (e.g., NKCC) in CFS patients who are exposed to stressors, then patients may suffer more frequent and protracted URIs that are accompanied by prolonged elevations in proinflammatory cytokines. Stress-associated reactivation of latent herpesviruses may also play a role in modulating the production of cytokines that underlie CFS symptom exacerbations.[119,120] Alternatively, distress increases may more directly influence cytokine dysregulation by way of neuroendocrine changes that, in turn, intensify physical symptoms. Importantly, for all of the possible paths, further increases in distress as a "reaction" to mounting symptoms creates a vicious cycle. Such a recursive system may act as a positive feedback loop, thereby accounting for the chronic nature of CFS and its refraction to interventions that focus solely on symptom reduction.

Our conceptual model for CFS was supported by data from our laboratory showing that distress levels in response to the stressor Hurricane Andrew were positively correlated with alterations in NK cells, elevated (compared to pre-storm values) circulating levels of the cytokines, exacerbation in CFS symptoms, and increases in sickness impact profile (SIP)–based illness burden scores among our CFS patients.[106] We found that CFS patients living in a hurricane exposure area (Dade County) had significantly greater severity of CFS symptom relapses (using clinician-rated fatigue levels and ability to engage in work-related activities) and significantly greater increases in illness burden as compared to age- and gender-matched CFS patients from the same clinical practice living in an adjacent geographical region that was not in the storm's path, namely, Broward/Palm Beach County. We also found that pre/post-hurricane NKCC changes were associated with pre/post-storm symptom severity changes, including cognitive symptoms, muscle weakness, and muscle pain. These data suggested that stressor-induced decrements in NKCC were associated with greater increases in the severity of cognitive difficulties, muscle weakness, and pain symptoms. A final regression analysis on NKCC indicated that appraisals in greater storm impact and low social support predicted the greatest pre/post-storm decrements in NKCC. Greater optimism and social support provisions were also associated with less elevations in TNF-α among storm victims.

CONCLUSIONS

The data summarized herein indicate that CFS is associated with immune abnormalities that can potentially account for physio- and psychopathological symptomatology. Assessment of immune status reveals a heterogeneity among CFS patients. Future research should further elucidate the cellular basis for immune dysfunction in CFS and its implications. Other compartments such as the CNS have to be assessed using similar techniques to those used with peripheral blood. Nonetheless, the studies in peripheral blood have been providing insight into the physio- and psychopathologies of CFS. Similar studies will prove useful for understanding the etiopathology of other CFS-related syndromes, such as multiple chemical sensitivity.

ACKNOWLEDGMENTS

This work was supported in part by a grant from the CFIDS Association of America, by NIH Center Grant No. 1UD1-AI 45940-02, and by funds from Neoprobe Corporation and Ciratech Corporation.

REFERENCES

1. SHANKS, N. *et al.* 1994. Alterations in central cathecolamines associated with immune responses in adult and aged mice. Brain Res. **666**(1): 77–87.
2. BESEDOVSKY, H. *et al.* 1983. The immune response evokes changes in brain noradrenergic neurons. Science **221**(4610): 564–566.
3. VASINA, I.G., E.P. FROLOV & N.G. SEREBRIAKOV. 1975. Sympathico-adrenal system activity in a primary immune response. Zh. Mikrobiol. Epidemiol. Immunobiol. **10**(9): 88–92.
4. BORANIC, M. 1990. The central nervous system and immunity. Lijec. Vjesn. **112**: 329–334.
5. BORANIC, M. *et al.* 1982. Immunological and neuroendocrine responses of rats to prolonged or repeated stress. Biomed. Pharmacother. **36**(1): 23–28.
6. BASSO, A.M., M. DEPIANTE-DEPAOLI & V.A. MOLINA. 1992. Chronic variable stress facilitates tumoral growth: reversal by imipramine administration. Life Sci. **50**(23): 1789–1796.
7. FOLEY, F.W. *et al.* 1992. A prospective study of depression and immune dysregulation in multiple sclerosis. Arch. Neurol. **49**(3): 238–244.
8. DE SOUZA, E.B. 1993. Corticotropin-releasing factor and interleukin-1 receptors in the brain-endocrine-immune axis: role in stress response and infection. Ann. N.Y. Acad. Sci. **697**: 9–27.
9. IRWIN, M. 1993. Stress-induced immune suppression: role of the autonomic nervous system. Ann. N.Y. Acad. Sci. **697**: 203–218.

10. WEISS, J.M., N. QUAN & S.K. SUNDAR. 1994. Widespread activation and consequences of interleukin-1 in the brain. Ann. N.Y. Acad. Sci. **741:** 338–357.
11. HEBERT, T.B. & S. COHEN. 1993. Depression and immunity: a meta-analytic review. Psychol. Bull. **113:** 472–486.
12. IRWIN, M. et al. 1990. Reduction of immune function in life stress and depression. Biol. Psychiatry **27:** 222–230.
13. IRWIN, M. et al. 1990. Major depressive disorder, alcoholism, and reduced natural killer cell cytotoxicity. Arch. Gen. Psychiatry **47:** 713–719.
14. SCHLEIFER, S.J. et al. 1989. Major depressive disorder: role of age, sex, severity, and hospitalization. Arch. Gen. Psychiatry **46:** 81–87.
15. LECHIN, F. et al. 1983. Distal colon motility and clinical parameters in depression. J. Affective Disord. **5:** 19–26.
16. LECHIN, F. et al. 1983. Distal colon motility as a predictor of antidepressant response to fenfluramine, imipramine, and clomipramine. J. Affective Disord. **5:** 27–35.
17. LECHIN, F. et al. 1985. Effects of clonidine on blood pressure, noradrenaline, cortisol, growth hormone, and prolactin plasma levels in low and high intestinal tone depressed patients. Neuroendocrinology **41:** 156–162.
18. LECHIN, F. et al. 1987. Role of stress in the exacerbation of chronic illness: effects of clonidine administration on blood pressure and plasma norepinephrine, cortisol, growth hormone, and prolactin concentrations. Psychoneuroendocrinology **12:** 117–129.
19. LECHIN, F. et al. 1989. Central neuronal pathways involved in depressive syndrome: experimental findings. *In* Neurochemistry and Clinical Disorders: Circuitry of Some Psychiatric and Psychosomatic Syndromes, pp. 65–89. CRC Press. Boca Raton, FL.
20. LECHIN, F. et al. 1994. Plasma neurotransmitters and cortisol in chronic illness: role of stress. J. Med. **25:** 181–192.
21. PATARCA, R., M.A. FLETCHER & N.G. KLIMAS. 1992. Immunological correlates of the chronic fatigue syndrome. *In* Chronic Fatigue Syndrome, pp. 1–21. American Psychiatric Press. Washington, D.C.
22. SOBEL, R.A. et al. 1988. The 2H4 (CD45R) antigen is selectively decreased in multiple sclerosis lesions. J. Immunol. **140:** 2210–2214.
23. BUCHWALD, D. et al. 1997. Markers of inflammation and immune activation in chronic fatigue and chronic fatigue syndrome. J. Rheumatol. **24**(2): 372–376.
24. PATARCA, R. et al. 1995. Dysregulated expression of soluble immune mediator receptors in a subset of patients with chronic fatigue syndrome: categorization of patients by immune status. J. Chronic Fatigue Syndrome **1:** 79–94.
25. PATARCA, R. et al. 1995. Interindividual immune status variation patterns in patients with chronic fatigue syndrome: association with the tumor necrosis factor system and gender. J. Chronic Fatigue Syndrome **2**(1): 13–19.
26. GOLDIE, A.S. et al. 1995. Natural cytokine antagonists and endogenous antiendotoxin core antibodies in sepsis syndrome. JAMA **274:** 172–177.
27. PATARCA, R. et al. 1995. Assessment of immune mediator expression levels in biological fluids and cells: a critical appraisal. Crit. Rev. Oncog. **6**(2): 117–149.
28. VOLLMER-CONNA, U. et al. 1998. Chronic fatigue syndrome: an immunological perspective. Aust. N. Z. J. Psychiatry **32**(4): 523–527.
29. SHENG, W.S. et al. 1996. Susceptibility to immunologically mediated fatigue in C57BL/6 versus Balb/c mice. Clin. Immunol. Immunopathol. **81**(2): 161–167.
30. ROOK, G.A. & A. ZUMLA. 1997. Gulf War syndrome: is it due to a systemic shift in cytokine balance towards a Th2 profile? Lancet **349**(9068): 1831–1833.
31. VOJDANI, A. & C. W. LAPP. 1999. Interferon-induced proteins are elevated in blood samples of patients with chemically or virally induced chronic fatigue syndrome. Immunopharmacol. Immunotoxicol. **21**(2): 175–202.
32. KLIMAS, N.G. & M.A. FLETCHER. 1999. Alteration of type 1/type 2 cytokine pattern following adoptive immunotherapy of patients with chronic fatigue syndrome (CFS) using autologous *ex vivo* expanded lymph node cells. Abstract: II International Conference on CFS, Brussels.
33. DINARELLO, C.A. 1991. Interleukin-1 and interleukin-1 antagonism. Blood **77**(8): 1627–1652.

34. PLATANIAS, L.C. & N.J. VOGELZANG. 1990. Interleukin-1: biology, pathophysiology, and clinical prospects. Am. J. Med. **89:** 621–629.
35. PATARCA, R. et al. 1994. Dysregulated expression of tumor necrosis factor in the chronic fatigue immune dysfunction syndrome: interrelations with cellular sources and patterns of soluble immune mediator expression. Clin. Infect. Dis. **18:** S147–S153.
36. LINDE, A. et al. 1992. Serum levels of lymphokines and soluble cellular receptors in primary EBV infection and in patients with chronic fatigue syndrome. J. Infect. Dis. **165:** 994–1000.
37. LLOYD, A. et al. 1992. Cell-mediated immunity in patients with chronic fatigue syndrome, healthy controls, and patients with major depression. Clin. Exp. Immunol. **87**(1)**:** 76–79.
38. PEAKMAN, M. et al. 1997. Clinical improvement in chronic fatigue syndrome is not associated with lymphocyte subsets of function or activation. Clin. Immunol. Immunopathol. **82**(1)**:** 83–91.
39. RASMUSSEN, A.K. et al. 1994. Chronic fatigue syndrome—a controlled cross-sectional study. J. Rheumatol. **21**(8)**:** 1527–1531.
40. MORTE, S. et al. 1989. Production of interleukin-1 by peripheral blood mononuclear cells in patients with chronic fatigue syndrome. J. Infect. Dis. **159:** 362.
41. STRAUS, S.E. et al. 1989. Circulating lymphokine levels in the chronic fatigue syndrome. J. Infect. Dis. **160**(6)**:** 1085–1086.
42. ARNASON, B.G.W. 1991. Nervous system—immune system communication. Rev. Infect. Dis. **13**(1)**:** S134–S137.
43. BERKENBOSCH, F. et al. 1987. Corticotropin-releasing factor–producing neurons in the RT activated by interleukin-1. Science **238:** 524–526.
44. BESEDOVSKY, H. et al. 1986. Immunoregulatory feedback between interleukin-1 and glucocorticoid hormones. Science **233:** 652–654.
45. SAPOLSKY, R. et al. 1987. Interleukin-1 stimulates the secretion of hypothalamic corticotropin-releasing factor. Science **233:** 522–524.
46. BERNTON, E.W. et al. 1987. Release of multiple hormones by a direct action of interleukin-1 on pituitary cells. Science **238:** 519–521.
47. RETTORI, V. et al. 1991. Interleukin 1a inhibits protaglandin E_2 release to suppress pulsatile release of luteinizing hormone, but not follicle-stimulating hormone. Proc. Natl. Acad. Sci. U.S.A. **88:** 2763–2767.
48. BERWAERTS, J., G. MOORKENS & R. ABS. 1998. Review of neuroendocrine disturbances in the chronic fatigue syndrome: indications for a role of the growth hormone–IGF-1 axis in the pathogenesis. J. Chronic Fatigue Syndrome **4**(4)**:** 81–92.
49. SHOHAM, S. et al. 1987. Recombinant tumor necrosis factor and interleukin 1 enhance slow-wave sleep. Am. J. Physiol. **253:** R142–R149.
50. HOLMES, G.P. et al. 1988. Chronic fatigue syndrome: a working cased definition. Ann. Intern. Med. **108:** 387–389.
51. MOLDOVSKY, H. 1989. Nonrestorative sleep and symptoms after a febrile illness in patients with fibrosis and chronic fatigue syndrome. J. Rheumatol. **16**(19)**:** 150–153.
52. VAN ELDIK, L.J. & D.B. ZIMMER. 1987. Secretion of S-100 from rat C6 glioma cells. Brain Res. **436:** 367–370.
53. GRIFFIN, W.S.T. et al. 1989. Brain interleukin 1 and S-100 immunoreactivity are elevated in Down's syndrome and Alzheimer's disease. Proc. Natl. Acad. Sci. U.S.A. **86:** 7611–7615.
54. DEJANA, E. et al. 1987. Modulation of endothelial cell function by different molecular species of interleukin-1. Blood **69:** 635–699.
55. CAVERZASIO, J., R. RIZZOLI & J.M. DAYER. 1987. Interleukin-1 decreases renal sodium reabsorption: possible mechanisms of endotoxin-induced natriuresis. Am. J. Physiol. **252:** 943–946.
56. GULICK, T. et al. 1989. Interleukin-1 and tumor necrosis factor inhibit cardiac myocyte beta-adrenergic responsiveness. Proc. Natl. Acad. Sci. U.S.A. **86:** 6753–6757.
57. CANNON, J.G. et al. 1997. Interleukin-1 beta, interleukin-1 receptor antagonist, and soluble interleukin-1 receptor type II secretion in chronic fatigue syndrome. J. Clin. Immunol. **17**(3)**:** 253–261.
58. SWANINK, C.M. et al. 1996. Lymphocyte subsets, apoptosis, and cytokines in patients with chronic fatigue syndrome. J. Infect. Dis. **173**(2)**:** 460–463.

59. BEUTLER, B. & A. CERAMI. 1988. Cachectin (tumor necrosis factor): a macrophage hormone governing cellular metabolism and inflammatory response. Endocr. Rev. **9:** 57–66.
60. KRIEGLER, M. *et al.* 1988. A novel form of TNF-cachectin in a cell surface cytotoxic transmembrane protein: ramifications for the complex physiology of TNF. Cell **53:** 45–53.
61. GUPTA, S. *et al.* 1997. Cytokine production by adherent and non-adherent mononuclear cells in chronic fatigue syndrome. J. Psychol. Res. **31**(1): 149–156.
62. WILT, S.G. *et al.* 1995. *In vitro* evidence for a dual role of tumor necrosis factor in human immunodeficiency virus type 1 encephalopathy. Ann. Neurol. **37:** 381–394.
63. DREISBACH, A.W. *et al.* 1998. Elevated levels of tumor necrosis factor alpha in postdialysis fatigue. Int. J. Artif. Organs **21**(2): 83–86.
64. PATARCA, R., K. GOODKIN & M.A. FLETCHER. 1995. Cryopreservation of peripheral blood mononuclear cells. *In* Manual of Clinical Laboratory Immunology. American Society of Microbiology.
65. DINARELLO, C. 1992. Interleukin-1 and tumor necrosis factor: effector cytokines in autoimmune diseases. Semin. Immunol. **4**(3): 133–145.
66. WATSON, J. & D. MOCHIZUKI. 1980. Interleukin-2: a class of T cell growth factor. Immunol. Rev. **51:** 257–278.
67. FLETCHER, M. & A.L. GOLDSTEIN. 1987. Recent advances in the understanding of the biochemistry and clinical pharmacology of interleukin-2. Lymphokine Res. **1:** 45–57.
68. MORGAN, D.A., F.W. RUSCETTI & R.C. GALLO. 1976. Selective *in vitro* growth of T lymphocytes from normal human bone marrows. Science **193:** 1007–1008.
69. MALKOVSKY, M. *et al.* 1987. Recombinant interleukin-2 directly augments the cytotoxicity of human monocytes. Nature **325:** 262–265.
70. TSUDO, M., T. ICHIYAMA & H. UCHINO. 1984. Expression of Tac antigen on activated normal human B cells. J. Exp. Med. **160:** 612–617.
71. CHENEY, P.R., S.E. DORMAN & D.S. BELL. 1989. Interleukin-2 and the chronic fatigue syndrome. Ann. Intern. Med. **110**(4): 321.
72. KIBLER, R. *et al.* 1985. Immune function in chronic active Epstein-Barr virus infection. J. Clin. Immunol. **5:** 46–54.
73. GOLD, D. *et al.* 1990. Chronic fatigue: a prospective clinical and virologic study. JAMA **264:** 48–53.
74. COHEN, N. *et al.* 1990. Soluble interleukin-2 receptor: detection and potential role in organ transplantation. Clin. Immunol. Newsl. **10**(12): 175.
75. PUI, C.H. 1989. Serum interleukin-2 receptor: clinical and biological implications. Leukemia **3**(5): 323–327.
76. VISSER, J. *et al.* 1998. CD4 T lymphocytes from patients with chronic fatigue syndrome have decreased interferon-gamma production and increased sensitivity to dexamethasone. J. Infect. Dis. **177**(2): 451–454.
77. PAUL, W.E. & & J. OHARA. 1987. B-cell stimulatory factor-1/interleukin-4. Annu. Rev. Immunol. **5:** 429–459.
78. KUEHN, R., K. RAJEWSKY & W. MUELLER. 1991. Generation and analysis of interleukin-4 deficient mice. Science **254:** 713–716.
79. CHAO, C.C. *et al.* 1990. Serum neopterin and interleukin-6 levels in chronic fatigue syndrome. J. Infect. Dis. **162:** 1412–1413.
80. CHAO, C.C. *et al.* 1991. Altered cytokine release in peripheral blood mononuclear cell cultures from patients with the chronic fatigue syndrome. Cytokine **3:** 292–298.
81. SEE, D.M. *et al.* 1997. *In vitro* effect of echinacea and ginseng on natural killer and antibody-dependent cell cytotoxicity in healthy subjects and chronic fatigue syndrome or acquired immunodeficiency syndrome. Immunopharmacology **35:** 229–235.
82. MIZEL, S.B. 1989. The interleukins. FASEB J. **3:** 2379–2388.
83. VAN SNICK, J. 1990. Interleukin-6: an overview. Annu. Rev. Immunol. **8:** 253–278.
84. PENTTILA, I.A. *et al.* 1998. Cytokine dysregulation in the post-Q-fever syndrome. Q. J. Med. **91**(8): 549–560.
85. STRAUS, S.E. *et al.* 1985. Persisting illness and fatigue in adults with evidence of Epstein-Barr virus infection. Ann. Intern. Med. **102:** 7–16.
86. JONES, J.F. *et al.* 1985. Evidence for active Epstein-Barr virus infection in patients with persistent, unexplained illnesses: elevated anti–early antigen antibodies. Ann. Intern. Med. **102:** 1–7.

87. BORYSIEWICZ, L.K. et al. 1986. Epstein-Barr virus–specific immune defects in patients with persistent symptoms following infectious mononucleosis. Q. J. Med. **58:** 111–121.
88. BUCHWALD, D. & A.L. KOMAROFF. 1991. Review of laboratory findings for patients with chronic fatigue syndrome. Rev. Infect. Dis. **13**(1): S12–S18.
89. AOKI, T. et al. 1987. Low natural syndrome: clinical and immunologic features. Nat. Immun. Cell Growth Regul. **6:** 116–128.
90. LLOYD, A., D.A. HANNA & D. WAKEFIELD. 1988. Interferon and myalgic encephalomyelitis. Lancet **1:** 471.
91. HO-YEN, D.O., D. CARRINGTON & A.A. ARMSTRONG. 1988. Myalgic encephalomyelitis and alpha-interferon. Lancet **1:** 125.
92. VOJDANI, A. et al. 1997. Elevated apoptotic cell population in patients with chronic fatigue syndrome: the pivotal role of protein kinase RNA. J. Intern. Med. **242**(6): 465–478.
93. DALAKAS, M.C. et al. 1998. Fatigue: definitions, mechanisms, and paradigms for study. Semin. Oncol. **25**(1, suppl. 1): 48–53.
94. JONES, T.H., S. WADLER & K.H. HUPART. 1998. Endocrine-mediated mechanisms of fatigue during treatment with interferon-alpha. Semin. Oncol. **25**(1, suppl. 1): 54–63.
95. PAVOL, M.A. et al. 1995. Pattern of neurobehavioral deficits with interferon alpha therapy for leukemia. Neurology **45:** 947–950.
96. DAVIS, J.M. et al. 1998. Immune system activation and fatigue during treadmill running: role of interferon. Med. Sci. Sports Exercise **30**(6): 863–868.
97. ZLOTNICK, A. et al. 1983. Characterization of the gamma interferon–mediated induction of antigen-presenting ability in P388D cells. J. Immunol. **131:** 2814–2820.
98. TARGAN, S. & N. STEBBING. 1982. In vitro interactions of purified cloned human interferons on NK cells: enhanced activation. J. Immunol. **129:** 934–935.
99. KNOP, J. et al. 1982. Interferon inhibits the suppressor T cell response of delayed hypersensitivity. Nature **296:** 757–759.
100. KLIMAS, N. et al. 1990. Immunologic abnormalities in chronic fatigue syndrome. J. Clin. Microbiol. **28**(6): 1403–1410.
101. BENNETT, A.L. et al. 1997. Elevation of bioactive transforming growth factor-beta in serum from patients with chronic fatigue syndrome. J. Clin. Immunol. **17**(2): 160–166.
102. BAGASRA, O., J.W. FITZHARIS & T.T. BAGASRA. 1988. Neopterin: an early marker of development of pre-AIDS conditions in HIV-seropositive individuals. Clin. Immunol. Newsl. **9:** 197–199.
103. PATARCA, R. 1997. Pteridines and neuroimmune function and pathology. J. Chronic Fatigue Syndrome **3**(1): 69–86.
104. FUCHS, D. et al. 1994. Nitric oxide synthase and antimicrobial armature of human macrophages. J. Infect. Dis. **169:** 224.
105. FUCHS, D., G. BAIER-BITTERLICH & H. WACHTER. 1995. Nitric oxide and AIDS dementia. N. Engl. J. Med. **333**(8): 521–522.
106. BAIER-BITTERLICH, G. et al. 1995. Effect of neopterin and 7,8-dihydroneopterin on tumor necrosis factor-alpha induced programmed cell death. FEBS Lett. **364:** 234–238.
107. LUTGENDORF, S. et al. 1995. Relationships of cognitive difficulties to immune measures, depression, and illness burden in chronic fatigue syndrome. J. Chronic Fatigue Syndrome **1**(2): 23–41.
108. LUTGENDORF, S. et al. 1995. Physical symptoms of chronic fatigue syndrome are exacerbated by the stress of Hurricane Andrew. Psychosom. Med. **57:** 310–323.
109. FUCHS, D. et al. 1990. Decreased serum tryptophan in patients with HIV-1 infection correlates with increased serum neopterin and with neurologic/psychiatric symptoms. J. AIDS **3:** 873–876.
110. IWAGAKI, H. et al. 1995. Decreased serum tryptophan in patients with cancer cachexia correlates with increased serum neopterin. Immunol. Invest. **24**(3): 467–478.
111. HEYES, M.P. et al. 1995. Quinolinic acid in tumors, hemorrhage, and bacterial infections of the central nervous system in children. J. Neurol. Sci. **133**(1–2): 112–118.
112. SAITO, K. 1995. Biochemical studies on AIDS dementia complex—possible contribution of quinolinic acid during brain damage. Rinsho Byori Jpn. J. Clin. Pathol. **43**(9): 891–901.

113. SHASKAN, E.G. 1992. Increased neopterin levels in brains of patients with human immunodeficiency virus type 1 infection. J. Neurochem. **59**(4): 1541–1546.
114. ANDONDONSKAJA-RENZ, B. & H. ZEITLER. 1984. Pteridines in plasma and in cells of peripheral blood tumor patients. *In* Biochemical and Clinical Aspects of Pteridines, pp. 295–311. de Gruyter. Berlin.
115. SONNERBORG, A. *et al.* 1990. Quantitative detection of brain aberrations in human immunodeficiency virus type 1–infected individuals by magnetic resonance imaging. J. Infect. Dis. **162**: 1245–1251.
116. BUCHWALD, D. *et al.* 1992. Chronic illness characterized by fatigue, neurologic and immunologic disorders, and active human herpesvirus 6 type infection. Ann. Intern. Med. **116**: 103–113.
117. GUPTA, S. & B. VAYUVEGULA. 1991. A comprehensive immunological analysis in chronic fatigue syndrome. Scand. J. Immunol. **33**(3): 319–327.
118. COHEN, S., D.A. TYRRELL & A.P. SMITH. 1991. Psychological stress and susceptibility to the common cold. N. Engl. J. Med. **325**(9): 606–612.
119. GLASER, R. & J.K. KIECOLT-GLASER. 1998. Stress-associated immune modulation: relevance to viral infections and chronic fatigue syndrome. Am. J. Med. **105**(3A): 35S–42S.
120. GLASER, R. *et al.* 1999. Stress-associated immune modulation: implications for infectious diseases? JAMA **281**(24): 2268–2270.

Mediators of Inflammation and Their Interaction with Sleep

Relevance for Chronic Fatigue Syndrome and Related Conditions

JANET M. MULLINGTON,[a,b] DUNJA HINZE-SELCH,[c] AND THOMAS POLLMÄCHER[d]

[b]*Department of Neurology, Beth Israel Deaconess Medical Center and Harvard Medical School, Boston, Massachusetts, USA*

[c]*Department of Psychiatry and Psychotherapy, Christian Albrechts University of Kiel, Kiel, Germany*

[d]*Max Planck Institute of Psychiatry, Clinical Institute, Munich, Germany*

> ABSTRACT: In humans, activation of the primary host defense system leads to increased or decreased NREM sleep quality, depending on the degree of early immune activation. Modest elevations of certain inflammatory cytokines are found during experimental sleep loss in humans and, in addition, relatively small elevations of cytokines are seen following commencement of pharmacological treatments with clozapine, a CNS active antipsychotic agent, known to have immunomodulatory properties. Cytokines such as TNF-α, its soluble receptors, and IL-6, present in the periphery and the CNS, comprise a link between peripheral immune stimulation and CNS-mediated behaviors and experiences such as sleep, sleepiness, and fatigue. The debilitating fatigue experienced in chronic fatigue syndrome and related diseases may also be related to altered cytokine profiles.

In animal research models, sleep is known to be very sensitive to stimulation with bacterial components and cytokine markers of early immune system activation, when applied both centrally and peripherally. Much of the animal research in this area has been reviewed in this volume.[1] In humans, it is also clear that activation of the primary host defense system leads to increased or decreased sleep quality, depending on the dose administered. In addition to host activation using biologic preparations or cytokines, medications may activate host defense mechanisms, which may in turn be related to alterations of human sleep-wake patterns. We will review here some of the effects of sleep loss on immune parameters and evidence for the effects of soluble mediators of inflammation on sleep and sleepiness. We will then turn to review sleep and host response changes associated with chronic fatigue syndrome and related conditions of fibromyalgia and multiple chemical sensitivity.

[a]Address for correspondence: Janet Mullington, Ph.D., Assistant Professor of Neurology, Harvard Medical School, Beth Israel Deaconess Medical Center, 330 Brookline, E/KS-220, Boston, MA 02215. Voice: 617-667-0434; fax: 617-667-1134.
  jmulling@caregroup.harvard.edu

SLEEP LOSS AND ALTERED IMMUNOLOGICAL MARKERS

Studies of sleep loss, both complete and partial sleep deprivation, have been conducted in experimental settings with healthy volunteers and some consistent findings have ensued. Circulating white blood cells, for instance, appear to be elevated during sleep loss.[2–4] The components of the innate immune system that are involved in the early host responses to infection, such as certain leukocyte populations, cytokines, and soluble cytokine receptors, are also sensitive to sleep loss. Monocytes, a major source of cytokines, have been shown to increase during acute sleep deprivation of 39 hours[4] and 64 hours.[3] In addition, cytokines such as interleukin-6 (IL-6) and tumor necrosis factor's soluble receptor p55[5] have been shown to increase in plasma over prolonged periods of sustained wakefulness.

Natural killer (NK) cells are like cytotoxic T lymphocytes, but without the ability to recognize antigen. They derive from bone marrow and have the ability to lyse tumor cells and virally infected cells. They are considered members of the innate immune system and are activated by IL-12, IL-15, and type 1 and 2 interferons. During sleep deprivation, they exhibit a short-lasting drop before rising in number[3,4] and they appear to continue to increase in activity throughout 64 hours of vigil.[3] Further evidence for the altered functional capacity of the innate immune system during sleep loss comes from findings that IL-2 production by LPS-stimulated T cells is reduced[4] and maximal lymphocyte proliferation to PHA is decreased at 48 hours of sleep loss.[6]

While it is clear that sleep loss alters several markers of the activation of the early immune response, we do not know whether these changes are secondary to subtle neuroendocrine or catecholamine changes associated with sleep loss or whether they are directly related to sleep loss itself. It is important therefore to investigate the effects of *in vivo* immune stimulation on sleep in controlled studies and, in addition, to examine these effects in the context of an accumulating sleep deficit.

EXPERIMENTAL HOST RESPONSE AND HUMAN SLEEP

Bacterial products have been used in human research for many years. Since the late 1970s, with the development of techniques that enabled the purification of the active components of gram-negative bacteria into preparations that could be safely used in human research, several lines of investigation have benefited greatly (for reviews, see ref. 7). These biologic preparations of lipopolysaccharide, or endotoxin, as it is commonly referred to, lead at low doses to effects such as short-lasting and mildly increased heart rate and body temperature, and rapid leukopenia followed by a leukocytosis, accompanied by symptoms including chills, headache, muscle ache, and sometimes nausea. The entire activation of the early host response to low-dose endotoxin lasts about 8 hours in total. The subjective symptoms experienced by the subject typically last about 2–3 hours.

The first investigation to use an endotoxin preparation to study human sleep was conducted at the Veterans Administration Hospital, Gainesville, Florida, by Ismet Karacan and colleagues. In their 1968 publication, they reported that, at doses that induced temperature increases of close to 2°C above baseline, rapid eye movement (REM) and non-rapid eye movement (NREM) sleep were suppressed, although

NREM showed a rebound in the second half of the night.[8] More than 20 years later, at the Max Planck Institute in Munich, Germany, using a more purified endotoxin preparation, Pollmächer and colleagues[9] examined the effects of low-dose endotoxin on human sleep, temperature, hypothalamic-pituitary axis hormones, and cytokines and found an increase in NREM sleep, mainly attributable to increased stage 2 sleep, and a decrease in REM sleep. Spectral analysis of NREM sleep EEG did not reveal any differences between placebo and endotoxin conditions with respect to delta power,[9] but did show increased alpha and beta power.[10] While the REM results are consistent with the earlier Karacan paper, the NREM results are contradictory. However, different preparations and pyrogenic potency of the endotoxin preparation used may explain the different findings. Both these contradictory findings and the fact that the animal literature showed more pronounced enhancements of deep NREM sleep than seen in the Pollmächer study led to further studies by the Munich group to examine dose-dependent differences of endotoxin on human sleep.

The dose-dependent studies of endotoxin's effect on human sleep demonstrate that stimulation sufficient to raise inflammatory cytokines, cortisol levels, and temperature by about 1.5°C is sleep-disruptive.[11] However, at levels that were subpyrogenic and failed to raise cortisol levels, but nonetheless increased the levels of inflammatory cytokines, increased amount and spectral intensity of slow wave sleep (SWS) ensued. A dose between these levels, producing temperature increases of about 0.6°C, produced no significant effects on nocturnal sleep, despite significant increases in inflammatory cytokines and cortisol. The human CNS therefore is keenly responsive to changes in peripheral cytokine levels.

The effects of IL-6 and granulocyte colony–stimulating factor (G-CSF) cytokines on human sleep have also been studied. While G-CSF does not elevate temperature, it does stimulate granulopoiesis and granulocyte function and has been shown to increase IL-1 receptor antagonist (IL-1ra) and sTNF-p55 and sTNF-p75 within 2 hours following subcutaneous injection.[12] In that study, TNF-α was reported to rise more slowly, showing a significant elevation over the control values by 8 hours following injection. These changes were persistent 2 hours later. Of particular interest was that, prior to TNF-α elevation, the soluble TNF receptors and IL-1ra were elevated, and deep NREM sleep (SWS) and EEG delta power were reduced. However, when TNF-α levels were elevated, between 5 and 7 A.M., SWS amount and delta power were elevated over placebo levels. These results again link moderate increases in TNF-α to a promotion of NREM amount and intensity. Moreover, these results suggest that increases in the circulating amounts of cytokine antagonists suppress NREM sleep.

IL-6 has been administered subcutaneously to healthy volunteers.[13] These investigators administered 0.5 μg/kg body weight, a dose that induced peak plasma levels of IL-6 of about 80 pg/mL, roughly equivalent to those seen following 0.4 ng/kg body weight of endotoxin.[9,11] Späth-Schwalbe and colleagues[13] found that NREM sleep was suppressed for the first half of the night and, during the second half of the night, there was a rebound. REM sleep, by contrast, was lower across the IL-6 night compared with placebo. Taken together, studies of endotoxin and cytokine administration are consistent in showing that NREM sleep is affected in a very dose-dependent manner, whereas REM sleep appears to be uniformly decreased by endotoxin or by inflammatory cytokines that induce similar levels of early immune system activation.

PHARMACOLOGICAL IMMUNOMODULATION AND SLEEP

Clozapine, an antipsychotic drug that is virtually free of parkinsonian-like side effects that are typical of other neuroleptics, leads to granulocytopenia in approximately 3% of patients and to life-threatening agranulocytosis in up to 1% of patients treated.[14] About 40–45% of patients who begin treatment with this medication experience transient fevers, usually in the second week of treatment.[15,16] These temperature increases within the first 2 weeks of treatment are associated with increased leukocyte counts and cytokine levels (TNF-α, sTNF-Rp55, sTNF-Rp75, sIL-2r, IL-6, and G-CSF). However, even in patients without clozapine-induced fever, plasma TNF-α, sTNF-Rp55, sTNF-Rp75, and sIL-2r were already elevated at 1 week after commencement of treatment and remained elevated at 5 weeks later. In those patients with fever, cytokine levels decreased to the levels of those without fever when they returned to normal body temperature. By contrast, IL-1ra failed to show any change from baseline through the 6-week treatment study period.[15,16] No changes were detected in these cytokines following initiation of treatment with haloperidol in psychiatric patients.[17]

The sleep patterns of patients initiating treatment with clozapine have been described by Hinze-Selch et al.,[18] who found an increase in NREM sleep stage 2 by the first week following initiation of treatment and continuing into the second week. This corresponds to the period where the cytokines measured in the Pollmächer et al.[15] study were also elevated. In a case study of a patient with clozapine-induced fever, Hinze-Selch et al.[19] reported that night sleep was disrupted during fever and these effects were gone by the time that the fever phase had passed at 3 weeks following initiation of treatment.

Taken together, the studies reviewed above suggest that the human CNS, and specifically the arousal system, is exquisitely sensitive to cytokine activation. The sleepiness and increased sleep seen between 1 and 2 weeks following initiation of clozapine treatment coincide with a time when TNF-α, a known somnogenic cytokine, is elevated approximately 60% over baseline levels, on average.

SLEEP AND SLEEPINESS: CYTOKINE CORRELATES

The lines of research discussed above lend support to the view that cytokines are important modulators of sleep and that their prevalence in circulation is altered by sleep loss. In addition to immunomodulation, it is clear that sleep loss affects neurobehavioral functioning. During total sleep deprivation, performance levels on vigilance testing drop steadily, particularly after 24 hours of continuous wakefulness.[3,20] Likewise, performance decrements accumulate during sustained partial sleep loss, or shortened sleep, and this accumulation seems to be without adaptation, at least when nocturnal sleep diet is cut in half for more than 7 days.[21] Sleepiness as manifested by sleep drive can be measured objectively with sleep latency testing in the laboratory, as well as testing the ability to resist sleep when conditions are optimal for sleep initiation. In addition, fatigue can be dissociated from sleepiness in patient symptoms and can also be objectively quantified in the laboratory.

Some data suggest that the cytokines most clearly associated with sleep enhancement may not be those most closely associated with daytime sleepiness and fatigue per se. While animal models have shown that TNF-α and IL-1β are potent somnogenic factors, we have demonstrated that sleep enhancement is seen only at low levels of host response stimulation.[11] Several studies have shown that sleepiness or sleep pressure is associated with increased IL-6 levels during wakefulness.[5,13,22,23] In a study of morning endotoxin challenge following a full night of sleep, Hermann and colleagues[22] found that, although the challenge did not lead to increased daytime sleep, it did result in increased subjective feelings of sleepiness. The time of peak IL-6 concentration in plasma corresponded to the time of greatest self-report of sleepiness. Furthermore, Korth et al.[24] and Hermann et al.[22] found that, when endotoxin was administered in the morning, IL-6 levels were actually negatively correlated with the amount of NREM sleep seen in a 30-min nap taken at 10 A.M. Späth-Schwalbe and colleagues[13] found that subjects reported more feelings of sleepiness and fatigue, felt less capable of concentration, were less activated, and had lower spirits following IL-6 injection than when they had received placebo.

Vgontzas and colleagues[25] induced an experimental sleep deficit to normal healthy volunteers by keeping them awake for 26 hours and then performed frequent blood sampling for the next 24 hours. For the first 14 hours, subjects continued to undergo sleep deprivation and then were permitted recovery sleep. During the wake portion of this frequent blood sampling period, IL-6 was elevated over predeprivation levels and, during recovery sleep, IL-6 rebounded and was actually lower than the baseline night values. More recently, IL-6 and TNF-p55 levels were found to increase steadily across 88 hours of sustained wakefulness, while TNF-α did not show significant change.[5]

While some studies suggest that IL-6 is involved in daytime sleepiness and fatigue, there is much work to be done to confirm such contentions. Based on animal work, we know that IL-1 and TNF-α are very much involved in mediating the host response effects on sleep[26] and that TNF-α exerts its main somnogenic effects via the TNF-p55 receptor[27] rather than its p75 receptor.[28] It is also clear that the effects of IL-1β on sleep are primarily exerted by the IL-1 type 1 receptor.[29] Effects of sleepiness during wake periods and fatigue lend themselves much more readily to study in controlled experiments with humans and, in fact, there is very little known about the effects of IL-6 on sleep in the animal model. In contrast to some of the human studies reviewed above, Opp and colleagues[30] found that IL-6 was not somnogenic in rabbits. Of course, such differences may also be species-specific.

SLEEP AND SLEEPINESS IN CHRONIC FATIGUE SYNDROME, FIBROMYALGIA, AND MULTIPLE CHEMICAL SENSITIVITY

It has been suggested that chronic fatigue syndrome (CFS), fibromyalgia (FM), and multiple chemical sensitivity (MCS) are related syndromes[31] and a 1999 consensus paper even went so far as to make recommendation that "... all 'solicitations' and 'requests for applications' issued by federal agencies for human research into any one of CFS, FM, or MCS direct investigators to screen for all three (regardless of their selection criteria, which need not be affected) and report their results in these terms."[32] Clearly, this approach would be helpful in data interpretation and cross-study integration, but also would be useful for improving diagnostic classifications.

CFS, FM, and MCS all show some degree of evidence of unrefreshing sleep and daytime fatigue. The sleep of these patients has been studied and signs of increased activation during sleep have been described, including increased alpha EEG activity during NREM sleep[33–37] as well as an increase in the fragmentation or wake after sleep onset of either the first half[38] or the whole nocturnal sleep period.[39–42] While chronic fatigue patients are highly aware of waking multiple times through the night, the fatigue that they experience is subjectively perceived to be preceded by disrupted sleep in only 20% of patients.[43]

The disrupted sleep experienced by CFS, FM, and MCS patients is frequently accompanied by pain and may be related to both disrupted slow wave sleep and altered neuroendocrine functioning. The connection between disrupted slow wave sleep and pain experienced on the subsequent day comes from studies of normal healthy volunteers who undergo experimental slow wave sleep disruption in the laboratory. Lentz *et al.*[44] studied healthy middle-aged women and disrupted deep NREM sleep by playing a loud tone when they went into this form of sleep on three consecutive nights. These procedures resulted in lowering the daytime pain threshold as well as increasing the subjective experience of fatigue and discomfort. Increased levels of pain have also been linked with elevated levels of substance P in fibromyalgia patients[45,46] and are also positively correlated with sleep disturbance in these patients.[45]

While the sleep disruption is very common, it cannot explain the pathophysiology of these disorders. To begin with, not every patient with FM, CFS, or MCS has disrupted nocturnal sleep, with or without the alpha-delta pattern. In addition, other patients and nonsymptomatic individuals may also exhibit the alpha-delta pattern in sleep EEG.[47,48] Still other sleep disorder patients have significantly fragmented sleep, yet do not experience the pain and fatigue to the extent experienced by these patients, and instead may experience frank daytime sleepiness and manifest uncontrollable lapses into sleep at inappropriate times during the day.

IMMUNE FUNCTION IN CFS, FM, AND MCS

Some evidence has accumulated suggesting that CFS, FM, and MCS are related to altered immune function. As many as 90% of these patients are women and over 80% have multiple allergic complications. The presence of allergy implies a shift to the TH2 profile of immune dysfunction. However, several studies have shown early inflammatory response profiles that are also abnormal. In contrast to Swanink *et al.*,[49] who found that endotoxin stimulated *ex vivo* production of TNF-α and that IL-1β was lower in CFS patients compared with healthy matched controls, Gupta *et al.*[50] found that spontaneous IL-6 production by isolated monocytes (primarily CD14+) and lymphocyte (primarily CD3+) spontaneous production of TNF-α were higher in patients with CFS. Both monocyte and lymphocyte spontaneous production of IL-10, a major anti-inflammatory cytokine, were reduced in the Gupta study. The increased IL-6 and TNF-α and decreased IL-10 seen in spontaneous production of isolated cells have been replicated by Borish *et al.*[51] Of note, one study has reported finding that serum IL-6 receptors and IL-1 receptor antagonist are elevated in fibromyalgia.[52] While these studies seem to suggest a link in pathophysiology between the immune system, sleep, and sleepiness, it is important to keep in mind that increases and decreases in circulating levels of cytokines or of cells stimulated *ex vivo* are only of limited speculative value without an interpretive context. For this reason, studies of *in vivo* stimulation are particularly important.

In a study designed to investigate the *in vivo* functioning of the inflammatory and HPA host response, Torpy *et al.*[53] administered a low dose of IL-6 to FM patients and control subjects. These investigators administered this dose subcutaneously and found that FM patients had a significantly delayed ACTH return to baseline levels and a higher heart rate when compared with control subjects. A mild fever response (to approximately 38°C) was found and there is no mention that it differed between groups. While the number of subjects is relatively small (7 FM and 7 control subjects received the IL-6 injection), there are no overwhelming findings. Although the heart rate differences are notable from the outset, they do not reach statistical significance. The IL-6 differences are only significant for the time taken to peak levels and there is, in fact, no significant difference between controls and FM patients following injection.

As reviewed above, we know that inflammatory cytokines such as TNF-α and IL-6 are associated with enhanced or disrupted sleep, depending on the dose. IL-6 may have a more tight association with sleepiness or fatigue rather than sleep pressure. Animal research has shown that the IL-1 system is also implicated in the sleep response to infection. The findings that subjective pain and substance P elevations are evident in these patients also implicate inflammatory system involvement in these patients.

Based on what is known in the literature associating sleep loss with inflammatory processes, the rise in pain and substance P in subjects who undergo sleep reduction through experimental sleep fragmentation, and the responsiveness of the sleep system to inflammatory stimulation, we suggest that sleep is an important factor in maintaining integrity of the host response system. Just how this operates is not yet well understood. However, the increased fragmentation of nocturnal sleep, the increased pain sensitivity, the altered immune response profile, and the increase in daytime fatigue so prevalent in disorders like CFS, FM, and MCS suggest that the understanding of these conditions might profit considerably from answers to the questions of how sleep and the neuroendocrine and neuroimmune systems interact. Understanding the interrelationships between these systems at a systemic level might help to elucidate the cause(s) for these diseases and might help to develop new and specific treatments.

ACKNOWLEDGMENTS

We would like to acknowledge NIH Grant No. MH 60641 for support to J. M. Mullington and the Volkswagenstiftung for support to T. Pollmächer.

REFERENCES

1. KRUEGER, J.M., F. OBÁL, JR., J. FANG *et al.* 2001. The role of cytokines in physiological sleep regulation. This volume.
2. KUHN, E., V. BRODAN, M. BRODANOVÁ & K. RYŠÁNEK. 1969. Metabolic reflection of sleep deprivation. Act. Nerv. Super. **11:** 165–174.

3. DINGES, D.F., S.D. DOUGLAS, L. ZAUGG et al. 1994. Leukocytosis and natural killer cell function parallel neurobehavioral fatigue induced by 64 hours of sleep deprivation. J. Clin. Invest. **93:** 1930–1939.
4. BORN, J., T. LANGE, K. HANSEN et al. 1997. Effects of sleep and circadian rhythm on human circulating immune cells. J. Immunol. **158:** 4454–4464.
5. SHEARER, W.T., J.M. REUBEN, J.M. MULLINGTON et al. 2000. Soluble tumor necrosis factor-alpha receptor I and interleukin-6 plasma levels in humans subjected to the sleep deprivation model of space flight. J. Allergy Clin. Immunol. In press.
6. PALMBLAD, J., B. PETRINI, J. WASSERMAN & T. ÅKERSTEDT. 1979. Lymphocyte and granulocyte reactions during sleep deprivation. Psychosom. Med. **41:** 273–278.
7. BRADE, H., S.M. OPAL, S.N. VOGEL & D.C. MORRISON, Eds. 1999. Endotoxin in Health and Disease. Dekker. New York.
8. KARACAN, I., S.M. WOLFF, R.L. WILLIAMS et al. 1968. The effects of fever on sleep and dream patterns. Psychosomatics **9:** 331–339.
9. POLLMÄCHER, T., W. SCHREIBER, S. GUDEWILL et al. 1993. Influence of endotoxin on nocturnal sleep in humans. Am. J. Physiol. **264:** R1077–R1083.
10. TRACHSEL, L., W. SCHREIBER, F. HOLSBOER & T. POLLMÄCHER. 1994. Endotoxin enhances EEG alpha and beta power in human sleep. Sleep **17:** 132–139.
11. MULLINGTON, J.M., C. KORTH, D. HERMANN et al. 2000. Dose-dependent effects of endotoxin on human sleep. Am. J. Physiol. **278:** R947–R955.
12. SCHULD, A., J. MULLINGTON, D. HERMANN et al. 1999. Effects of granulocyte colony–stimulating factor on night sleep in humans. Am. J. Physiol. **276:** R1149–R1155.
13. SPÄTH-SCHWALBE, E., K. HANSEN, F. SCHMIDT et al. 1998. Acute effects of recombinant human interleukin-6 on endocrine and central nervous sleep functions in healthy men. J. Clin. Endocrinol. Metab. **83:** 1573–1579.
14. ALVIR, J.M.J., A. LIEBERMAN, A.Z. SAFFERMAN et al. 1993. Clozapine-induced agranulocytosis: incidence and risk factors in the United States. N. Engl. J. Med. **329:** 162–167.
15. POLLMÄCHER, T., D. HINZE-SELCH & J. MULLINGTON. 1996. Effects of clozapine on plasma cytokine and soluble cytokine receptor levels. J. Clin. Psychopharmacol. **16:** 403–409.
16. POLLMÄCHER, T., T. FENZEL, J. MULLINGTON & D. HINZE-SELCH. 1997. The influence of clozapine treatment on plasma granulocyte colony–stimulating factor (G-CSF) levels. Pharmacopsychiatry **30:** 118–121.
17. POLLMÄCHER, T., D. HINZE-SELCH, T. FENZEL et al. 1997. Plasma levels of cytokines and soluble cytokine receptors during treatment with haloperidol. Am. J. Psychiatry **154:** 1763–1765.
18. HINZE-SELCH, D., J. MULLINGTON, A. ORTH et al. 1997. Effects of clozapine on sleep: a longitudinal study. Biol. Psychiatry **42:** 260–266.
19. HINZE-SELCH, D., J. MULLINGTON & T. POLLMÄCHER. 1995. Sleep during clozapine-induced fever in a schizophrenic patient. Biol. Psychiatry **38:** 690–693.
20. DINGES, D.F. 1992. Probing the limits of functional capability: the effects of sleep loss on short-duration tasks. *In* Sleep, Arousal, and Performance, pp. 176–188. Birkhäuser. Basel/Boston.
21. DINGES, D.F., G. MAISLIN, A. KUO et al. 1999. Chronic sleep restriction: neurobehavioral effects of 4 hr, 6 hr, 8 hr TIB. Sleep **22:** S115–S116.
22. HERMANN, D.M., J. MULLINGTON et al. 1998. Endotoxin-induced changes in sleep and sleepiness during the day. Psychoneuroendocrinology **23:** 427–437.
23. VGONTZAS, A.N., D.A. PAPANICOLAOU, E.O. BIXLER et al. 1997. Elevation of plasma cytokines in disorders of excessive daytime sleepiness: role of sleep disturbance and obesity. J. Clin. Endocrinol. Metab. **82:** 1313–1316.
24. KORTH, C., J. MULLINGTON, W. SCHREIBER & T. POLLMÄCHER. 1996. Influence of endotoxin on daytime sleep in humans. Infect. Immun. **64:** 1110–1115.
25. VGONTZAS, A.N., D.A. PAPANICOLAOU, E.O. BIXLER et al. 1999. Circadian interleukin-6 secretion and quantity and depth of sleep. J. Clin. Endocrinol. Metab. **84:** 2603–2607.
26. TAKAHASHI, S., L. KAPAS, J. FANG & J.M. KRUEGER. 1999. Somnogenic relationships between tumor necrosis factor and interleukin-1. Am. J. Physiol. **276:** R1132–R1140.

27. FANG, J., Y. WANG & J.M. KRUEGER. 1997. Mice lacking the TNF 55 kDa receptor fail to sleep more after TNF-α treatment. J. Neurosci. **17:** 5949–5955.
28. LANCEL, M., J. CRONLEIN, P. MULLER-PREUSS & F. HOLSBOER. 1995. Lipopolysaccharide increases EEG delta activity within non-REM sleep and disrupts sleep continuity in rats. Am. J. Physiol. **268:** R1310–R1318.
29. FANG, J., Y. WANG & J.M. KRUEGER. 1998. Effects of interleukin-1β on sleep are mediated by the type I receptor. Am. J. Physiol. **274:** R655–R660.
30. OPP, M.R., F. OBÁL, JR., A.B. CADY et al. 1989. Interleukin-6 is pyrogenic, but not somnogenic. Physiol. Behav. **45:** 1069–1072.
31. BUCHWALD, D. & D. GARRITY. 1994. Comparison of patients with chronic fatigue syndrome, fibromyalgia, and multiple chemical sensitivities. Arch. Intern. Med. **154:** 2049–2053.
32. BARTHA, L., W. BAUMZWEIGER, D.S. BUSCHER et al. 1999. Multiple chemical sensitivity: a 1999 consensus. Arch. Environ. Health **54:** 147–149.
33. MOLDOFSKY, H., P. SCARISBRICK, R. ENGLAND & H. SMYTHE. 1975. Musculoskeletal symptoms and NREM sleep disturbances in patients with "fibrositis syndrome" and healthy subjects. Psychosom. Med. **37:** 341–351.
34. MOLDOFSKY, H., P. SASKIN & F.A. LUE. 1988. Sleep and symptoms in fibrositis syndrome after a febrile illness. J. Rheumatol. **15:** 1701–1704.
35. SASKIN, P., H. MOLDOFSKY, & F.A. LUE. 1986. Sleep and posttraumatic rheumatic pain modulation disorder (fibrositis syndrome). Psychosom. Med. **48:** 319–323.
36. WHELTON, C.L., I. SALIT & H. MOLDOFSKY. 1992. Sleep, Epstein-Barr virus infection, musculoskeletal pain, and depressive symptoms in chronic fatigue syndrome. J. Rheumatol. **19:** 939–943.
37. MACFARLANE, J.G., B. SHAHAL, C. MOUSLY & H. MOLDOFSKY. 1996. Periodic K-alpha sleep EEG activity and periodic limb movements during sleep: comparisons of clinical features and sleep parameters. Sleep **19:** 200–204.
38. SHAVER, J.L.F., M. LENTZ, C.A. LANDIS et al. 1997. Sleep, psychological distress, and stress arousal in women with fibromyalgia. Res. Nurs. Health **20:** 247–257.
39. MOLONY, R.R., D.M. MACPEEK, P.L. SCHIFFMAN et al. 1986. Sleep, sleep apnea, and the fibromyalgia syndrome. J. Rheumatol. **13:** 797–800.
40. BRANCO, J., A. ATALAIA & T. PAIVA. 1994. Sleep cycles and alpha-delta sleep in fibromyalgia syndrome. J. Rheumatol. **21:** 1113–1117.
41. JENNUM, P., A.M. DREWES, A. ANDREASEN & K.D. NIELSON. 1993. Sleep and other symptoms in primary fibromyalgia and in healthy controls. J. Rheumatol. **20:** 1756–1759.
42. BELL, I.R., R.R. BOOTZIN, C. RITENBAUGH et al. 1996. A polysomnographic study of sleep disturbance in community elderly with self-reported environmental chemical odor intolerance. Biol. Psychiatry **40:** 123–133.
43. MORRISS, R.K., A.J. WEARDEN & L. BATTERSBY. 1997. The relation of sleep difficulties to fatigue, mood, and disability in chronic fatigue syndrome. J. Psychosom. Res. **42:** 597–605.
44. LENTZ, M.J., C.A. LANDIS, J. ROTHERMEL & J.L.F. SHAVER. 1999. Effects of selective slow wave sleep disruption on musculoskeletal pain and fatigue in middle aged women. J. Rheumatol. **26:** 1586–1592.
45. SCHWARTZ, M.J., M. SPÄTH, H. MÜLLER-BARDORFF et al. 1999. Relationship of substance P, 5-hydroxyindole acetic acid, and tryptophan in serum of fibromyalgia patients. Neurosci. Lett. **259:** 196–198.
46. RUSSELL, I.J., M. ORR, B. LITTMAN et al. 1994. Elevated cerebrospinal fluid levels of substance P in patients with the fibromyalgia syndrome. Arthritis Rheum. **37:** 1593–1601.
47. SCHEULER, W., D. STINSHOFF & S. KUBICKI. 1983. The alpha-sleep pattern: differentiation from other sleep patterns and effect of hypnotics. Neuropsychobiology **10:** 183–189.
48. BADER, G.G., T. KAMPE, T. TAGDAE et al. 1997. Descriptive physiological data on a sleep bruxism population. Sleep **20:** 982–990.
49. SWANINK, C.M., J.H. VERCOULEN, J.M. GALAMA et al. 1996. Lymphocyte subsets, apoptosis, and cytokines in patients with chronic fatigue syndrome. J. Infect. Dis. **173:** 460–463.

50. GUPTA, S., S. AGGARWAL, D. SEE & A. STARR. 1997. Cytokine production by adherent and non-adherent mononuclear cells in chronic fatigue syndrome. J. Psychiatr. Res. **31:** 149–156.
51. BORISH, L., K. SCHMALING, J.D. DiCLEMENTI *et al.* 1998. Chronic fatigue syndrome: identification of distinct subgroups on the basis of allergy and psychologic variables. J. Allergy Clin. Immunol. **102:** 222–230.
52. MAES, M., I. LIBBRECHT, F. VAN HUNSEL *et al.* 1999. The immune-inflammatory pathophysiology of fibromyalgia: increased serum soluble gp130, the common signal transducer protein of various neurotrophic cytokines. Psychoneuroendocrinology **24:** 371–383.
53. TORPY, D.J., D.A. PAPANICOLAOU, A.J. LOTSIKAS *et al.* 2000. Responses of the sympathetic nervous system and the hypothalamic-pituitary-adrenal axis to interleukin-6: a pilot study in fibromyalgia. Arthritis Rheum. **43:** 872–880.

The Role of Cytokines in Physiological Sleep Regulation

JAMES M. KRUEGER,[a,b] FERENC OBÁL, JR.,[c] JIDONG FANG,[b] TAKESHI KUBOTA,[b] AND PING TAISHI[b]

[b]*Department of VCAPP, Washington State University, Pullman, Washington 99164, USA*

[c]*Department of Physiology, University of Szeged, Albert Szent-Györgyi Medical Center, Szeged, Hungary*

> ABSTRACT: Several growth factors (GFs) are implicated in sleep regulation. It is posited that these GFs are produced in response to neural activity and affect input-output relationships within the neural circuits where they are produced, thereby inducing a local state shift. These GFs also influence synaptic efficacy. All the GFs currently identified as sleep regulatory substances are also implicated in synaptic plasticity. Among these substances, the most extensively studied for their role in sleep regulation are interleukin-1β (IL-1) and tumor necrosis factor α (TNF). Injection of IL-1 or TNF enhances non-rapid eye movement sleep (NREMS). Inhibition of either IL-1 or TNF inhibits spontaneous sleep and the sleep rebound that occurs after sleep deprivation. Stimulation of the endogenous production of IL-1 and TNF enhances NREMS. Brain levels of IL-1 and TNF correlate with sleep propensity; for example, after sleep deprivation, their levels increase. IL-1 and TNF are part of a complex biochemical cascade regulating sleep. Downstream events include nitric oxide, growth hormone releasing hormone, nerve growth factor, nuclear factor kappa B, and possibly adenosine and prostaglandins. Endogenous substances moderating the effects of IL-1 and TNF include anti-inflammatory cytokines such as IL-4, IL-10, and IL-13. Clinical conditions altering IL-1 or TNF activity are associated with changes in sleep, for example, infectious disease and sleep apnea. As our knowledge of the biochemical regulation of sleep progresses, our understanding of sleep function and of many clinical conditions will improve.

Over the past decade, there has been intense investigation of the biochemical mechanisms of sleep. These studies have led to new insights as to how the brain is organized to produce sleep and to testable ideas concerning the function of sleep. Modern science cannot yet provide a definitive answer to the question, "Why do we sleep?" The enigma of sleep function, unless solved, will likely hinder a complete understanding of other important brain outputs such as memory, emotion, perception, thought, and even consciousness. Regardless, our understanding of the humoral mechanisms of sleep has progressed considerably. This essay will focus on how the cytokines, interleukin-1β (IL-1) and tumor necrosis factor α (TNF), are involved in

---

[a]Address for correspondence: Department of VCAPP, P.O. Box 646520, Washington State University, Pullman, WA 99164-6520. Voice: 509-335-8212; fax: 509-335-4650.
krueger@vetmed.wsu.edu

TABLE 1. Criteria that a putative sleep regulatory substance should fulfill

(1) The substance should induce physiological sleep.

(2) The substance and its receptors should be present in the animal.

(3) The concentration or turnover of the substance or its receptor should vary with the sleep-wake cycle.

(4) Induction of the substance should induce sleep.

(5) Inactivation of the substance or its receptor should reduce spontaneous sleep.

(6) Inactivation of the substance or its receptor should reduce sleep induced by somnogenic stimuli such as sleep deprivation, infectious disease, and mild increases in ambient temperature.

(7) Other biological actions of the substance should be separable, in part, from its sleep-promoting actions.

NOTE: Adapted from reference 1; of the substances illustrated in FIGURE 1, IL-1, TNF, NO, GHRH, and PGD$_2$ have met these criteria. The endogenous inhibitors of sleep illustrated in FIGURE 1, for example, IL-4, IL-10, etc., could also be considered sleep regulator substances; in that case, some of the criteria would be changed to the opposite direction of effect. For example, Opp has shown that CRH has met similar criteria and refers to CRH as a waking substance.[58]

physiological sleep regulation and how this work has contributed to ideas of sleep function.

HUMORAL REGULATION OF NON-RAPID EYE MOVEMENT SLEEP (NREMS)

Many of the molecules involved in NREMS regulation are illustrated in FIGURE 1. These molecules work in concert with each other; there are negative and positive feedback loops within this sleep regulatory system. Further, there are serial steps as well as parallel pathways leading to NREMS. Several investigators have made lists of criteria that a putative sleep regulatory substance should fulfill (see TABLE 1). Of the substances shown in FIGURE 1, IL-1, TNF, nitric oxide (NO), growth hormone releasing hormone (GHRH), and prostaglandin D$_2$ (PGD$_2$) have met all reasonable criteria thus far presented. Briefly, the evidence relating IL-1 and TNF to these criteria follows.[1]

Injection of either IL-1 or TNF enhances the amount of time spent in NREMS. These effects can be rather large. For instance, rabbits given IL-1 at dark onset sleep about 3 extra hours during the first 12 hours after the injection. Normal sleep architecture is maintained after IL-1 or TNF treatment; thus, animals continue to cycle through periods of wakefulness, NREMS, and rapid eye movement sleep (REMS). Animals are easily aroused and the circadian rhythm of sleep continues in IL-1- or TNF-treated animals. Autonomic changes normally associated with sleep-wake cycles such as changes in brain temperature that occur as animals enter either NREMS or REMS persist in IL-1- or TNF-treated animals.[2] IL-1 and TNF are effective whether given directly into the brain or after intraperitoneal or intravenous injections. IL-1 and TNF have been somnogenic in every species thus far tested: these include rats, mice, monkeys, cats, and rabbits. IL-1 and TNF also induce an enhancement of electroencephalographic (EEG) slow waves.[1] Indistinguishable enhancements of EEG slow waves occur during the deep sleep following prolonged wakefulness and are thought to reflect the intensity of sleep.[3] IL-1 and TNF thus appear, by a variety of measures, to induce physiological sleep. However, high doses of IL-1 inhibit sleep rather than promote it. This action could result from the upregulation of negative feedback pathways such as the corticotropin-releasing hormone (CRH)–glucocorticoid axis. IL-1 stimulates CRH production and CRH promotes wakefulness.

Both IL-1 and TNF and their receptors are present in normal brain (reviewed in ref. 1). There are diurnal rhythms of IL-1 mRNA and TNF mRNA and their proteins in rat brain;[4–7] highest levels correlate with the onset of the light period, which in rats is the time of day when NREMS is maximum. After sleep deprivation, IL-1 mRNA and TNF mRNA increase in the brain.[4] Further, excessive food intake, a condition associated with excess NREMS, is also associated with an increase in IL-1 mRNA in the hypothalamus. In cats, cerebrospinal fluid levels of IL-1 also vary with the sleep-wake cycle.[8] In humans, plasma levels of IL-1 are highest at the onset of sleep[9] and circulating levels of TNF correlate with EEG slow-wave activity.[10] Collectively, these data strongly support the notion that levels of IL-1 and TNF vary with the sleep-wake cycle.

Induction of the synthesis of IL-1 or TNF also induces excess NREMS. Thus, microbial substances such as muramyl peptides, viral double-stranded RNA, and lipopolysaccharide all induce IL-1 and TNF production and sleep.[11] The acute phase response during infectious disease is associated with an upregulation of IL-1, TNF, and NREMS. Sleep apnea, a disease associated with sleepiness, is also associated with an upregulation of TNF.[12]

Inactivation of either IL-1 or TNF reduces spontaneous NREMS. For instance, anti-IL-1 or anti-TNF antibodies or IL-1 or TNF soluble receptors inhibit spontaneous sleep.[1,11] These effects can be large; for example, after administration of high doses of the soluble TNF receptor, NREMS is reduced by about 30% for the next 6 hours of recording.[13] Similarly, endogenous substances that inhibit the actions of IL-1 (e.g., α melanocyte-stimulating hormone) inhibit spontaneous sleep.[14] Substances that inhibit the production of either IL-1 or TNF (e.g., IL-4, IL-10, IL-13, or transforming growth factor-β-1) inhibit NREMS.[15] Some of the inhibitors have also been shown to inhibit the sleep rebound that would normally occur after sleep deprivation (e.g., the IL-1 and TNF soluble receptors). Mice lacking either the type I IL-1 receptor[16] or the 55-kDa TNF receptor[17] have less spontaneous sleep than corresponding controls. Mild increases in ambient temperature (Tamb) promote NREMS; if TNF is blocked, the Tamb-induced NREMS responses are attenuated.[18]

Both IL-1 and TNF are pleiotropic—for instance, both are pyrogens. However, both IL-1 and TNF induce increases of NREMS at doses lower than those needed to induce fever. Further, at slightly higher doses that are both somnogenic and pyrogenic, these actions can be separated. For example, coadministration of an antipyretic with IL-1 blocks IL-1-induced fever, but not IL-1-induced NREMS.[19] Conversely, blocking NO synthase using arginine analogs blocks IL-1-induced sleep responses, but not IL-1-induced fever.[20] It is not known whether the many additional biological actions of IL-1 and TNF can be separated from their effects on sleep.

Although both IL-1 and TNF appear to be involved in physiological sleep regulation, other cytokines likely participate in sleep regulation. Thus, acidic fibroblast growth factor, epidermal growth factor, interferon α, IL-18, IL-2, and neurotrophins 1, 2, 3, and 4 all have the capacity to promote NREMS.[1,11] Whether these cytokines have a role in physiological sleep regulation has not been studied. It seems likely that in the future even more substances will be implicated in the biochemical regulation of sleep. A major challenge for sleep research will be to decipher these complex events. Currently, it appears that IL-1 and TNF play a central role in sleep regulation.

DOWNSTREAM BIOCHEMICAL EVENTS INVOLVED IN IL-1 AND TNF INDUCTION OF NREMS

The regulation of all physiological processes such as sleep involves multiple regulatory and effector substances. IL-1 and TNF induce the upregulation and downregulation of many substances thought to be stimuli for the sleep-wake cycle. Both IL-1 and TNF induce activation of the gene transcription factor, nuclear factor kappa B (NFκB). Conversely, NFκB upregulates both IL-1 and TNF and thereby forms a positive feedback loop. Nerve growth factor (neurotrophin-1) shares a similar relationship with NFκB. Inhibition of NFκB, using an inhibitor peptide of NFκB transport from the cytoplasm to the nucleus, inhibits sleep.[21] Further, activation of NFκB, which involves the phosphorylation of IκB and its dissociation from NFκB, is enhanced in the cerebral cortex by sleep deprivation.[22] The promoter region of the genes of many substances thought to be involved in sleep regulation contains an NFκB binding domain. Thus, the adenosine A1 receptor, cyclooxygenase-2 (Cox-2), and NO synthase (NOS) are upregulated by NFκB (FIG. 1).

Positive feedback loops are characteristic of nonlinear systems of amplification. The presence of these positive feedback loops requires the presence of dampening systems. There are many substances in the brain that can inhibit the positive feedback loops illustrated in FIGURE 1. For example, IL-1 induces production of CRH; CRH, in turn, inhibits IL-1 production. CRH also inhibits sleep and this effect is dependent on inhibition of IL-1.[23] Cox-2 is involved in the synthesis of both sleep-promoting prostaglandin D_2 (PGD_2) and sleep-inhibiting PGE_2; PGE_2 inhibits IL-1 production.

Both IL-1 and TNF also induce release of GHRH. GHRH is somnogenic[24] and this pathway may be somewhat independent of NFκB mechanisms, thereby forming a parallel somnogenic pathway (FIG. 1). If rats are pretreated with an anti-GHRH antibody, their NREMS responses induced by IL-1 are greatly attenuated.[25] Anti-GHRH also attenuates spontaneous sleep.[26] GHRH is part of the somatotrophic axis and many of the regulatory steps known for the regulation of pituitary GH secretion also seem to be in place for sleep regulation. GHRHergic neurons projecting to the median eminence are involved in pituitary GH release. Other GHRHergic neurons project to the preoptic anterior hypothalamus (POA) and basal forebrain (BF) areas;[27] these areas are well characterized as being involved in sleep regulation.[28] The effects of GHRH on sleep are likely mediated via these areas. If GHRH is given to hypophysectomized rats, they still exhibit NREMS responses.[29] Microinjection of GHRH into these areas enhances NREMS, whereas microinjection of a GHRH antagonist peptide inhibits sleep and the sleep rebound that occurs after sleep deprivation.[30] Both somatostatin[31] and insulin-like growth factor-1[32] (which is also an anti-inflammatory cytokine) inhibit sleep and inhibit GHRH. Transgenic mice overexpressing GH in the brain, and thus underexpressing GHRH, have less NREMS than corresponding controls.[33] A dwarf strain of rats that have dysfunctional GHRH receptors also have less NREMS than controls.[1] Collectively, there is strong evidence for the involvement of GHRH in physiological NREMS regulation. It seems likely that the somnogenic actions of IL-1 and TNF are, in part, mediated by GHRH.

Finally, in reference to FIGURE 1, only substances involved in NREMS are illustrated. A partially independent biochemical cascade for REMS regulation could be made; it would include the addition of vasoactive intestinal peptide and prolactin.

SLEEP AND BRAIN ORGANIZATION

Many of the NREMS regulatory substances such as GHRH, IL-1, adenosine, NO, and PGD_2 can induce NREMS if applied directly to sleep regulatory circuits such as the POA-BF areas. However, in response to sleep loss, the production of IL-1, TNF, brain-derived neurotropic factor (BDNF; also called neurotrophin-2), adenosine, and possibly other molecules illustrated in FIGURE 1 is enhanced in other brain areas such as the cerebral cortex. These and other findings have led to a reconsideration of how the brain is organized to produce sleep. It has raised simple questions that are difficult to answer. For example: What is it exactly that sleeps? Is sleep an emergent property of a population of neurons or is it a cellular property of neurons? The latter would be very difficult to define since there is no set of cellular properties that lend themselves to defining sleep at a higher level of organization.

Several major activational systems exist in the brain. Further, several sleep regulatory networks such as the POA-BF areas for NREMS regulation and the pons for REMS are well documented. These findings form the basis for the dominant paradigm in sleep research: the concept that sleep is imposed upon the brain by specific neural networks. However, recent evidence challenges this paradigm by suggesting that sleep is not imposed upon the brain by a small group of neurons, nor is it a phenomenon of the whole brain.[34] No neuronal circuit *necessary* for sleep has been identified. Countless lesions and poststroke investigations lead to the simple conclusion: if an animal or person survives the injury, it sleeps. Dolphins have high amplitude EEG slow waves characteristic of deep NREMS only on one half the brain at a time.[35] Further, unihemispheric deprivation of sleep results in sleep rebound on the half of the brain deprived of sleep, but not on the other half.[36] Birds can detect predators during unihemispheric NREMS, and the occurrences of unihemispheric sleep vary as a function of predation risk.[37] Evidence was obtained in monkeys that electrophysiological signs of sleep occur in the association cortex sooner than in the primary visual cortex.[38] In humans, there is an anteroposterior gradient in the power of low-frequency activity in the EEG during the first sleep cycles.[39] The sleep deprivation-induced increases in slow-wave activity are larger in the frontal derivations than in parietal derivations.[40] Rats also exhibit larger increases in slow-wave activity after sleep deprivation in the frontal derivations than in occipital derivations.[41] The distribution of activation during sleep, whether measured by EEG techniques or functional magnetic resonance imaging (fMRI), is dependent upon the distribution of activity during prior wakefulness. Thus, unilateral stimulation of the somatosensory cortex during wakefulness results in enhanced slow-wave activity in the stimulated area during subsequent NREMS.[42] Similarly, Drummond et al.[43,44] using fMRI reached the conclusion that the localized effects of sleep loss are dependent, in part, on the specific cognitive task performed during prior wakefulness. Such data suggest that sleep can be differentially stimulated in various areas of the brain depending on prior neural activity. This concept is a significant departure from the long-held view that sleep is dependent upon duration (rather than activity) of prior wakefulness. This concept is also consistent with the observations that stimuli, such as mild increases in ambient temperature,[45] excessive food intake,[46] or certain stressors,[47] enhance sleep without prior sleep loss. Such considerations have led several investigators to conclude that sleep is a distributed process of the brain with small highly interconnected groups of neurons forming the fundamental units of sleep organization.[34,48,49]

SLEEP FUNCTION

The notion that sleep is a fundamental property of neuronal groups consisting of relatively few highly interconnected neurons [see Edelman[50] for an extensive discourse on the concept of neuronal groups] led directly to the question of sleep function. Theories of sleep function fall into two classes: those positing that sleep serves to maintain, repair, or consolidate synapses and those focusing on bodily functions. We focus here on the synaptic plasticity notions since the bodily function theories fail to explain why the loss of vigilance associated with sleep (which considered by itself is maladaptive) is necessary. In contrast, synaptic theories of sleep function all indirectly imply the following: if work is being done on synapses, then the brain needs to be taken "off line" so that a mismatch of environmental input to organism output does not occur.

Moruzzi[51] first stated that sleep serves a synaptic function. However, his concept was formulated within the context of the idea that use of synapses led to their wear and tear, and thus sleep, thought to be a period of synaptic quiescence, was needed as a synaptic repair period. Within the field of memory, different ideas of synaptic efficacy had already developed. Thus, in 1949, Hebb[52] had proposed that synaptic efficacy (the Hebbian terminology is synaptic weights, which can be positive or negative) is enhanced by synaptic use and this action thereby forms the physical substrate of memory. More modern research has provided overwhelming evidence in support of Hebb's ideas.[53] Thus, the microcircuitry of the brain remains dynamic throughout life and is, to a large extent, determined by use and disuse of synapses.[53,54] As a consequence, some mechanism is required to maintain synapses responsible for innate memories as well as acquired memories. For instance, circuits involved in species-specific behaviors, the synaptic organization responsible for co-ordinating homostatic processes, or synapses responsible for memories formed years before recall may be seldom used. Such synapses need stimulation to remain functional and we previously termed the pattern of synaptic activation for such events a synaptic superstructure.[34] We proposed that stimulation of such a synaptic superstructure is a function of sleep. Further, sleep would also contribute to the efficacy of synapses intensely used or newly formed during wakefulness, thereby helping, for instance, memory consolidation.

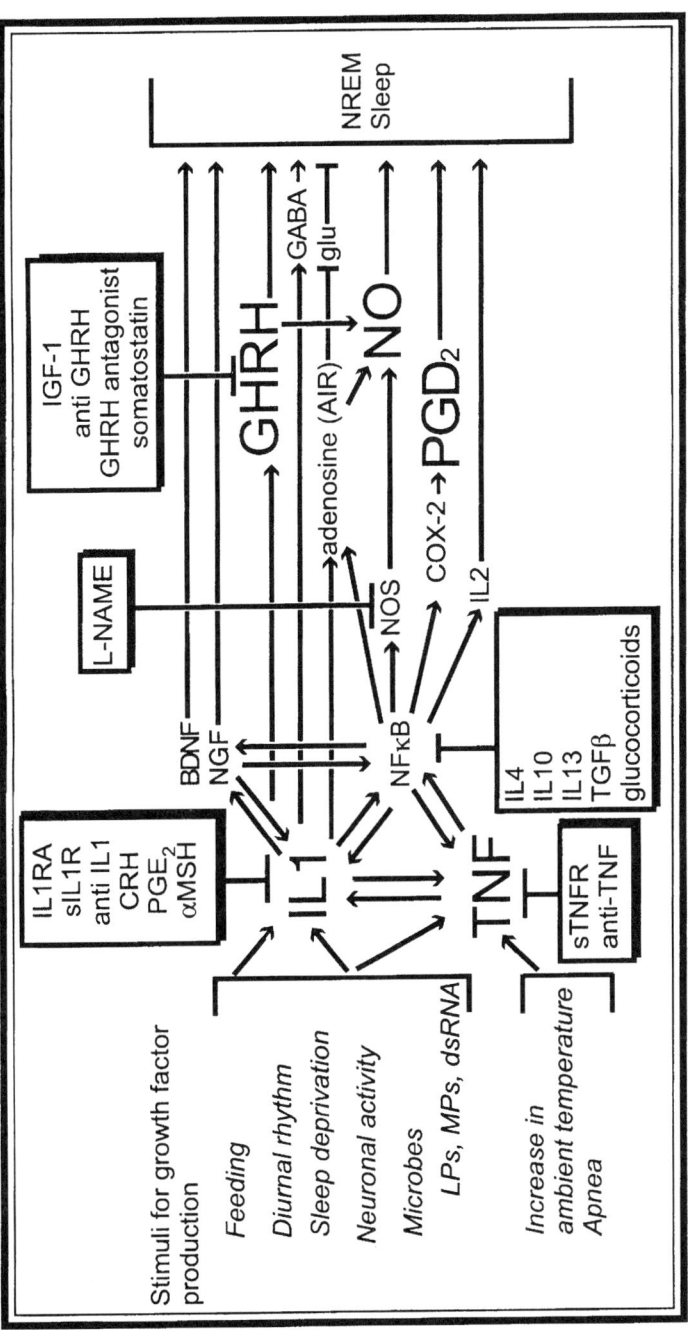

FIGURE 1. See following page for caption.

TABLE 2. Putative sleep regulatory substances involved in synaptic plasticity

Interleukin-1	Nuclear factor kappa B
Tumor necrosis factor	Brain-derived neurotropic factor
Nitric oxide	Nerve growth factor
Adenosine	Fibroblast growth factor
Prostaglandins	Epidermal growth factor

NOTE: Citations for the effect of each of these substances on sleep and plasticity are easily found using Pub-Med. The release/synthesis of all the substances listed is enhanced by neuronal activity.

We have proposed that, when neurons are activated, the associated changes in membrane potentials, neurotransmitter release, ionic conductance, etc., stimulate the production of sleep regulatory substances (FIG. 1; TABLE 2). These substances are growth factors and, as such, alter expression of genes involved in synaptic function and thereby alter the microcircuitry of the brain as a function of neural use. These substances also have additional actions; they affect membrane potentials[55] and other cellular functions, such as intracellular Ca^{++} concentration, of nearby neurons and thereby alter input-output relationships of neurons. Thus, synapses that were not activated by the initial train of events are secondarily activated with a time delay due to the production and diffusion times of upregulated growth factors (see ref. 34 for a model). As a consequence, the input-output activity patterns of the neural groups are changed and thereby divorce the outputs from environmental input.

We have hypothesized that, when neuronal groups are in the state in which their outputs are divorced in time from environmental inputs, they are asleep.[34] To return these groups to an awake state, the substances discussed above that dampen the

---

FIGURE 1. Sleep regulatory system. Extensive evidence exists showing that the substances illustrated are involved in sleep regulation (see text). These substances affect the production or action of one another. Collectively, these actions form the biochemical cascade illustrated. Arrows (→) indicate activation or enhanced production; ⊣ indicates an inhibitory effect. Substances in boxes inhibit NREMS, while other substances enhance NREMS. Many of those substances that promote sleep are growth factors (e.g., IL1, TNF, BDNF, NGF, IL2, NO, PGs, adenosine, NFκB) and are upregulated by neuronal activity (e.g., IL1, TNF, BDNF, NGF, adenosine, NO). We have hypothesized that sleep mechanisms involve these neuron-activity-dependent substances and that sleep function is related to synaptic efficacy (see text). Abbreviations: LPs, lipopolysaccharides; MPs, muramyl peptides; dsRNA, double-stranded RNA; IL1RA, interleukin-1 receptor antagonist; sIL1R, soluble IL1 receptor; anti-IL1, anti-IL1 antibodies; CRH, corticotropin-releasing hormone; PGE_2, prostaglandin E_2; αMSH, α melanocyte-stimulating hormone; IL1, interleukin-1; TNF, tumor necrosis factor; sTNFR, soluble TNF receptor; anti-TNF, anti-TNF antibodies; BDNF, brain-derived neurotrophic factor; NGF, nerve growth factor; NFκB, nuclear factor kappa B; IL4, interleukin-4; IL10, interleukin-10; IL13, interleukin-13; TGFβ, transforming growth factor β; L-NAME, an arginine analog; NOS, nitric oxide synthase; COX-2, cyclooxygenase-2; IL2, interleukin-2; IGF-1, insulin-like growth factor 1; anti-GHRH, anti-GHRH antibodies; GHRH, growth hormone releasing hormone; NO, nitric oxide; PGD_2, prostaglandin D_2; A1R, the adenosine A1 receptor; GABA, γ-aminobutyric acid; glu, glutamic acid.

positive feedback loops illustrated in FIGURE 1 would serve this purpose. Further, we view the loss of responsiveness to environmental stimuli (sleep-associated unconsciousness) as a graded function of the number of neural groups in the "sleep state". Sleep is thus a statistical property of a population of neural groups in different states.

Regardless of such considerations, there is sufficient evidence to conclude that cytokines such as TNFα or IL-1β are involved in physiological sleep regulation. Further, it seems clear that the fatigue of certain pathologies is associated with an overexpression of cytokines. For example, chronic fatigue syndrome is associated with an increase in TNFα.[56] Other conditions such as rheumatoid arthritis are also associated with increased TNFα. Further treatment of rheumatoid arthritic patients with an inhibitor of TNFα, the 75-kDa TNF soluble receptor, reduces the fatigue associated with the disease.[57] It is tempting to speculate that perhaps similar treatment might be beneficial to chronic fatigue syndrome and chemical intolerant patients.

ACKNOWLEDGMENTS

This work was supported in part by the National Institutes of Health (Grant Nos. NS25378, NS27250, NS31453, and HD36520).

REFERENCES

1. KRUEGER, J.M. *et al.* 1999. Humoral regulation of physiological sleep: cytokines and GHRH. J. Sleep Res. **8**(suppl. 1): 53–59.
2. WALTER, J. *et al.* 1986. Brain temperature changes coupled to sleep states persist during interleukin-1-enhanced sleep. Am. J. Physiol. **250**: R96–R103.
3. PAPPENHEIMER, J.R. *et al.* 1975. Extraction of sleep-promoting factor S from cerebrospinal fluid and from brains of sleep-deprived animals. J. Neurophysiol. **38**: 1299–1311.
4. TAISHI, P. *et al.* 1998. Sleep-associated changes in interleukin-1β mRNA in the brain. J. Interferon Cytokine Res. **18**: 793–798.
5. BREDOW, S. *et al.* 1997. Diurnal variations of tumor necrosis factor α mRNA and α-tubulin mRNA in rat brain. Neuroimmunomodulation **4**: 84–90.
6. FLOYD, R.A. & J.M. KRUEGER. 1997. Diurnal variation of TNF α in the rat brain. Neuroreport **8**: 915–918.
7. NGUYEN, K.T. *et al.* 1998. Exposure to acute stress induces brain interleukin-1β protein in the rat. J. Neurosci. **18**: 2239–2246.
8. LUE, F.A. *et al.* 1988. Sleep and cerebrospinal fluid interleukin-1-like activity in the cat. Int. J. Neurosci. **42**: 179–183.
9. MOLDOFSKY, H. *et al.* 1986. The relationship of interleukin-1 and immune functions to sleep in humans. Psychosom. Med. **48**: 309–318.
10. DARKO, D.F. *et al.* 1995. Sleep electroencephalogram delta-frequency amplitude, night plasma levels of tumor necrosis factor α, and human immunodeficiency virus infection. Proc. Natl. Acad. Sci. U.S.A. **92**: 12080–12084.
11. KRUEGER, J.M. & J.A. MAJDE. 1994. Microbial products and cytokines in sleep and fever regulation. Crit. Rev. Immunol. **14**: 355–379.
12. VGONTZAS, A.N. *et al.* 2000. Sleep apnea and daytime sleepiness and fatigue: relation to visceral obesity, insulin resistance, and hypercytokinemia. J. Clin. Endocrinol. Metab. **85**: 1151–1158.
13. TAKAHASHI, S. *et al.* 1995. Inhibition of tumor necrosis factor in the brain suppresses rabbit sleep. Pflüg. Arch. **431**: 155–160.
14. OPP, M.R. *et al.* 1988. Effects of α-MSH on sleep, behavior, and brain temperature: interactions with IL 1. Am. J. Physiol. **255**: R914–R922.

15. KUBOTA, T. *et al.* 2000. Interleukin-13 and transforming growth factor-β1 inhibit spontaneous sleep in rabbits. Am. J. Physiol. **279:** R786–R792.
16. FANG, J. *et al.* 1998. Effects of interleukin-1β on sleep are mediated by the type I receptor. Am. J. Physiol. **274:** R655–R660.
17. FANG, J. *et al.* 1997. Mice lacking the TNF 55 kDa receptor fail to sleep more after TNFα treatment. J. Neurosci. **17:** 5949–5955.
18. TAKAHASHI, S. & J.M. KRUEGER. 1997. Inhibition of tumor necrosis factor prevents warming-induced sleep responses in rabbits. Am. J. Physiol. **272:** R1325–R1329.
19. KRUEGER, J.M. *et al.* 1984. Sleep-promoting effects of endogenous pyrogen (interleukin-1). Am. J. Physiol. **246:** R994–R999.
20. KAPÁS, L. *et al.* 1994. Inhibition of nitric oxide synthesis suppresses sleep in rabbits. Am. J. Physiol. **266:** R151–R157.
21. KUBOTA, T. *et al.* 2000. A nuclear factor-kappa B (NF-κB) inhibitor peptide inhibits spontaneous and interleukin-1β-induced sleep. Am. J. Physiol. **279:** R404–R413.
22. CHEN, Z. *et al.* 1999. Nuclear factor-κB-like activity increases in murine cerebral cortex after sleep deprivation. Am. J. Physiol. **276:** R1812–R1818.
23. OPP, M. *et al.* 1989. Corticotropin-releasing factor attenuates interleukin 1–induced sleep and fever in rabbits. Am. J. Physiol. **257:** R528–R535.
24. OBÁL, F., JR. *et al.* 1988. Growth hormone–releasing factor enhances sleep in rats and rabbits. Am. J. Physiol. **255:** R310–R316.
25. OBÁL, F., JR. *et al.* 1995. Growth-hormone-releasing hormone mediates the sleep-promoting activity of interleukin-1 in rats. Neuroendocrinology **61:** 559–565.
26. OBÁL, F., JR. *et al.* 1992. Growth hormone–releasing hormone antibodies suppress sleep and prevent enhancement of sleep after sleep deprivation. Am. J. Physiol. **263:** R1078–R1085.
27. SAWCHENKO, P.E. *et al.* 1985. The distribution of growth-hormone-releasing factor (GRF) immunoreactivity in the central nervous system of the rat: an immunohistochemical study using antisera directed against rat hypothalamic GRF. J. Comp. Neurol. **237:** 100–115.
28. SZYMUSIAK, R. 1995. Magnocellular nuclei of the basal forebrain: substrates of sleep and arousal regulation. Sleep **18:** 478–500.
29. OBÁL, F., JR. *et al.* 1996. Effects of systemic GHRH on sleep in intact and hypophysectomized rats. Am. J. Physiol. **270:** E230–E237.
30. ZHANG, J. *et al.* 1999. Intrapreoptic microinjection of GHRH or its antagonist alters sleep in rats. J. Neurosci. **19:** 2187–2194.
31. BERANEK, L. *et al.* 1999. Central administration of the somatostatin analog octreotide induces captopril-insensitive sleep responses. Am. J. Physiol. **277:** R1297–R1304.
32. OBÁL, F. *et al.* 1999. Insulin-like growth factor-1 (IGF-1)–induced inhibition of growth hormone secretion is associated with sleep suppression. Brain Res. **818:** 267–274.
33. ZHANG, J. *et al.* 1996. Non-rapid eye movement sleep is suppressed in transgenic mice with a deficiency in the somatotropic system. Neurosci. Lett. **220:** 97–100.
34. KRUEGER, J.M. & F. OBÁL. 1993. A neuronal group theory of sleep function. J. Sleep Res. **2:** 63–69.
35. MUKHAMETOV, L.M. *et al.* 1977. Interhemispheric asymmetry of the electroencephalographic sleep patterns in dolphins. Brain Res. **134:** 581–584.
36. OLEKSENKO, A.I. *et al.* 1992. Unihemispheric sleep deprivation in bottlenose dolphins. J. Sleep Res. **1:** 40–44.
37. RATTENBORG, N. *et al.* 1999. Half-awake to the risk of predation. Nature **397:** 397–398.
38. PIGAREV, I.N. *et al.* 1997. Evidence for asynchronous development of sleep in cortical areas. Neuroreport **8:** 2557–2560.
39. WERTH, E. *et al.* 1997. Fronto-occipital EEG power gradients in human sleep. J. Sleep Res. **6:** 102–112.
40. CAJOCHEN, C. *et al.* 1999. Frontal predominance of a relative increase in sleep delta and theta EEG activity after sleep loss in humans. Sleep Res. Online **2:** 65–69.
41. SCHWIERIN, B. *et al.* 1999. Regional differences in the dynamics of the cortical EEG in the rat after sleep deprivation. Clin. Neurophysiol. **110:** 869–875.
42. KATTLER, H. *et al.* 1994. Effect of unilateral somatosensory stimulation prior to sleep on the sleep EEG in humans. J. Sleep Res. **3:** 159–164.

43. DRUMMOND, A. *et al.* 2000. Altered brain response to verbal learning following sleep deprivation. Nature **403:** 655–657.
44. DRUMMOND, A. *et al.* 1999. Sleep deprivation–induced reduction in cortical functional response to serial subtraction. Neuroreport **10:** 3745–3748.
45. OBÁL, F., JR. 1984. Thermoregulation and sleep. Exp. Brain Res. Suppl. **8:** 157–172.
46. HANSEN, M.K. *et al.* 1998. Cafeteria diet–induced sleep is blocked by subdiaphragmatic vagotomy in rats. Am. J. Physiol. **274:** R168–R174.
47. JOUVET, M. 1994. Paradoxical sleep mechanisms. Sleep **17:** S77–S83.
48. KAVANAU, J.L. 1994. Sleep and dynamic stabilization of neural circuitry: a review and synthesis. Behav. Brain Res. **63:** 111–126.
49. BENINGTON, J.H. & H.C. HELLER. 1995. Restoration of brain energy metabolism as the function of sleep. Prog. Neurobiol. **45:** 347–360.
50. EDELMAN, G.M. 1987. Neural Darwinism. Basic Books. New York.
51. MORUZZI, G. 1972. The sleep-waking cycle. Rev. Physiol. **64:** 2–165.
52. HEBB, D.O. 1949. The Organization of Behavior. Wiley. New York.
53. BAUDRY, J.L. *et al.* 2000. Advances in Synaptic Plasticity. MIT Press. Cambridge, MA.
54. PURVES, D. 1994. Neural Activity and the Growth of the Brain. Cambridge University Press. London/New York.
55. LUK, W.P. *et al.* 1999. Adenosine: a mediator of interleukin-1β-induced hippocampal synaptic inhibition. J. Neurosci. **19:** 4238–4244.
56. MOSS, R.B. *et al.* 1999. TNF-alpha and chronic fatigue syndrome. J. Clin. Immunol. **19:** 314–316.
57. FRANKLIN, C.M. 1999. Clinical experience with soluble TNF p75 receptor in rheumatoid arthritis. Semin. Arthritis Rheum. **29:** 172–181.
58. CHANG, F.C. *et al.* 1998. Blockade of corticotropin-releasing hormone receptors reduces spontaneous waking in the rat. Am. J. Physiol. **275:** R793–R802.

Cytokine-Induced Sickness Behavior: Mechanisms and Implications

ROBERT DANTZER[a]

INRA-INSERM U394, 33077 Bordeaux Cedex, France

ABSTRACT: Sickness behavior refers to a coordinated set of behavioral changes that develop in sick individuals during the course of an infection. At the molecular level, these changes are due to the brain effects of proinflammatory cytokines such as interleukin-1 (IL-1) and tumor necrosis factor alpha (TNFα). Peripherally released cytokines act on the brain via a fast transmission pathway involving primary afferent nerves innervating the bodily site of inflammation and a slow transmission pathway involving cytokines originating from the choroid plexus and circumventricular organs and diffusing into the brain parenchyma by volume transmission. At the behavioral level, sickness behavior appears to be the expression of a central motivational state that reorganizes the organism priorities to cope with infectious pathogens. There is evidence that the sickness motivational state can interact with other motivational states and respond to nonimmune stimuli probably by way of sensitization and/or classical conditioning. However, the mechanisms that are involved in plasticity of the sickness motivational state are not yet understood.

INTRODUCTION

Nonspecific symptoms of infection and inflammation include fever and profound physiological and behavioral changes. Sick individuals experience weakness, malaise, listlessness, and inability to concentrate. They become depressed and lethargic, show little interest in their surroundings, and stop eating and drinking. This constellation of nonspecific symptoms is collectively referred to as "sickness behavior". Due to their commonality, sickness symptoms are frequently ignored by physicians. They are considered as an uncomfortable, but rather banal, component of the pathogen-induced debilitation.

This view is, however, totally inadequate. The behavioral symptoms of sickness represent, together with the fever response, a highly organized strategy of the organism to fight infection.[1] In physiological terms, fever corresponds to a new homeostatic state that is characterized by a raised set point of body temperature regulation. A feverish individual feels cold at usual environmental temperatures. Therefore, the feverish person not only seeks warmer temperatures, but also enhances heat production (increased thermogenesis) and reduces heat loss (decreased thermolysis). The higher body temperature that is achieved during fever stimulates proliferation of immune cells and is unfavorable for the growth of many bacterial and viral patho-

---

[a]Address for correspondence: INSERM U394, Rue Camille Saint-Saens, 33077 Bordeaux Cedex, France. Voice: (33) 5 57 57 37 25; fax: (33) 56 98 90 29.
   robert.dantzer@bordeaux.inserm.fr

gens. In addition, the reduction of zinc and iron plasma levels that occurs during fever decreases the availability of these vital elements for growth and multiplication of microorganisms. The adaptive nature of the fever response is apparent from studies showing that organisms infected with a bacteria or virus and unable to mount an appropriate fever response because they are kept in a cold environment or treated with an antipyretic drug have a lower survival rate than organisms that develop a normal fever.[2]

The amount of energy that is required to increase body temperature during the febrile process is quite high since, in human beings, metabolic rate needs to be increased by 13% for a rise of 1°C in body temperature. Because of the high metabolic cost of fever, there is little room for activities other than those favoring heat production (e.g., shivering) and minimizing thermal losses (e.g., rest, curl-up posture, piloerection).

In recent years, evidence has rapidly accumulated to demonstrate that the necessary synchrony between metabolic, physiological, and behavioral components of the systemic response to infection is dependent on the same molecular signals as those that are already responsible for the local inflammatory response. These signals are proinflammatory cytokines, such as interleukin-1 (IL-1), interleukin-6 (IL-6), tumor necrosis factor α (TNFα), and interferons (IFNs), that are released by activated monocytes and macrophages during the course of an infection. These cytokines act on the brain in two successive waves: a first wave that is triggered by activation of primary afferent neurons innervating the body site where the inflammatory reaction takes place and a second wave that involves slowly diffusing cytokines from the circumventricular organs and choroid plexus to brain targets such as the amygdaloid complex.

Although sickness behavior is a normal response of the host to pathogens that are recognized by the innate immune system, there is evidence that sickness behavior can be triggered by nonimmune stimuli, in the same way that sickness behavior can alter the organism response to environmental stressors.

CYTOKINES INDUCE SICKNESS BEHAVIOR

Systemic or central infusion of recombinant cytokines induces the full-blown repertoire of nonspecific symptoms of sickness in both experimental animals and human beings. The same effects are obtained in response to the administration of molecules that induce the synthesis of endogenous cytokines [e.g., lipopolysaccharide (LPS), the active fragment of endotoxin from gram-negative bacteria].

The behavior of animals injected with LPS or cytokines at the periphery or into the lateral ventricle of the brain has been studied extensively.[3] Rats injected with LPS or IL-1β after drinking a new taste solution develop a conditioned aversion to the taste of that solution.[4,5] Conditioned taste aversions have also been established to TNFα. However, treatment with IFNα fails to induce conditioned taste aversion.[6] The reasons for these differences between cytokines are still unclear.

Decreased social exploration of juvenile conspecifics has been used as a convenient way to assess sickness behavior in laboratory rodents. It involves olfactory sampling of the partner and is normally used for social recognition. It offers the advantage of being reproducible and quantifiable. The use of juvenile conspecifics helps to keep at a minimum the emergence of other behavioral patterns such as sexual behavior or aggression normally occurring with adult partners. Systemic administration of LPS, IL-1β, and TNFα to adult laboratory animals, rats, or mice consistently decreases the time spent in exploration of juveniles.[7–9]

Another important component of sickness behavior is the decreased intake of food that develops in sick individuals. Systemic administration of IL-1β and TNFα consistently suppresses feeding. This effect has been observed using various measurements of food intake under *ad libitum* as well as deprived conditions.[10,11] In contrast to the decrease in social exploration that takes about 2 hours to develop, the suppression of food intake occurs within 1 hour following treatment.

NEUROANATOMICAL BASIS OF SICKNESS BEHAVIOR

Our understanding of the way that sickness behavior is organized in the brain is based on several methodological approaches. Molecular biology studies have demonstrated that peripheral cytokines induce the synthesis and release of cytokines in the brain. LPS, for instance, induces the expression of IL-1α, IL-1β, and TNFα, followed by that of IL-6.[12,13] The main cellular sources of IL-1 are represented by microglial cells and perivascular and meningeal macrophages.[14] These locally produced cytokines are responsible for the central components of the host response to infection, as demonstrated by pharmacology experiments making use of cytokine antagonists or cytokine receptor antagonists. For instance, administration of the IL-1 receptor antagonist (IL-1ra) into the lateral ventricle of the brain to block brain IL-1 receptors abrogated the depressing effect of peripherally administered IL-1 on social exploration in rats exposed to a juvenile.[15] Using expression of the early gene *c-fos* as a marker of neuronal activation in those brain areas that are activated by stressors, neuroanatomists have identified the brain targets of peripheral immune stimuli. Wan *et al.*[16] were the first authors to show that intraperitoneal injection of LPS activates the primary projection area of the vagus nerve in the brain, which is represented by the nucleus tractus solitarius, and the secondary projections of this nerve, including the parabrachial nucleus, the hypothalamic paraventricular and supraoptic nuclei, the central nucleus of the amygdala, and the bed nucleus of the stria terminalis. A subdiaphragmatic section of the vagus nerves abrogated the expression of Fos in these brain areas. The key role of the vagus nerve in the transmission of peripheral immune signals to the brain was further confirmed by the demonstration that vagotomy attenuates the behavioral actions of peripheral cytokines[17,18] and abrogates the induction of IL-1β in the brain in response to peripheral LPS or IL-1β.[19,20]

The abdominal vagus nerve has the important peculiarity of being associated with immune cells that express IL-1β in response to local inflammation.[21] This locally produced IL-1β binds to vagal fibers to increase vagal discharge activity. Glutamate is released at the level of the nucleus tractus solitarius (NTS) where vagal fibers terminate.[22] Glutamate acts on catecholaminergic neurons of the NTS that project to the paraventricular and preoptic nuclei.[23,24] The central nucleus of the amygdala can be reached via this pathway or, more probably, via the parabrachial nuclei.[25] These pathways appear to be responsible for the activating effects of inflammatory stimuli on the hypothalamic-pituitary-adrenal (HPA) axis and their depressing effects on behavior. However, the pyrogenic activity of inflammatory stimuli involves still another pathway represented by prostaglandin synthesis by cyclooxygenase-2 around blood vessels.[26]

The brain production of IL-1β in response to peripheral inflammatory stimuli is first restricted to the choroid plexus and circumventricular organs.[27] It then slowly diffuses to the brain side of the blood-brain barrier by volume transmission. Direct activation of neurons by slowly diffusing IL-1β takes place in the basolateral amygdala and the area postrema. Projections from the basolateral amygdala mediate the depressing effects of IL-1β on social exploration, whereas those from the area postrema contribute to activation of the HPA axis.[28] The observation that a late (4 hours post-LPS) infusion of IL-1ra into the lateral ventricle of the brain attenuates the depressing effects of systemic LPS on social exploration concomitantly with an abrogation of Fos expression in the central amygdala and bed nucleus of the stria terminalis points to the role of these two structures in cytokine-induced behavioral depression.[28]

In summary, activation of afferent nerve fibers by peripherally released cytokines represents a fast pathway of transmission of immune signals from the periphery to the brain. This pathway certainly sensitizes the brain target areas to the action of brain-produced cytokines that relay and amplify the action of peripheral cytokines.

MOTIVATIONAL ASPECTS OF SICKNESS BEHAVIOR

Sickness behavior is usually viewed by physicians as the result of debilitation and physical weakness that inevitably occur in an organism whose all resources are engaged in a defensive process against pathogens. An alternative hypothesis is that sickness behavior is the expression of a highly organized strategy that is critical to the survival of the organism. If it is the case, then it follows that sick individuals should be able to reorganize their behavior depending on its consequences and the internal and external constraints they are exposed to. This flexibility is characteristic of what psychologists call a motivation. A motivation can be defined as a central state that reorganizes perception and action. A typical motivational state is fear. In order to escape a potential threat, a fearful individual must be attentive to everything that is occurring in his/her environment. At the same time, he/she must be ready to engage in the most appropriate defensive behavioral pattern that he/she has available in his/her behavioral repertoire. In other terms, a motivational state does not trigger an unflexible behavioral pattern. It enables one to uncouple perception from action and therefore to select the appropriate strategy depending on the eliciting situation.[29]

The first evidence that sickness behavior is the expression of a motivational state rather than the consequence of weakness was provided by Miller.[30] He showed that rats injected with endotoxin stopped bar-pressing for water, but, when given water, drank it, although to a lesser extent than normally. This effect was not specific to thirst since the endotoxin treatment also reduced bar-pressing for food and even blocked responding in rats trained to press a bar for the rewarding effects of electrical stimulation in the lateral hypothalamus. Interestingly enough, when rats were trained to turn off an aversive electrical stimulation in this brain area, endotoxin also reduced the rate of responding, but to a lesser extent than bar-pressing for a rewarding brain stimulation. However, when rats were placed in a rotating drum that they could stop for brief periods by pressing a lever, endotoxin treatment resulted in an increase rather than a decrease in their response rate. The mere fact that endotoxin treatment could decrease or increase behavioral output depending on its consequences gave strong support to the motivational interpretation of the behavioral effects of such a treatment.

An example of behavioral reorganization in response to sickness is provided by the effects of LPS on macronutrient intake. When rats are given the opportunity to select components of their diet, their selection pattern reflects the organism's nutritional and energetic requirements. To determine whether this selection pattern is altered during sickness, rats were submitted to a dietary self-selection protocol in which they had free access to carbohydrate, protein, and fat diets for 4 hours a day.[31] After a 10-day habituation to this regimen, they were injected with LPS or IL-1β. Under the effect of this treatment, they decreased their total food intake, but reorganized their self-selection pattern so as to ingest relatively more carbohydrate and less protein, whereas fat intake remained unchanged. This change in macronutrient intake contrasts with the increased fat intake that occurs in rats exposed to cold. Although eating fat would be a better way for feverish animals to cope with their increased energy requirements, it would not be of much use since cytokines have adverse metabolic effects resulting in increased lipolysis and hypertriglyceridemia. Under these conditions, an increased intake of fat would actually be counterproductive since it would further enhance hyperlipidemia without positively contributing to lipid metabolism.

An important characteristic of a motivational state is that it competes with other motivational states for behavioral output. The normal expression of behavior requires a hierarchical organization of motivational states that is continuously updated according to circumstances. When an infection occurs, the sick individual is at a life or death juncture and his/her physiology and behavior must be altered so as to overcome the disease. However, this is a relatively long-term process that needs to make room for more urgent needs when necessary. It is easy to imagine the following: if a sick person lying in his/her bed hears a fire alarm ringing in his/her house and sees flames and smoke coming out of the basement, he/she should be able to momentarily overcome his/her sickness behavior to escape danger. In motivational terms, fear competes with sickness, and fear-motivated behavior takes precedence over sickness behavior. An example of this competition between fear and sickness is provided by the observation that the depressing effects of IL-1β on behavior of mice are more pronounced when experimental animals are tested in the safe surroundings of their home cage than when they are placed into a new environment.

Another example of the motivational aspects of sickness behavior is the effect of cytokines on maternal behavior. If fitness is the key issue, it is evident that dams should care for their infants despite sickness. In motivational terms, the components of maternal behavior that are crucial for the survival of the progeny should be more resilient, that is, less sensitive to the depressing effects of pyrogens, than those behavioral patterns that are less important. In accordance with this prediction, administration of LPS to lactating mice did not disrupt pup retrieval, but impaired nest-building.[32] However, LPS treatment was less effective in depressing nest-building when the dams and their litters were exposed to 4°C, increasing the fitness value of nest-building, than when dams were tested at 20°C.

To show that sickness does not interfere with the subject's ability to adjust his/her behavioral strategies with regard to his/her needs and capacities, Aubert *et al.*[33] assessed the effects of LPS on food hoarding and food consumption in rats receiving or not a food supplement in addition to the amount of food they obtained in the situation. Rats were trained to get food for 30 min in an apparatus consisting of a cage connected to an alley with free food at its end. In this apparatus, rats normally bring back to their home cage the food that is available at the end of the alley and the amount of food they hoard is lower when they receive a food supplement than when they have no supplement. In response to LPS, food intake was decreased to the same extent whether rats received a food supplement or not. However, food hoarding was less affected in rats that did not receive a food supplement compared to rats provided with the food supplement. These results indicate that the internal state of sickness induced by LPS is more effective in suppressing the immediate response to food than the anticipatory response to future needs.

SENSITIZATION AND CONDITIONING OF CYTOKINE-INDUCED SICKNESS BEHAVIOR

Repeated injections of TNFα lead to different results depending on the interval between injections.[34] In animals injected with a subeffective dose of the cytokine, administration of TNFα at 1–7 days later was associated with a lowered response or a lack of response. However, lengthening the interval to 14–29 days resulted in an enhancement of the sickness response.

Instances of cross-sensitization between cytokines and nonimmune stressors have been reported, using the pituitary-adrenal response as an endpoint. Adult rats injected with a single dose of IL-1β and exposed 1 to 2 weeks later to a novel environment displayed a heightened reactivity of the pituitary-adrenal axis to novelty.[35] Similar long-lasting (1–12 weeks) sensitization of the pituitary-adrenal axis response to IL-2 has been reported in humans.[36] In the first case, the enhanced reactivity of the HPA axis has been shown to be mediated by an increased expression of vasopressin in the hypothalamic neurons that normally predominantly express corticotropin-releasing hormone (CRH).[35]

The possibility that sickness behavior can be triggered by nonimmune stimuli has been studied using mainly behavioral conditioning. Most of the studies have focused on the febrile response to LPS. In a typical experiment carried out in rats, LPS was used as an unconditioned stimulus in a taste aversion model using the taste of a saccharin solution as the unconditioned stimulus. LPS induced an initial fall in body temperature followed by an increase. The same pattern, although less marked, was observed in rats reexposed to the saccharin taste solution at 2 weeks after conditioning.[37] Conditioning of the febrile response has also been observed in mice exposed to a camphor odor paired with administration of the interferon inducer poly I:C.[38] In this study, one conditioning session was sufficient for conditioning-increased body temperature in young and old mice, and this conditioned response was quickly extinguished following a second reexposure to the conditioned stimulus. The possibility that conditioning extends to other components of the sickness response has been examined in a number of studies. Rats responded to saccharin paired with LPS by displaying a conditioned decrease in food intake,[39] as well as a conditioned suppression of splenocyte IL-2 production and splenic norepinephrine content concomitantly with a conditioned enhancement of plasma corticosterone levels.[40] All components of the sickness response to LPS are not conditionable to the same extent since rats reexposed to saccharin paired with LPS displayed a conditioned febrile response, but not the typical increased slow-wave sleep and decreased REM sleep observed in LPS-treated animals on the conditioning day.[41] However, since this experiment was carried out during the light portion of the dark-light cycle, the possibility that the somnogenic components of the acute phase response are conditionable was retested by reexposing rats to the saccharin taste solution during the dark portion of the light-dark cycle.[42] This resulted in a conditioned increase in slow-wave sleep, but no change in REM sleep. All these findings appear at first glance to provide a demonstration of the conditionability of the sickness response. However, the interpretation of this phenomenon is not as straightforward as it appears a priori, especially since, at least in the case of body temperature, conditioned changes in body temperature were observed in rats exposed to saccharin paired with lithium chloride instead of LPS.[37] Thus, there is clearly a need for further investigation of the modalities and specificity of conditioning influences on sickness behavior.

PSYCHOPATHOLOGICAL IMPLICATIONS OF THE EXISTENCE OF A MOTIVATIONAL STATE OF SICKNESS

The demonstration that the immune system is able to influence behavior and mental states has important implications for our understanding of the relationships between psychological factors and disease. In the case of cancer, for example, such psychological features as the feelings of hopelessness and helplessness that are commonly associated with the onset and progression of the disease might be secondary to the effects on the central nervous system of factors released from immune or tumor cells during the early stage of the neoplastic process. The same possibility applies to the relationship between psychological factors and autoimmune diseases. The possible causal role of cytokines in the mental and behavioral symptoms that occur in various pathological conditions has hardly been investigated, except in a few cases, such as infection and fever, cachexia, AIDS dementia complex, chronic fatigue syndrome, and depression.

There is already evidence demonstrating that proinflammatory cytokines are responsible for the development of subjective and behavioral symptoms of sickness during infection with a bacterial or viral pathogen. For instance, patients treated with IFNα show fever, anorexia, fatigue, headache, myalgia, and arthralgia. These symptoms culminate in lethargy and withdrawal from the surroundings. The same symptoms are observed in volunteers injected with low doses of LPS. The possibility that the release of cytokines accounts for more subtle changes in cognition and performance has been assessed by Smith *et al.*[43] On the basis of earlier work showing that infection with upper respiratory viruses decreased the efficiency with which psychomotor tasks were performed, volunteers of both sexes were injected with IFNα. Volunteers injected with the larger dose were significantly slower at responding in a reaction time task when they were uncertain when the target stimulus would appear. Simultaneously, they displayed hyperthermia and experienced feelings of illness.

However, they were not impaired on a pursuit tracking task or syntactic reasoning task. These effects were similar to the alterations in performance observed in patients with influenza.[43]

The possibility that proinflammatory cytokines have relatively specific effects on cognitive processes has been further investigated in animal models. IL-1β, but not IL-6, impaired spatial navigation learning in rats.[44] A similar deficit in spatial learning was observed in mice injected with IL-1β or infected with the pathogenic agent *Legionella pneumophila*.[45] Interference of cytokines with formation of new memories has also been demonstrated in an autoshaping task in which rats learned to press a lever that was introduced into the cage before food delivery.[46] These effects of cytokines appear to be independent of their pyrogenic activity since they were observed whether body temperature increased or decreased in response to the treatment under study.

There has been much speculation on the possible pathogenic role of cytokines in chronic fatigue syndrome (CFS). Always feeling tired is a common complaint of patients afflicted with a viral infection and represents the core symptom of the so-called postviral fatigue syndrome. CFS patients feel the same, but in the absence of any persistent viral infection.[47] Their symptoms are real, pervasive, and often incapacitating. The fact that a substantial proportion of these patients fulfill criteria for major depression and other psychiatric illness does not facilitate the classification of this disorder. Whatever the case, and in view of the similarities between the subjective effects of cytokines and the symptoms reported by CFS patients, many researchers have looked for possible overproduction of cytokines in this condition. Elevated plasma levels of proinflammatory cytokines have been reported in a number of studies of CFS patients,[48,49] but these results have not been found in other studies.[50–52] Such inconsistent results can be easily explained by heterogeneity of the clinical population under study, technical problems associated with the detection of cytokines in biological fluids, and the poor correlation between plasma levels of cytokines and local activity of these mediators. A better way of assessing peripheral cytokine function is to study the ability of peripheral blood mononuclear cells (PBMC) to produce cytokines when put in culture and stimulated with adequate stimuli. Using such a strategy, a few authors have found evidence that chronic fatigue is associated with low-level activation of the immune system.[53–55] However, it is important to note that abnormalities, if any, of the cytokine network are not necessarily present at the periphery, but might instead affect preferably cytokines that are expressed in the central nervous system.

Besides their commonality in CFS patients, lack of energy and loss of interest are very frequent in depressed patients. These symptoms are actually incorporated in the basic description of depressive episodes. The tenth revision of the International Classification of Disease begins with the statement that "the subject suffers from a lowering of mood, reduction of energy, and decrease in activity. Capacity for enjoyment, interest, and concentration are impaired, and marked tiredness after even minimum effort is common." The possibility that activation of peripheral blood monocytes and T lymphocytes plays a role in the pathophysiology of major depression has been proposed by Maes *et al.*[56] In addition to the evidence pointing out the profound effects of cytokines on behavior and the HPA axis, this hypothesis is based on the observation of an increased production of cytokines by monocytes and T lymphocytes of depressed patients. For example, elevated levels of acute phase proteins and increased concentrations of IL-6 and its soluble receptor have been found in the plasma of subjects with major depression and there was a close relationship between IL-6 levels and acute phase proteins. However, more research is still needed before a specific role of immune products in the pathogenesis of depressive symptoms can be accepted.[57] The observed immune alterations appear to be a trait rather than a state marker of depression since they persist even when depressive symptoms regress. Further, the possible contribution of antidepressant treatment to the changes in immune functions observed in depressed patients remains to be established.

If the evidence in favor of an association between depression and an acute phase response is still contradictory, it is clear that administration of cytokines to non-psychiatric patients can induce true depressive episodes. Cytokines are commonly administered in the medical treatment of malignancies and chronic viral infection. The flu-like symptoms that develop very early in all of the patients are followed more or less rapidly by depressed mood and alterations in cognition. Severe depression occurs in about one-third of the patients. Patients treated with IL-2 become clinically depressed after a few days of treatment, whereas patients treated with IFNα become depressed after a few weeks.[58] The risk of developing a depressive episode is positively correlated to the score of depressed mood at the initiation of treatment, despite the fact that the initial scores are within the normal range.[59] There is preliminary evidence that the mood changes induced by IFNα immunotherapy can be prevented by pretreatment with fluoxetine.[60]

The possibility of a role of cytokines in depression has also been studied in animal models of depression. In the absence of any knowledge on the causal factors of depression, most animal models of depression are based on behavioral and pharmacological analogies. At the behavioral level, the two main symptoms that are usually considered include the deficit in escape/avoidance learning and the anhedonia, or more precisely the diminished capacity to experience pleasure, which are typically displayed by experimental animals exposed to uncontrollable electric shocks. At the pharmacological level, chronic (but not acute) treatment with antidepressant drugs blocks the development of these symptoms. A number of studies provide some evidence for a role of cytokines in animal models of depression. Intracerebroventricular administration of the IL-1 receptor antagonist (IL-1ra), which blocks the access of endogenous IL-1 to its receptors, attenuated the escape-avoidance deficit induced by inescapable electric shock in rats.[61] In a different series of experiments, cytokine treatment was found to induce anhedonia in rats, as evidenced by decreased responding for rewarding lateral hypothalamic self-stimulation in response to IL-2 and LPS, but not to IL-1β and IL-6,[62] and attenuated preference for a saccharin solution in response to LPS.[63] This last effect was antagonized by chronic (but not acute) treatment with the antidepressant drug imipramine.[63] The behavioral effects of LPS were attenuated by pretreatment with chronic (but not acute) imipramine.[63] The atypical antidepressant drug tianeptine had the same action. It attenuated the effects of LPS and IL-1β injected peripherally on behavior and pituitary-adrenal activity, but it failed to alter the behavioral effects of LPS and IL-1β when these molecules were injected into the lateral ventricle of the brain.[64]

Since chemical intolerance overlaps considerably with somatization and depression, the possibility that cytokines play a role in the associated symptomatology certainly warrants specific investigations. Positive results were recently reported in a small-scale study comparing middle-aged women with chemical intolerance to depressed women and a normal control group.[65] Circulating levels of neopterin, a marker of inflammation and monocyte/macrophage activation, did not differ between groups, but were positively correlated with chemical intolerance and somatization scales.

CONCLUSIONS

Sufficient evidence is now available to accept the concept that cytokines are interpreted by the brain as molecular signals of sickness. Sickness can actually be considered as a motivation, that is, a central state that organizes perception and action in face of this particular threat that is represented by infectious pathogens. A sick individual does not have the same priorities as a well one, and this reorganization of priorities is mediated by the effects of cytokines on a number of peripheral and central targets. The elucidation of the mechanisms that are involved in these effects should give new insight on the way that sickness and recovery processes are organized in the brain.

ACKNOWLEDGMENTS

This work was supported by INSERM, INRA, Université de Bordeaux II, Pôle Médicament Aquitaine, the European Community (Biomed CT97-2492, TMR CT97-0149), and NIH (MH51569-02 and DK49311).

REFERENCES

1. HART, B.L. 1988. Biological basis of the behavior of sick animals. Neurosci. Biobehav. Rev. **12:** 123–137.
2. KLUGER, M.J. 1979. Fever: Its Biology, Evolution, and Function. Princeton University Press. Princeton, NJ.
3. KENT, S., R.M. BLUTHÉ, K.W. KELLEY et al. 1992. Sickness behavior as a new target for drug development. Trends Pharmacol. Sci. **13:** 24–28.
4. TAZI, A., R. DANTZER, F. CRESTANI et al. 1988. Interleukin-1 induces conditioned taste aversion in rats: a possible explanation for its pituitary-adrenal stimulating activity. Brain Res. **473:** 369–371.
5. TAZI, A., F. CRESTANI & R. DANTZER. 1990. Aversive effects of centrally injected interleukin-1 are independent of its pyrogenic activity. Neurosci. Res. Commun. **7:** 159–165.
6. SEGALL, M.A. & L.S. CRNIC. 1990. A test of conditioned taste aversion with mouse interferon-α. Brain Behav. Immun. **4:** 223–231.
7. BLUTHÉ, R.M., R. DANTZER & K.W. KELLEY. 1992. Effects of interleukin-1 receptor antagonist on the behavioral effects of lipopolysaccharide in rat. Brain Res. **573:** 318–320.
8. BLUTHÉ, R.M., F. CRESTANI, K.W. KELLEY et al. 1992. Mechanisms of the behavioral effects of interleukin-1: role of prostaglandins and CRF. Ann. N.Y. Acad. Sci. **650:** 268–275.
9. BLUTHÉ, R.M., M. PAWLOWSKI, S. SUAREZ et al. 1994. Synergy between tumor necrosis factor α and interleukin-1 in the induction of sickness behavior in mice. Psychoneuroendocrinology **19:** 197–207.

10. KENT, S., J.L. BRET-DIBAT, K.W. KELLEY et al. 1995. Mechanisms of sickness-induced decreases in food-motivated behavior. Neurosci. Biobehav. Rev. **20:** 171–175.
11. PLATA-SALAMAN, C.R. 1993. Cytokines and ingestive behavior: methods and overview. Methods Neurosci. **17:** 151–168.
12. GATTI, S. & T. BARTFAI. 1993. Induction of tumor necrosis factor-α mRNA in the brain after peripheral endotoxin treatment: comparison with interleukin-1 family and interleukin-6. Brain Res. **624:** 291–295.
13. LAYÉ, S., P. PARNET, E. GOUJON et al. 1994. Peripheral administration of lipopolysaccharide induces the expression of cytokine transcripts in the brain and pituitary of mice. Mol. Brain Res. **27:** 157–162.
14. VAN DAM, A.M., M. BROUNS, S. LOUISSE et al. 1992. Appearance of interleukin-1 in macrophages and ramified microglia in the brain of endotoxin-treated rats: a pathway for the induction of nonspecific symptoms of sickness. Brain Res. **588:** 291–296.
15. KENT, S., R.M. BLUTHÉ, R. DANTZER et al. 1992. Different receptor mechanisms mediate the pyrogenic and behavioral effects of interleukin-1. Proc. Natl. Acad. Sci. U.S.A. **89:** 9117–9120.
16. WAN, W., L. WETMORE, C.M. SORENSEN et al. 1994. Neural and biochemical mediators of endotoxin and stress-induced *c-fos* expression in the rat brain. Brain Res. Bull. **34:** 7–14.
17. BLUTHÉ, R.M., V. WALTER, P. PARNET et al. 1994. Lipopolysaccharide induces sickness behavior in rats by a vagal mediated mechanism. C. R. Acad. Sci. Paris Sci. Vie **317:** 499–503.
18. BLUTHÉ, R.M., B. MICHAUD, K.W. KELLEY et al. 1996. Vagotomy attenuates behavioral effects of interleukin-1 injected peripherally, but not centrally. Neuroreport **7:** 1485–1488.
19. LAYÉ, S., R.M. BLUTHÉ, S. KENT et al. 1995. Subdiaphragmatic vagotomy blocks induction of IL-1β mRNA in mice brain in response to peripheral LPS. Am. J. Physiol. **268:** R1327–R1331.
20. HANSEN, M.K., P. TAISHI, Z. CHEN et al. 1998. Vagotomy blocks the induction of interleukin-1 beta (IL-1 beta) mRNA in the brain of rats in response to systemic IL-1 beta. J. Neurosci. **18:** 2247–2253.
21. GOEHLER, L.E., R.P. GAYKEMA, K.T. NGUYEN et al. 1999. Interleukin-1 beta in immune cells of the abdominal vagus nerve: a link between the nervous and immune systems? J. Neurosci. **19:** 2799–2806.
22. MASCARUCCI, P., C. PEREGO, S. TERRAZZINO et al. 1998. Glutamate release in the nucleus tractus solitarius induced by peripheral lipopolysaccharide and interleukin-1 beta. Neuroscience **86:** 1285–1290.
23. ERICSSON, A., K.J. KOVACS & P.E. SAWCHENKO. 1994. A functional anatomical analysis of central pathways subserving the effects of interleukin-1 on stress-related neuroendocrine neurons. J. Neurosci. **14:** 897–913.
24. SAWCHENKO, P.E. & L.W. SWANSON. 1982. The organization of noradrenergic pathways from the brain stem to the paraventricular and supraoptic nuclei in the rat. Brain Res. **257:** 275–325.
25. TKACS, N. & J. LI. 1999. Immune stimulation induces Fos expression in brain stem amygdala afferents. Brain Res. Bull. **48:** 223–231.
26. CAO, C., K. MATSUMURA, K. YAMAGATA et al. 1997. Involvement of cyclooxygenase-2 in LPS-induced fever and regulation of its mRNA by LPS in the rat brain. Am. J. Physiol. **272:** R1712–R1725.
27. KONSMAN, J.P., K.W. KELLEY & R. DANTZER. 1999. Temporal and spatial relationships between lipopolysaccharide-induced expression of Fos, interleukin-1β, and inducible nitric oxide synthase in rat brain. Neuroscience **89:** 535–548.
28. KONSMAN, J.P. 2000. Immune-to-brain communication: a functional neuroanatomical analysis. Ph.D. thesis, Gröningen University/Bordeaux II University, Gröningen/Bordeaux.
29. BOLLES, R.C. 1970. Species-specific defense reactions and avoidance learning. Psychol. Rev. **77:** 32–48.
30. MILLER, N.E. 1964. Some psychophysiological studies of motivation and of the behavioral effects of illness. Bull. Br. Psychol. Soc. **17:** 1–20.

31. AUBERT, A., G. GOODALL & R. DANTZER. 1995. Compared effects of cold ambient temperature and cytokines on macronutrient intake in rats. Physiol. Behav. **57:** 869–873.
32. AUBERT, A., G. GOODALL, R. DANTZER et al. 1997. Differential effects of lipopolysaccharide on pup retrieving and nest building in lactating mice. Brain Behav. Immun. **11:** 107–118.
33. AUBERT, A., K.W. KELLEY & R. DANTZER. 1997. Differential effects of lipopolysaccharide on food hoarding behavior and food consumption in rats. Brain Behav. Immun. **11:** 229–238.
34. HAYLEY, S., K. BREBNER, S. LACOSTA et al. 1999. Sensitization to the effects of tumor necrosis factor-alpha: neuroendocrine, central monoamine, and behavioral variations. J. Neurosci. **19:** 5654–5665.
35. TILDERS, F.J.H. & E.D. SCHMIDT. 1999. Cross-sensitization between immune and non-immune stressors: a role in the etiology of depression? Adv. Exp. Biol. Med. **461:** 179–197.
36. DENICOFF, K.D., T.M. DURKIN, M.T. LOTZE et al. 1989. The neuroendocrine effects of interleukin-2 treatment. J. Clin. Endocrinol. Metab. **69:** 402–410.
37. BULL, D.F., R. BROWN, M.G. KING et al. 1991. Modulation of body temperature through taste aversion conditioning. Physiol. Behav. **49:** 1229–1233.
38. HIRAMOTO, R.N., V.K. GHANTA, C.F. ROGERS et al. 1991. Conditioning the elevation of body temperature, a host defensive reflex response. Life Sci. **49:** 93–99.
39. EXTON, M.S., D.F. BULL & M.G. KING. 1995. Behavioral conditioning of lipopolysaccharide-induced anorexia. Physiol. Behav. **57:** 401–405.
40. JANZ, L.L., J. GREEN-JOHNSON, L. MURRAY et al. 1996. Pavlovian conditioning of LPS-induced responses: effects on corticosterone, splenic NE, and IL-2 production. Physiol. Behav. **59:** 1103–1109.
41. BULL, D.F., M.S. EXTON & A.J. HUSBAND. 1994. Acute-phase immune response: lipopolysaccharide-induced fever and sleep alterations are not simultaneously conditionable in the rat during the inactive (light) phase. Physiol. Behav. **56:** 143–149.
42. EXTON, M.S., D.F. BULL, M.G. KING et al. 1995. Modification of body temperature and sleep state using behavioral conditioning. Physiol. Behav. **57:** 723–729.
43. SMITH, A., D. TYRRELL, K. COYLE et al. 1988. Effects of interferon alpha in man: a preliminary report. Psychopharmacology **96:** 414–416.
44. OITZL, M.S., H. VAN OERS, B. SCHÖBITZ et al. 1993. Interleukin-1β, but not interleukin-6, impairs spatial navigation learning. Brain Res. **613:** 160–163.
45. GIBERTINI, M., C. NEWTON, H. FRIEDMAN et al. 1995. Spatial learning impairment in mice infected with *Legionella pneumophila* or administered exogenous interleukin-1β. Brain Behav. Immun. **9:** 113–128.
46. AUBERT, A., C. VEGA, R. DANTZER et al. 1995. Pyrogens specifically disrupt the acquisition of a task involving cognitive processing in the rat. Brain Behav. Immun. **9:** 129–148.
47. KENDELL, R.E. 1991. Chronic fatigue, viruses, and depression. Lancet **337:** 160–162.
48. CANNON, J.G., J.B. ANGEL, R.W. BALL et al. 1999. Acute phase response and cytokine secretion in chronic fatigue syndrome. J. Clin. Immunol. **19:** 414–421.
49. MOSS, R.B., A. MERCANDETTI & A. VOJDANI. 1999. TNF-alpha and chronic fatigue syndrome. J. Clin. Immunol. **19:** 314–316.
50. LAMANCA, J.J., S.A. SISTO, X.D. ZHOU et al. 1999. Immunological responses in chronic fatigue syndrome following a graded exercise test to exhaustion. J. Clin. Immunol. **19:** 135–142.
51. ZHANG, Q., X.D. ZHOU, T. DENNY et al. 1999. Changes in immune parameters seen in Gulf War veterans, but not in civilians with chronic fatigue syndrome. Clin. Diagn. Lab. Immunol. **6:** 6–13.
52. BUCHWALD, D., M.H. WENER, T. PEARLMAN et al. 1997. Markers of inflammation and immune activation in chronic fatigue and chronic fatigue syndrome. J. Rheumatol. **24:** 372–376.
53. GUPTA, S., S. AGGARWAL, D. SEE et al. 1997. Cytokine production by adherent and non-adherent mononuclear cells in chronic fatigue syndrome. J. Psychiatr. Res. **31:** 149–156.
54. CANNON, J.G., J.B. ANGEL, L.W. ABAD et al. 1997. Interleukin-1 beta, interleukin-1 receptor antagonist, and soluble interleukin-1 receptor type II secretion in chronic fatigue syndrome. J. Clin. Immunol. **17:** 253–261.

55. CHAO, C.C., E.N. JANOFF, S. HU *et al.* 1991. Altered cytokine release in peripheral blood mononuclear cell cultures from patients with the chronic fatigue syndrome. Cytokine **3:** 292–295.
56. MAES, M., R. SMITH & S. SCHARPE. 1995. The monocyte-T-lymphocyte hypothesis of major depression. Psychoneuroendocrinology **20:** 111–116.
57. DANTZER, R., L. VITKOVIC, E.E. WOLLMAN & R. YIRMIYA. 1999. Cytokines and depression: fortuitous or causative association? Mol. Psychiatry **4:** 328–332.
58. CAPURON, L., A. RAVAUD & R. DANTZER. 2000. Early depressive symptoms in cancer patients receiving interleukin–2 and/or interferon alpha-2b therapy. J. Clin. Oncol. **18:** 2143–2151.
59. CAPURON, L. & A. RAVAUD. 1999. Prediction of the depressive effects of interferon alpha therapy by the patient's initial affective state. N. Engl. J. Med. **340:** 1370.
60. MILLER, A.H., C.M. PARIANTE & B.D. PEARCE. 1999. Effects of cytokines on glucocorticoid receptor expression and function: glucocorticoid resistance and relevance to depression. Adv. Exp. Med. Biol. **461:** 107–116.
61. MAIER, S.F. & L. WATKINS. 1995. Intracerebroventricular interleukin-1 receptor antagonist blocks the enhancement of fear conditioning and interference with escape produced by inescapable shock. Brain Res. **695:** 279–282.
62. ANISMAN, H. & Z. MERALI. 1999. Anhedonic and anxiogenic effects of cytokine exposure. Adv. Exp. Biol. Med. **461:** 199–234.
63. YIRMIYA, R. 1996. Endotoxin produces a depressive-like episode in rats. Brain Res. **711:** 163–174.
64. CASTANON, N., R.M. BLUTHÉ & R. DANTZER. 2000. Chronic treatment with the atypical antidepressant tianeptine attenuates sickness behavior induced by peripheral, but not central lipopolysaccharide and interleukin-1β in the rat. Psychopharmacology. In press.
65. BELL, I.R., R. PATARCA, C.M. BALDWIN *et al.* 1998. Serum neopterin and somatization in women with chemical intolerance, depressives, and normals. Neuropsychobiology **38:** 13–18.

Potential Mechanisms in Chemical Intolerance and Related Conditions

DANIEL J. CLAUW

Georgetown Chronic Pain and Fatigue Research Center, and Division of Rheumatology, Immunology, and Allergy, Department of Medicine, Georgetown University Medical Center, Washington, District of Columbia 20007, USA

ABSTRACT: The symptom of chemical intolerance may occur in isolation, but often occurs in conjunction with other chronic symptoms such as pain, fatigue, memory disturbances, etc. This frequent clustering of symptoms in individuals has led to the definition of several chronic multisymptom syndromes, such as multiple chemical sensitivity, fibromyalgia, chronic fatigue syndrome, and Gulf War illnesses. The aggregate research into these syndromes has suggested some unifying mechanisms that contribute to symptomatology. Multiple lines of evidence suggest that there is aberrant function of numerous efferent neural pathways, such as the autonomic nervous system and hypothalamic-pituitary axes, in subsets of individuals with these conditions. There is perhaps the greatest evidence for abnormal sensory processing in these syndromes, with a low "unpleasantness threshold" for multiple types of sensory stimuli. Psychological and behavioral factors are known to play a significant role in initiating or perpetuating symptoms in some persons with these illnesses. In the field of pain research, the interrelationship between physiologic and psychologic factors in symptom expression has been well studied. Using both established and novel methodologies, studies have suggested that psychologic factors such as hypervigilance and expectancy are playing a relatively minor role in most individuals with fibromyalgia and that clear evidence exists of physiologic amplification of sensory stimuli. These studies need to be extended to more sensory tasks and to larger numbers of subjects with related conditions. It is of note, though, that existing data on this spectrum of illnesses would suggest that there may be greater psychologic contributions to symptomatology if an illness is defined in part by behavior (e.g., avoidance of chemical exposures) rather than on the basis of symptoms alone.

INTRODUCTION

Chemical intolerance is a common symptom, affecting 10–20% of the U.S. population.[1] Like other somatic symptoms, chemical intolerance frequently occurs as an isolated symptom that is intermittently present and causes little or no functional disability. However, the symptom of chemical intolerance also may be more intense, frequent, and/or accompanied by other symptoms and may result in severe disability. The resulting syndrome has frequently been termed multiple chemical sensitivity (MCS).

Multiple chemical sensitivity is one of several somatic syndromes that have been clinically characterized. Virtually nothing regarding these somatic syndromes is agreed upon. There is disagreement about the appropriate semantic terms that we should use to describe these conditions, whether these conditions have a primarily physiological or psychological origin, and whether these are truly disabling conditions.[2–6]

In part because there is no agreed upon case definition for MCS, very little research into this condition has been done, and the studies that have been performed are difficult to interpret. Because of this, this review will focus on research in two related conditions that have well-established definitions, fibromyalgia (FM) and chronic fatigue syndrome (CFS). Several studies have been performed establishing that considerable clinical overlap exists between MCS, FM, and CFS, in that approximately one-half of the individuals who meet criteria for one of these conditions will also meet criteria for one or both of the others.[7–11] In addition, many other systemic and regional syndromes fall within this spectrum.

This review will use the term chronic multisymptom illnesses (CMI), coined in a recent Centers for Disease Control and Prevention study, to describe this constellation of symptoms and syndromes.[12] The focus of this manuscript will be on mechanisms that are likely to be involved in symptom expression, as well as "lessons learned" from the work to date in this area.

DEFINITION AND CLINICAL FEATURES OF CHRONIC SYSTEMIC MULTISYMPTOM ILLNESSES

The most commonly recognized systemic conditions that fall within the CMI spectrum include FM, CFS, MCS, and somatoform disorders. There are also a variety of less frequent conditions that share considerable homology with these illnesses. Other illnesses within this spectrum affect only one organ system or portion of the body, with the seminal features being pain and/or dysfunction in this region (e.g., migraine or tension headaches, irritable bowel syndrome, temporomandibular joint dysfunction etc.).[13,14]

Fibromyalgia

FM is the second most common rheumatologic disorder, behind osteoarthritis.[15,16] In contrast to the three other disorders noted above, which are defined entirely on the basis of symptoms, the diagnostic criteria for this illness also require a physical finding on examination: diffuse tenderness. To fulfill the criteria for FM established in 1990, an individual must have both chronic widespread pain involving all four quadrants of the body (and the axial skeleton) and the presence of 11 of 18 "tender points" on examination.[15]

Although tender points were originally felt to make the criteria for FM more robust than an entirely symptom-based definition, in retrospect there are considerable problems with tender points.[17] A tender point is defined as an anatomic site where an individual complains of pain when approximately four kilograms of pressure is applied. Although early studies suggested that FM patients experienced tenderness only in these discrete regions, recent data show that individuals with FM display increased sensitivity to pain throughout the body.[18–20] There is nothing inherently abnormal about tender points because many people have some, with the mean value in the general population ranging from one to four, depending on the methodologies employed.[16,21] Thus, tender points (e.g., the midtrapezius region, epicondyles, etc.) appear to merely represent regions of the body where everyone is more tender.

More importantly, though, tender points are probably not a good measure of tenderness. For example, several population-based studies have demonstrated that the number of tender points that an individual has is highly correlated with a number of measures of distress.[22] However, distress is not an inherent feature of persons who are tender because, when a pressure-pain threshold is performed concurrently with both a tender point determination and dolorimetry/algometry (a pressure gauge with a rubber stopper attached), the tender point count correlates with measures of distress; this is much less so with the dolorimeter value.

There are several other problems associated with tender points. For example, the requirement for having 11 of 18 tender points in order to fulfill the American College of Rheumatology (ACR) criteria for FM is largely responsible for FM being a condition that is exceedingly more prevalent in females. The other component of the ACR definition, chronic pain in all four quadrants of the body plus the axial skeleton, only occurs in approximately 1.5 times as many females as males in the population. However, females are approximately 9 times more likely than males to have 11/18 tender points. Also, tenderness is influenced by many factors besides female gender, such as time in menstrual cycle, increasing age, poor aerobic fitness, and mood disorders, all tending to increase cutaneous pressure sensitivity. Thus, any criteria that require a certain number of tender points to establish the diagnosis of FM will be skewed toward identifying older females with poor aerobic fitness and a high level of distress.

Population-based studies using these ACR criteria for FM have also been very instructive. These studies have shown that pain and tenderness occur as a continuum in the general population; thus, some individuals rarely experience pain, some experience continuous widespread pain, and others have occasional pain.[16,23] There is no bimodal distribution, with a group of patients who are very tender and another group who has a "normal" pain threshold. These same characteristics are seen when examining the frequency or severity of nearly any somatic symptom in the population, including chemical intolerance, fatigue, etc.

Chronic Fatigue Syndrome

CFS is another of the CMI that have been well studied. Although the symptom of chronic fatigue affects 5–10% of the general population, CFS as currently defined is much less common.[24,25] The current definition for CFS requires that the affected individual display severe chronic fatigue without a defined cause, as well as the presence of four of eight of the following symptoms: myalgias, arthralgias, sore throat, tender nodes, cognitive difficulty, headache, postexertional malaise, or sleep disturbance.[26] This definition was only recently adopted, in part because some objective findings required in previous criteria (e.g., pharyngitis, lymphadenopathy) were in fact uncommonly noted in CFS. More frequently, the patient with CFS experiences a sore throat rather than inflammation of the pharynx, and tender nodes rather than enlargement of the lymph nodes. The new CFS definition includes five (or eight) pain-based symptoms, reinforcing the fact that diffuse pain (without accompanying abnormalities in the peripheral tissues) is also common in this condition. Besides the "defining symptoms" noted in the criteria, there are a variety of other symptoms seen with increased frequency in CFS. These are extremely similar to those noted for FM.[13,27,28] The demographics of CFS are also similar to FM, with a strong female predominance.[26]

A brief review of the history of CFS is helpful to understand how early clinical impressions regarding potential attribution of symptoms can aberrantly influence research directions. Because the cardinal features of CFS resemble those of an infectious illness (e.g., myalgias, sore throat, fatigue) and because this illness has frequently been described as beginning in an epidemic, the study of this entity has been focused on identifying an infectious agent that causes the illness. None has been identified. Although emerging evidence suggests that CMI may be *triggered* by an infectious agent, in most individuals the chronic symptoms of these conditions are unlikely to be caused by an active infection.

Recent epidemiologic studies have even cast doubt on the notion that CFS commonly occurs as an epidemic. Fukuda and colleagues at the Centers for Disease Control and Prevention (CDC) investigated an epidemic of CFS reported by a physician in a rural Michigan town.[24] Residents of two towns within the epidemic region were selected as the cases, and residents of two distant towns were selected as controls. There were two noteworthy results. First, no difference was found in the prevalence of prolonged fatigue (8%) or CFS (2%) between the two groups of residents. This calls into question the validity of many reports of apparent epidemics of CMI because it shows that a pseudo-epidemic can result when there is active surveillance for a disorder with a high background rate of undiagnosed individuals in the population.

Another reason that the viral/immune theory of CFS has come into question is the lack of specificity of the studies suggesting that these factors are causal. Early work demonstrated that many individuals with CFS had evidence of an enhanced antibody response to Epstein-Barr Virus (EBV).[29] In fact, for a brief period, the terms used to describe this condition suggested that the EBV virus was the sole cause of this entity. Subsequent reports showed that many CFS patients lacked evidence of EBV reactivity and that many others displayed elevated antibody titers to a number of other viruses, including HHV-6, CMV, varicella, as well as various enteroviruses and retroviruses.[30] The finding of elevations of serum antibodies to numerous ubiquitous infectious agents in CFS obviously weakens the role for any single virus in the chronic phase of the disease. Moreover, substantial data show that global increases in humoral immune responses are seen in a number of chronic stress states and that neurohormonal changes account for these and other immune aberrations.[31,32]

Somatoform Disorders

Somatoform disorders are a group of classified psychiatric disorders defined by the presence of physical symptoms that are not fully explained by a known medical condition. These disorders include somatization disorder, hypochondriasis, conversion disorder, and pain disorder.[33] Somatization disorder, formerly called Briquet's syndrome, is diagnosed when an individual has multiple somatic complaints, which begin before age 30, for which medical attention has been sought, but the complaints are not due to a known physical disorder. To meet criteria for this disorder, the individual must have at least eight unexplained symptoms over a lifetime. As defined, this condition is quite uncommon (0.1% to 1.0% of the population). However, a less severe form of somatization is diagnosed when an individual displays one or more unexplained symptoms for greater than six months; this form is much more common (affecting approximately 4% of the population). This illness has been variously termed subsyndromal somatization disorder and undifferentiated somatoform disorder (DSM-IV).[34] Therefore, if the symptoms of FM or CFS are considered *unexplained*, most individuals who meet criteria for one of these illnesses will also meet criteria for a somatoform disorder.

Just as with FM and CFS, there is considerable controversy regarding somatoform disorders. This controversy generally takes a different form than that surrounding FM and CFS. For example, there has been little "burden of proof" placed on proponents of the concept of somatoform disorders because by definition these conditions are acknowledged to have a psychiatric rather than a physical basis. This is problematic because there are multiple objective physiologic abnormalities noted in individuals with FM and CFS that might explain symptomatology. Thus, it becomes difficult to characterize these symptoms as physiologically unexplained.[35,36] Moreover, even undeniably psychiatric disorders, such as schizophrenia and major depression, are characterized by symptoms that are no longer considered biologically unexplained, as we learn that these illnesses are likely to be mediated in large part by central neurochemical imbalances.

However, just as with FM and CFS, there have been research findings in the investigation of somatoform disorders that are of irrefutable value. Perhaps the most important are that somatic symptoms are very common, cluster in the population, and exert a tremendous cost in terms of both health care and related disability.[37] For example, it is estimated that about 25% of patients attending a primary care clinic will meet criteria for subsyndromal somatization disorder, and up to 50% of primary care visits are for somatic complaints within this spectrum.[38–40] Patients with somatization disorder (the most severe form of somatoform disorders) use 10 times the mean outpatient and inpatient medical services as those in the general population.[41] Given the high percentage of outpatient and inpatient visits that are due to symptoms within this spectrum, the economic costs of somatoform disorders—or any other semantic term that is clearly chosen—are substantial.

Other "Miscellaneous" Systemic Disorders

A number of other systemic conditions fall within this spectrum. Multiple chemical sensitivity (MCS) and the closely related symptom of chemical intolerance are examples. Although no accepted definition of this entity exists, most use some variation of the criteria proposed by Cullen and require (1) symptoms in multiple organ systems in response to multiple substances and (2) a change in behavior in response to these symptoms. Of particular note is the requirement that an individual change his or her behavior in order to meet diagnostic criteria. Although this requirement for behavior change was likely felt to be important to judge the severity of the chemical intolerance, there are probably significant implications of this requirement. Since studies suggest that nearly 20% of individuals in the population experience occasional chemical intolerance and only a small percentage of these change their behavior in response to this symptom, those who change their behavior are not likely to be representative of the larger group. It is possible, if not likely, that this accounts for the very high rate of psychiatric comorbidity in individuals who meet criteria for MCS, even in population-based samples.[42]

Other CMI are not defined on the basis of symptoms or signs, but instead by an environmental exposure that is alleged to cause the illness. We have previously referred to these conditions as "exposure syndromes"[14] and these include Gulf War illnesses, sick-building syndrome, and illnesses seen in women with silicone breast implants, just to name a few.[43–46] Usually, the clinical features and laboratory abnormalities described for these illnesses are difficult to distinguish from those of FM, CFS, MCS, and somatoform disorders.

POTENTIAL MECHANISMS

Several potential mechanisms have been reproducibly noted in one or more CMI. Reproducible abnormalities that have been noted in these conditions are presented and placed within a theoretical construct that unites many findings, which at first glance appear disparate. In the model of illness proposed, there is a group of individuals who are genetically predisposed to develop this entire spectrum of illnesses. These illnesses may develop indolently or abruptly and, in the latter instances, typically follow exposure to a stressor or series of stressors. These stressors may be physical, immune, emotional, or chemical, or could act by other mechanisms that disrupt the body's homeostasis. A number of factors, including the environment in which the person is exposed to the stressor, genetic factors, and exposure to prior stressors, may play a role in determining which individuals are most susceptible to develop these illnesses when exposed to stress.

Once an individual develops these illnesses, there is typically evidence of one or more of the following: (1) sensory amplification, (2) attenuated hypothalamic-pituitary function, (3) lability of the autonomic nervous system, and (4) psychological and behavior factors. In this paradigm, changes in the immune system and in the peripheral tissues are de-emphasized because there are data suggesting that these anomalies occur because of these central alterations in the stress system.

Genetic or Familial Predisposition

There is some evidence of familial aggregation for nearly all of the illnesses within this spectrum, although often these data are inferential rather than definitive. Several prospective studies have suggested that relatives of FM patients display higher than expected rates of FM.[47–49] Family members of patients with FM also display a high frequency of a number of conditions related to FM, including irritable bowel syndrome, migraine headaches, and mood disorders.[47] Many of these allied conditions, such as migraine headaches, have also been noted independently to have a familial predilection.[50]

Triggering Events

FM is arguably the best studied of the CMI regarding precipitating factors or "triggers". Like many illnesses, the expression of CMI may occur when a person who is genetically predisposed comes in contact with certain environmental exposures that can trigger the development of symptoms. Many environmental exposures are generally accepted triggers of FM, all of which fall into the general category of stressors. Examples of stressors that have been shown to lead to the development of FM include physical trauma (especially to the axial skeleton), infections (e.g., parvovirus, hepatitis C), emotional distress (acute or chronic), endocrine disorders (e.g., hypothyroidism), and immune stimulation, which may also occur in a variety of autoimmune disorders.[8,15,47,51–53]

As with other illnesses, patients with CMI may frequently have inaccurate attributions regarding the cause of their symptoms. A study of CFS demonstrated this phenomenon.[54] One hundred and thirty-four consecutive patients who met CDC criteria for CFS were seen by an infectious disease specialist and had a comprehensive evaluation, including serologic studies for infectious agents postulated to cause this illness. These individuals also completed self-report questionnaires, which examined the number and type of stressful events that had occurred in the year before the diagnosis of CFS. Although 72% of these patients felt they had an infectious cause of illness, the evaluation revealed that 52% had no serological evidence of infection and only 20% had evidence of probable or definite infection. In contrast, 85% of the CFS patients reported at least one major stressful event in the year before the diagnosis of CFS (the average was 1.7 such events/patient), compared with only 6% of a control group (average of 0.1 events/control).

The epidemic of Gulf War illnesses that occurred in troops deployed to the Persian Gulf in 1990–1991 affords an excellent example of how CMI may be triggered. To review, in 1990–1991 the United States deployed approximately 700,000 troops to the Persian Gulf to liberate Kuwait from Iraqi occupation. Fortunately, there were relatively few combat-related injuries and diseases during this conflict, but up to 45% of deployed veterans (as compared to 15% of nondeployed veterans) developed a constellation of symptoms and syndromes including muscle and joint pain, fatigue, memory problems, headaches, and gastrointestinal complaints.[12] This experience was not unique to U.S. troops because veterans of this conflict from the United Kingdom experienced a similar increase in this spectrum of illness.[55] Several expert panels have been convened to examine these illnesses. There is agreement that this is not a single illness, but rather a constellation of symptoms and syndromes very similar to that seen in FM and CFS. Only a single population-based study has identified a single environment associated with a higher risk of developing CMI (a series of vaccinations given to U.K. troops), whereas numerous other studies have demonstrated no link between single environmental exposures and the development of illness. Given that similar symptom complexes have recently been retrospectively noted after nearly every war, many believe that it is not any single stressor that led to the increase in CMI after war, but instead the exposure to a large number of different types of stressors over a relatively short period of time.[56,57]

Mechanisms Potentially Responsible for Continued Symptoms

FIGURE 1 depicts the abnormalities in afferent, central, and efferent neural function that may play a role in CMI. The model proposed posits that many of the symptoms and clinical features that occur in CMI occur because of past or present exposure to a variety of stressors. With respect to chemical intolerance, the stress

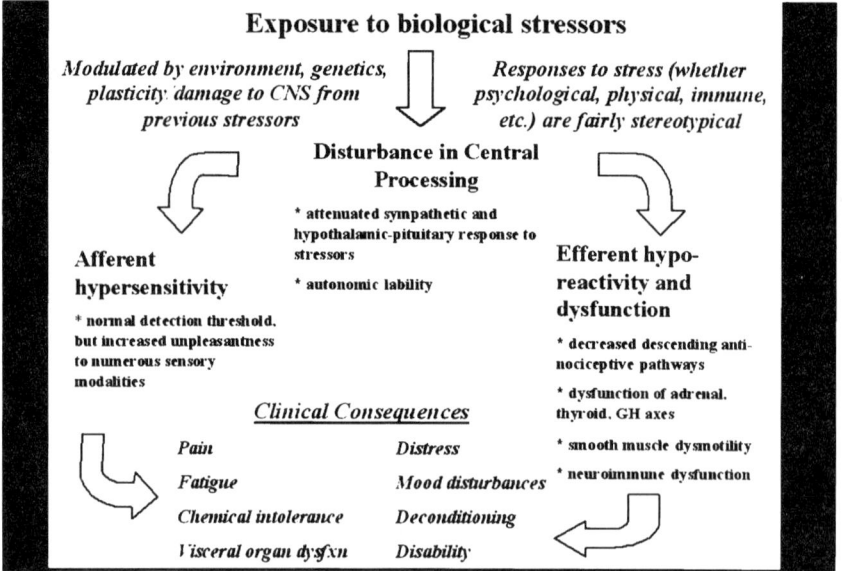

FIGURE 1. Proposed pathogenesis of CMI. In the case of chemical intolerance, the "stressor" might be the chemical or the individual's perception that he/she is being exposed to a harmful exposure.

could be the actual chemical that an individual is sensitive to, or the distress that occurs when an individual is exposed to something they perceive as harmful.

There are many reasons why the stress response may be functioning abnormally in these conditions. These include an inherited abnormality in the activity of this system and/or an acquired abnormality in function that might occur with repeated exposure to stressors. Several observations regarding the stress response, however, must be emphasized because of the potential importance to the proposed hypothesis:

1. Several authors have noted the following: although this system is adaptive in animals and early human species, *it may be maladaptive in the twentieth century.* In everyday life, this system is much more likely to be activated by daily events that have no threat to survival (e.g., sitting in traffic) than for the intended purposes of this system (e.g., to protect against predators, starvation, etc.).[58,59]

2. *The environment in which an organism is exposed to a stressor is of tremendous importance in determining the biological response*, in both animals and humans. Stressors perceived as inescapable or unavoidable, or which are accompanied by lack of predictability or support, evoke the strongest adverse biological consequences.[59–62] This could conceivably explain why victims of trauma, such as motor vehicle accidents, appear to have a much higher rate of development of FM and myofascial pain than those that are responsible for the accident.[53]

3. *Early life stressors can have a permanent and profound impact on the subsequent biological response to stress in animals because of the plasticity of the nervous system.* Studies in rodents have demonstrated that exposure to endotoxin, trauma, or separation in the neonatal period can all lead to permanent changes in the subsequent biological response to stress, extending throughout the life of the animal.[59,60,63,64] This plasticity may be due to changes in the number of neurons or circuits and/or to increases or decreases in gene expression, leading to permanent changes in molecules that define the function of the system.[65,66] This permanent effect of early stressors could explain why individuals who develop FM, CFS, somatoform disorders, irritable bowel syndrome (IBS), and other disorders in this spectrum display a higher than expected incidence of childhood physical and sexual abuse.[67-69]

4. *Within any species, there are genetic differences in the activity of the biological stress response.*[58,70] It is possible that the genetic predisposition to develop this spectrum of disorders is actually due to inherited differences in the activity of the stress response.

Afferent Abnormalities in Sensory Processing

Because FM is defined on the basis of sensory hypersensitivity, sensory function has been extensively studied in this condition. Several investigators have moved beyond determinations of tender point counts and dolorimeter values in FM to more extensively examine the basis for widespread pain and tenderness in this condition. Such studies have demonstrated that FM patients cannot *detect* electrical, pressure, or thermal stimuli at lower levels than normals, but the point at which these stimuli cause pain or unpleasantless is lower.[71,72] Other studies have examined regional differences in pain sensitivity and have demonstrated that, although tender points are anatomic locations that are more sensitive to pressure, these regions are actually less responsive to both electrical and thermal stimuli than "control points".[71] As previously noted, the increased sensitivity to pain extends throughout the entire body and occurs in response to thermal and electrical, as well as pressure, stimuli. In studies examining the precise location of the hyperalgesia in FM, it appears as though the largest difference is below the level of the skin, but not exclusively muscle.[73]

Some data exist on the pharmacologic treatment of FM patients that may offer insight into the mechanism(s) involved in pain transmission. In arguably the most comprehensive of such studies, Sorenson *et al.* examined the responsiveness of FM patients to morphine, lidocaine, and subanesthetic doses of ketamine.[74] They found that most subjects responded to one or more of these substances, although to different combinations of these medications, and the rate of placebo response was low. They suggested that spinal or supraspinal mechanisms are involved in pain maintenance in this condition and that this may be due to heterogeneous processes.

Other modulating influences have been examined to elucidate the precise mechanism(s) involved in pain transmission. One possible link between the systemic symptoms that these individuals experience and the diffuse pain seen in this condition is the sympathetic nervous system. There is emerging evidence that FM may be characterized by a decrease in the activity of descending, antinociceptive pathways that begin in subcortical structures, including the locus coeruleus, and descend into the spinal cord. Under normal conditions, these pathways are tonically active and inhibit the upward transmission of pain. Kosek *et al.* demonstrated that isometric contraction of muscle exerted the expected analgesic effect on the pressure pain threshold in normal subjects, whereas FM patients responded to this maneuver with a paradoxically lowered pain threshold.[75] Other investigators studied the effect of a tonic painful stimulus on pain threshold in FM patients and found that, in contrast to controls, there was no increase in pain threshold.[76] They suggested that this indicated a lack of descending noxious inhibitory control (DNIC) mechanisms in the FM patients.

Other investigators have used "functional" brain imaging in persons with FM to substantiate the notion that there may be a disturbance in pain processing in this condition. In these studies, persons with this condition were studied at baseline rather than with response to a painful (or other) stimulus. Mountz *et al.* collected SPECT data on females with FM and found evidence for regional differences in blood flow in areas involved in pain transmission, such as the caudate nucleus.[77]

Although nearly all of the research on sensory processing in FM has focused on the processing of pain, some data suggest a more generalized disturbance in sensory processing. For example, data suggest that FM patients experience an increased sensitivity to loud noises and, anecdotally, these individuals are also more sensitive to bright lights, odors, drugs, and chemicals. These symptoms of generalized sensitivity to multiple stimuli in FM and other CMI would favor a more generalized hypersensitivity to sensory stimuli than to just certain stimuli (e.g., tactile in FM, chemical in MCS, etc.).

Other investigations have attempted to identify specific neurochemical abnormalities that may be associated with abnormal pain transmission. In arguably the most important biologic studies performed in this illness, several groups have demonstrated that patients with FM have concentrations of SP approximately threefold higher in cerebrospinal fluid (CSF) than normal controls.[78–81] Substance P (SP) is a pronociceptive peptide stored in the secretory granules of sensory nerves and released upon axonal stimulation. A remarkable consistency is found among the results of these groups of investigators and, in all cases, there is very little overlap in SP levels between the FM patients and normal controls.

The meaning of these elevated CSF SP levels in FM is not entirely clear. The SP could theoretically be derived from overactive peripheral nociceptive fibers or from central neurons. An elevated CSF SP is not specific for FM because this finding has also been noted in patients with osteoarthritis of the hip and chronic low-back pain. It is likely that these findings are related to the presence of pain because persons with CFS do not display this finding.[82] Russell has demonstrated that these SP levels in FM are stable, or rise over time, and do not change in response to an acute painful stimulus. Also, the same magnitude of elevation of CSF SP is found in FM patients with and without psychiatric comorbidities.[81] Animal models suggest that SP and excitatory amino acids (EAA) acting synergistically at the level of the dorsal column of the spinal cord contribute to the development of allodynia (a diffuse state of heightened sensitivity to normally nonpainful stimuli as seen in FM). In these models, EAA act rapidly to acutely change the pain threshold, whereas SP acts more slowly and is likely more operative in chronic pain states.

Several other substances are known to have prominent effects on nociception that may be abnormal in FM. For example, norepinephrine has an antinociceptive function centrally and the level of its principal metabolite, 3-methoxy-4-hydroxyphenethylene [MHPG], is low in the CSF of FM patients.[83] This finding again supports the possibility that descending antinociceptive influences from the autonomic nervous system could be a potential mechanism for the allodynia and hyperalgesia seen in FM. It is also of note that some of the most effective drugs in treating central pain syndromes such as FM act by augmenting central adrenergic activity.

Finally, there is some evidence to justify a role for low central levels of serotonin in several disorders within this spectrum. Data exist that suggest a generalized defect in serotonin synthesis or metabolism in FM, indicated by low levels of serotonin and its precursor, L-tryptophan, in the serum, as well as low levels of the principal metabolite, 5-HIAA, in the CSF (serotonin is undetectable in the CSF of humans).[83,84]

Efferent Hypothalamic-Pituitary Dysfunction

Substantial data indicate that the hypothalamic-pituitary axes (HPA) function abnormally in subsets of persons with FM and related disorders.[85] Each of these disorders differs somewhat with respect to the precise perturbations and, in all instances, hypothalamic function is only "abnormal" in a small subset of subjects. In FM, most studies have revealed low 24-h free urinary cortisol, exaggerated ACTH release in response to CRH challenge, and abnormal diurnal rhythmicity of secretion of cortisol and other hormones. Adrenal insufficiency also occurs in response to exercise in FM because cortisol levels paradoxically fall rather than rise in response to physical exertion.[86] This postexercise adrenal insufficiency, as well as the decreased sympathetic response to exercise noted below, might in some way contribute to the severe postexertional pain and fatigue that both FM and CFS patients experience. These changes in the HPA axis are opposite to those seen in melancholic depression, which is characterized by chronically increased stress system activity.[61]

Changes have also been noted in the growth hormone axis that suggest abnormal hypothalamic function. Insulin-like growth factor-1 (IGF-1) is produced in the liver, primarily in response to growth hormone (GH), and is responsible for many of the biological activities of GH. Bennett has demonstrated that IGF-1 is very low in about one-quarter of FM patients.[87] The defect in GH secretion that leads to the low IGF-1 appears to be hypothalamic in origin because these individuals fail to secrete GH in response to a variety of stimulations.[87] Although administration of recombinant GH to this subset of FM patients has been demonstrated to be of clinical benefit, the expense of this treatment and the likelihood that other less expensive treatments may be of similar efficacy have limited the use of this modality.

Efferent Autonomic Nervous System Dysfunction

There are also identifiable abnormalities in autonomic nervous system function in many of the disorders in this spectrum. Just as with studies of neuroendocrine function, though, only a subset of FM patients will have "abnormal" autonomic function, depending on how this is defined. In summary, various studies have demonstrated that subsets of persons with FM, as well as other similar disorders such as CFS, display low baseline sympathetic tone and an inability to respond to stressors.[86,88,89] The clinical manifestations that are related to autonomic dysfunction are not entirely clear, but may include orthostatic intolerance (e.g., as in neurally mediated hypotension), vasomotor instability, and visceral dysfunction.

Dysautonomia has likewise been documented in CFS, IBS, and migraine headaches.[90–93] Although the autonomic nervous system has not been as extensively studied in CFS as it has in FM, several groups have demonstrated similar types of abnormalities in autonomic nervous system function in this disorder. For example, as in FM, patients with CFS are found to have a higher than expected rate of neurally mediated hypotension on tilt-table testing.[94] Again, the absolute percentage of individuals who have abnormal tests appears to be very dependent on a number of factors, including patient selection (especially with respect to medication usage and deconditioning) and the tilt-table testing protocol used. In another study, CFS patients were run through a battery of tests assessing various components of autonomic function and were found to have significantly more abnormalities than expected.[95]

In IBS, there have been several studies suggesting abnormalities in both central sympathetic and parasympathetic influences; some have suggested that the specific abnormalities in the autonomic nervous system can predict certain types of symptoms (e.g., diarrhea or constipation-predominant).[96–98] Defects in autonomic function have also been delineated in migraine, with the aggregate data in these studies suggesting that there is baseline sympathetic hypofunction, as well as instability of the sympathetic response.[99–102] Furthermore, studies in both IBS and migraine suggest that there is a dissociation between the symptoms of pain and of autonomic dysfunction, which supports our hypotheses regarding the independence of the axes of the stress response.[90,92,99,102–104]

Psychiatric, Psychological, and Behavioral Factors

As noted previously, the symptoms of CMI and those of psychiatric disorders overlap significantly. Although some contend that *all* of these symptoms are "supratentorial" in origin, others counter that the rate of psychiatric comorbidities in these conditions is similar to any chronic disease.[3,105,106] A review of the accumulated data in these conditions supports a few consistent observations:

1. Approximately 20–40% of individuals with FM or CFS seen in tertiary care centers have an identifiable *current* mood disorder such as depression or anxiety disorder.[3,106,107] Some studies have suggested that the frequency of psychiatric comorbidity is lower in individuals identified in primary care practices or in the general population, whereas other studies have found equally high percentages.[108,109] Regardless of the precise percentage of individuals with psychiatric comorbidities, at least 60% of individuals with FM or CFS have no identifiable concurrent psychiatric condition. Thus, there must be nonpsychiatric mechanisms capable of causing all of the symptoms seen in these disorders.

2. The *lifetime* history of mood disorders in individuals with FM or CFS is high, averaging about 40–70% over several studies.[106,107,110] These data are among those used by Hudson and colleagues to posit that there is a spectrum of disorders, including FM, migraines, irritable bowel, and affective disorders, that may share a common genetic predisposition and underlying pathogenic mechanisms. Again, though, some of these differences in the lifetime history of depression may be due to health-care-seeking behaviors because lower

lifetime incidences of affective disorders are typically noted in individuals with FM who are identified in the general population.[23,109]

3. A myriad of complex psychosocial factors play a significant role in some individuals with these illnesses, as with nearly any chronic medical illness. These include behavioral pathways, such as sick role behavior and maladaptive coping mechanisms; cognitive pathways such as victimization and loss of control; and social pathways, such as interference with role functioning and deterioration of social or other support networks. Psychosocial factors are known to play a particularly prominent role in the transition from acute pain to chronic pain and disability. As pain, fatigue, chemical intolerance, or a plethora of symptoms occur over time, it is not uncommon for problems to emerge for the individual such as job loss, financial constraints, distancing of friends, etc. If patients' responses to these problems are maladaptive, such as avoidance of work, friends, financial responsibilities, and physical activity, the patient may become distressed and overwhelmed by the pain and its negative impact on life. Increased stress, learned helplessness, depression, increased anxiety, anger, distrust, entitlement, and somatization can all emerge and worsen symptoms, probably by interrelated physiologic and psychologic mechanisms. All of these factors can be important in dictating how individuals report symptoms, how and when they seek health care, and how they respond to therapy. This may also explain why cognitive-behavioral therapy, which addresses many of these issues, has generally been effective in the treatment of individuals with FM, as well as nearly any other chronic medical condition.[111]

FIGURE 2 summarizes the relationship between physiologic factors and psychobehavioral factors in this spectrum of illness. In the model presented, psychological factors can play no role, or the major role, in symptom expression in CMI. At the far left of the figure, psychobehavioral factors play a minor role. Examples of individuals in this category would be those with recent onset of symptoms, or those with chronic symptoms and adequate social support, control of their environment, and coping strategies. At the far right of the figure, psychobehavioral factors are playing a major role. These would include those with prominent psychological distress as the driving force of their physiologic dysfunction, individuals with psychiatric co-morbidities, or those whose symptoms overwhelm their ability to continue to function normally. These latter factors are seen much more commonly in individuals who attend tertiary care clinics and, conversely, individuals found with these syndromes in the general population, or in primary care, are less likely to have such factors.

LESSONS LEARNED—RELEVANCE TO CHEMICAL INTOLERANCE

Importance of Case Definition

Problems with early definitions of FM and chronic CFS should serve as lessons for future attempts to develop such a definition for MCS/CI. Subtle changes in the criteria (e.g., adding the requirement for tender points to the FM definition) can be of profound importance.

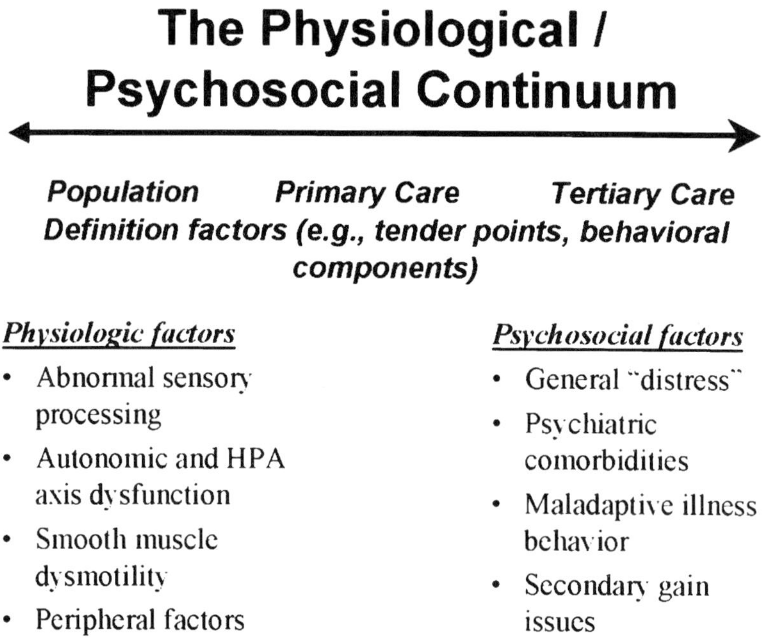

The Physiological / Psychosocial Continuum

⬅————————————————————➡

Population   **Primary Care**   **Tertiary Care**
Definition factors (e.g., tender points, behavioral components)

Physiologic factors
- Abnormal sensory processing
- Autonomic and HPA axis dysfunction
- Smooth muscle dysmotility
- Peripheral factors

Psychosocial factors
- General "distress"
- Psychiatric comorbidities
- Maladaptive illness behavior
- Secondary gain issues

FIGURE 2. Relationship between physiologic and psychobehavioral factors in CMI. Some individuals with these conditions may have primarily physiologic factors responsible for symptom expression, whereas in others psychological and behavioral factors play a more prominent role. Certain factors such as the type of sample being used (e.g., population-based versus tertiary care) or how the illness is defined may predict the relative importance of psychological/behavioral factors.

Problems with Ascertainment Bias

Although there is no current definition for MCS/CI, most investigators use some variation of the Cullen criteria, which require that an individual change his or her behavior in order to be defined as having this illness. It is important to recognize that this may lead to an increased rate of psychiatric comorbidities in the population being studied. The same bias will likely be introduced when health-care seekers being seen in tertiary care centers serve as the study population.

Psychophysical Characteristics of Sensory Paradigms

Future studies of chemical intolerance could test the processing of multiple types of sensory information, using different modes of stimulus presentation. Researchers in the processing of pain, visual, and auditory information have been working through the most appropriate paradigms to minimize the effects of psychological factors.

Focus on Mechanisms That Could Be Responsible for the Entire Spectrum of Complaints

Although patients with MCS frequently have CI as their primary complaint, compelling evidence exists for a more widespread defect in the processing of many types of sensory stimuli. Thus, it is not likely that models with a narrow focus, on nasal mechanisms for example, will ultimately be of paramount importance.

REFERENCES

1. KREUTZER, R., R.R. NEUTRA & N. LASHUAY. 1999. Prevalence of people reporting sensitivities to chemicals in a population-based survey. Am. J. Epidemiol. **150:** 1–12.
2. HADLER, N.M. 1996. Is fibromyalgia a useful diagnostic label? Clevel. Clin. J. Med. **63**(2): 85–87.
3. MANU, P., T.J. LANE & D.A. MATTHEWS. 1993. Chronic fatigue and chronic fatigue syndrome: clinical epidemiology and aetiological classification. Ciba Found. Symp. **173:** 23–31; 31–42 (discussion).
4. BOHR, T. 1996. Problems with myofascial pain syndrome and fibromyalgia syndrome [editorial]. Neurology **46:** 593–597.
5. BARSKY, A.J. & J.F. BORUS. 1999. Functional somatic syndromes. Ann. Intern. Med. **130:** 910–921.
6. WESSELY, S., C. NIMNUAN & M. SHARPE. 1999. Functional somatic syndromes: one or many? Lancet **354:** 936–939.
7. GOLDENBERG, D.L. 1991. Fibromyalgia, chronic fatigue syndrome, and myofascial pain syndrome. Curr. Opin. Rheumatol. **3:** 247–258.
8. RUSSO, J., W. KATON, M. SULLIVAN et al. 1994. Severity of somatization and its relationship to psychiatric disorders and personality. Psychosomatics **35:** 546–556.
9. BUCHWALD, D. & D. GARRITY. 1994. Comparison of patients with chronic fatigue syndrome, fibromyalgia, and multiple chemical sensitivities. Arch. Intern. Med. **154:** 2049–2053.
10. ZIEM, G. & A. DONNAY. 1995. Chronic fatigue, fibromyalgia, and chemical sensitivity: overlapping disorders. Arch. Intern. Med. **155:** 1913–1913.
11. SLOTKOFF-MARX, A.T., D.A. RADULOVIC & D.J. CLAUW. 1997. The relationship between multiple chemical hypersensitivity and fibromyalgia. Scand. J. Rheumatol. **26:** 364–367.
12. FUKUDA, K., R. NISENBAUM, G. STEWART et al. 1999. Chronic mutlisymptom illness affecting Air Force veterans of the Gulf War. JAMA **280:** 981–988.
13. CLAUW, D.J. 1995. Fibromyalgia: more than just a musculoskeletal disease. Am. Fam. Phys. **52:** 843–851.
14. CLAUW, D.J. & G.P. CHROUSOS. 1997. Chronic pain and fatigue syndromes: overlapping clinical and neuroendocrine features and potential pathogenic mechanisms. Neuroimmunomodulation **4:** 134–153.
15. WOLFE, F., H.A. SMYTHE, M.B. YUNUS et al. 1993. The American College of Rheumatology 1990 criteria for the classification of fibromyalgia: report of the Multicenter Criteria Committee. Arthritis Rheum. **33:** 160–172.
16. WOLFE, F., K. ROSS, J. ANDERSON et al. 1995. The prevalence and characteristics of fibromyalgia in the general population. Arthritis Rheum. **38:** 19–28.
17. COHEN, M.L. & J.L. QUINTNER. 1993. Fibromyalgia syndrome, a problem of tautology. Lancet **342:** 906–909.
18. GRANGES, G. & G. LITTLEJOHN. 1993. Pressure pain threshold in pain-free subjects, in patients with chronic regional pain syndromes, and in patients with fibromyalgia syndrome. Arthritis Rheum. **36:** 642–646.
19. YUNUS, M.B. 1992. Towards a model of pathophysiology of fibromyalgia: aberrant central pain mechanisms with peripheral modulation. J. Rheumatol. **19:** 846–850.

20. MIKKELSSON, M., P. LATIKKA, H. KAUTIAINEN *et al.* 1992. Muscle and bone pressure pain threshold and pain tolerance in fibromyalgia patients and controls. Arch. Phys. Med. Rehabil. **73:** 814–818.
21. CROFT, P., J. SCHOLLUM & A. SILMAN. 1994. Population study of tender point counts and pain as evidence of fibromyalgia. BMJ **309:** 696–699.
22. WOLFE, F. 1997. The relation between tender points and fibromyalgia symptom variables: evidence that fibromyalgia is not a discrete disorder in the clinic. Ann. Rheum. Dis. **56:** 268–271.
23. WOLFE, F., K. ROSS, J. ANDERSON & I.J. RUSSELL. 1995. Aspects of fibromyalgia in the general population: sex, pain threshold, and fibromyalgia symptoms. J. Rheumatol. **22:** 151–156.
24. FUKUDA, K., L. WILSON & J. DOBBINS. 1994. A community-based study of unexplained prolonged and chronic fatiguing illness in a rural area of Michigan. *In* AACFS 1994 Proceedings.
25. BUCHWALD, D., P. UMALI, J. UMALI *et al.* 1995. Chronic fatigue and the chronic fatigue syndrome: prevalence in a Pacific Northwest health care system. Ann. Intern. Med. **123:** 81–88.
26. FUKUDA, K. *et al.* 1994. Chronic fatigue syndrome: a comprehensive approach to its definition and study. Ann. Intern. Med. **121:** 953–959.
27. KOMAROFF, A.L. 1993. Clinical presentation of chronic fatigue syndrome. Ciba Found. Symp. **173:** 43–54; 54–61 (discussion).
28. MCKENZIE, R. & S.E. STRAUS. 1995. Chronic fatigue syndrome. Adv. Intern. Med. **40:** 119–153.
29. STRAUS, S.E. 1993. Studies of herpesvirus infection in chronic fatigue syndrome. Ciba Found. Symp. **173:** 132–139; 139–145 (discussion).
30. ABLASHI, D.V. 1994. Viral studies of chronic fatigue syndrome. Clin. Infect. Dis. **18**(S1): S130–S133.
31. KIECOLT-GLASER, J.K., J.T. CACIOPPO, W.B. MALARKEY & R. GLASER. 1992. Acute psychological stressors and short-term immune changes: what, why, for whom, and to what extent? Psychosom. Med. **54:** 680–685.
32. STEIN, M., S. KELLER & S. SCHLEIFER. 1985. Stress and immunomodulation: the role of depression and neuroendocrine function. J. Immunol. **135:** 827s–833s.
33. KATON, W., E. LIN, M. VON KORFF *et al.* 1991. Somatization: a spectrum of severity. Am. J. Psychiatry **148:** 34–40.
34. AMERICAN PSYCHIATRIC ASSOCIATION. 1994. Diagnostic and Statistical Manual of Mental Disorders.
35. QUINTNER, J.L. 1995. Somatisation disorder: a major public health issue [letter; comment]. Med. J. Aust. **163:** 558; 558–559 (discussion).
36. BELL, I.R. 1994. Somatization disorder: health care costs in the decade of the brain. Biol. Psychiatry **35:** 81–83.
37. BARSKY, A.J. & J.F. BORUS. 1995. Somatization and medicalization in the era of managed care. JAMA **274:** 1931–1934.
38. KIRMAYER, L.J. & J.M. ROBBINS. 1991. Three forms of somatization in primary care: prevalence, co-occurrence, and sociodemographic characteristics. J. Nerv. Ment. Dis. **179:** 647–655.
39. KROENKE, K. & A.D. MANGELSDORF. 1989. Common symptoms in primary care: incidence, evaluation, therapy, and outcome. Am. J. Med. **86:** 262–266.
40. KROENKE, K., R.L. SPITZER, J.B. WILLIAMS *et al.* 1994. Physical symptoms in primary care: predictors of psychiatric disorders and functional impairment. Arch. Fam. Med. **3:** 774–779.
41. SMITH, G.R., R. MONSON & D. RAY. 1986. Patients with multiple unexplained symptoms: their characteristics, functional health, and health care utilization. Arch. Intern. Med. **146:** 69–72.
42. BRUNO, R.L., R. SAPOLSKY, J.R. ZIMMERMAN & N.M. FRICK. 1995. Pathophysiology of a central cause of post-polio fatigue. Ann. N.Y. Acad. Sci. **753:** 257–275.
43. NIH WORKSHOP PANEL. 1994. The Persian Gulf experience and health. JAMA **272:** 391–396.

44. BRIDGES, A.J., C. CONLEY, G. WANG et al. 1993. A clinical and immunologic evaluation of women with silicone breast implants and symptoms of rheumatic disease [see comments]. Ann. Intern. Med. **118:** 929–936.
45. GOTHE, C.J., C. MOLIN & C.G. NILSSON. 1995. The environmental somatization syndrome. Psychosomatics **36:** 1–11.
46. CHESTER, A.C. & P.H. LEVINE. 1994. Concurrent sick building syndrome and chronic fatigue syndrome: epidemic neuromyasthenia revisited. Clin. Infect. Dis. **18**(S1): S43–S48.
47. HUDSON, J.I., D.L. GOLDENBERG, H.G. POPE, JR. et al. 1992. Comorbidity of fibromyalgia with medical and psychiatric disorders. Am. J. Med. **92:** 363–367.
48. STORMORKEN, H. & F. BROSSTAD. 1992. Fibromyalgia: family clustering and sensory urgency with early onset indicate genetic predisposition and thus a "true" disease. Scand. J. Rheumatol. **21:** 207.
49. PELLEGRINO, M.J., G.W. WAYLONIS & A. SOMMER. 1989. Familial occurrence of primary fibromyalgia. Arch. Phys. Med. Rehabil. **70:** 61–63.
50. MESSINGER, H.B., E.L.H. SPIERINGS, A.J.P. VINCENT & J. LEBBINK. 1991. Headache and family history. Cephalgia **11:** 13–18.
51. BUSKILA, D., L. NEUMANN, G. VAISBERG et al. 1997. Increased rates of fibromyalgia following cervical spine injury: a controlled study of 161 cases of traumatic injury. Arthritis Rheum. **40:** 446–452.
52. WAYLONIS, G.W. & R.H. PERKINS. 1994. Post-traumatic fibromyalgia: a long-term follow-up. Am. J. Phys. Med. Rehabil. **73:** 403–412.
53. GREENFIELD, S., M.A. FITZCHARLES & J.M. ESDAILE. 1992. Reactive fibromyalgia syndrome. Arthritis Rheum. **35:** 678–681.
54. SALIT, I. 1994. Precipitating events in CFS. *In* AACFS 1994 Proceedings.
55. UNWIN, C., N. BLATCHLEY, W. COKER et al. 1999. Health of UK servicemen who served in the Persian Gulf War. Lancet **353:** 169–178.
56. HYAMS, K.C., F.S. WIGNALL & R. ROSWELL. 1996. War syndromes and their evaluation: from the U.S. Civil War to Persian Gulf War. Ann. Intern. Med. **125:** 398–405.
57. CLAUW, D.J. 1998. The "Gulf War syndrome": implications for rheumatologists. J. Clin. Rheum. **4:** 173–174.
58. MEANEY, M.J., S. BHATNAGAR, S. LAROCQUE et al. 1993. Individual differences in the hypothalamic-pituitary-adrenal stress response and the hypothalamic CRF system. Ann. N.Y. Acad. Sci. **697:** 70–85.
59. ROMERO, L.M., P.M. PLOTSKY & R.M. SAPOLSKY. 1993. Patterns of adrenocorticotropin secretagogue release with hypoglycemia, novelty, and restraint after colchicine blockade of axonal transport. Endocrinology **132:** 199–204.
60. VIAU, V., S. SHARMA, P.M. PLOTSKY & M.J. MEANEY. 1993. Increased plasma ACTH responses to stress in nonhandled compared with handled rats require basal levels of corticosterone and are associated with increased levels of ACTH secretagogues in the median eminence. J. Neurosci. **13:** 1097–1105.
61. CHROUSOS, G.P. & P.W. GOLD. 1992. The concepts of stress and stress system disorders: overview of physical and behavioral homeostasis. JAMA **267:** 1244–1252.
62. GOLD, P.W., F. GOODWIN & G.P. CHROUSOS. 1988. Clinical and biochemical manifestations of depression: relationship to the neurobiology of stress (part 1). N. Engl. J. Med. **319:** 348–353.
63. STEIN-BEHRENS, B.A., W.J. LIN & R.M. SAPOLSKY. 1994. Physiological elevations of glucocorticoids potentiate glutamate accumulation in the hippocampus. J. Neurochem. **63:** 596–602.
64. SAPOLSKY, R.M. 1996. Why stress is bad for your brain. Science **273:** 749–750.
65. STEIN-BEHRENS, B., M.P. MATTSON, I. CHANG et al. 1994. Stress exacerbates neuron loss and cytoskeletal pathology in the hippocampus. J. Neurosci. **14:** 5373–5380.
66. GLASER, R., W.P. LAFUSE, R.H. BONNEAU et al. 1993. Stress-associated modulation of proto-oncogene expression in human peripheral blood leukocytes. Behav. Neurosci. **107:** 525–529.
67. WALLING, M.K., M.W. O'HARA, R.C. REITER et al. 1994. Abuse history and chronic pain in women: II. A multivariate analysis of abuse and psychological morbidity. Obstet. Gynecol. **84:** 200–206.

68. SPACCARELLI, S. 1994. Stress, appraisal, and coping in child sexual abuse: a theoretical and empirical review. Psychol. Bull. **116:** 340–362.
69. BENDIXEN, M., K.M. MUUS & B. SCHEI. 1994. The impact of child sexual abuse—a study of a random sample of Norwegian students. Child Abuse Neglect **18:** 837–847.
70. STERNBERG, E.M. 1993. Hyperimmune fatigue syndromes: diseases of the stress response? J. Rheumatol. **20**(3): 418–421.
71. LAUTENBACHER, S., G.B. ROLLMAN & G.A. MCCAIN. 1994. Multi-method assessment of experimental and clinical pain in patients with fibromyalgia. Pain **59:** 45–53.
72. ARROYO, J.F. & M.L. COHEN. 1993. Abnormal responses to electrocutaneous stimulation in fibromyalgia. J. Rheumatol. **20:** 1925–1931.
73. KOSEK, E., J. EKHOLM & P. HANSSON. 1995. Increased pressure pain sensibility in fibromyalgia patients is located deep to the skin, but not restricted to muscle tissue. Pain **63:** 335–339.
74. SORENSON, J., A. BENGTSSON, E. BACKMAN et al. 1995. Pain analysis in patients with fibromyalgia: effects of intravenous morphine, lidocaine, and ketamine. Scand. J. Rheumatol. **24:** 360–365.
75. KOSEK, E., J. EKHOLM & P. HANSSON. 1996. Modulation of pressure pain thresholds during and following isometric contraction in patients with fibromyalgia and in healthy controls. Pain **64:** 415–423.
76. LAUTENBACHER, S. & G.B. ROLLMAN. 1997. Possible deficiencies of pain modulation in fibromyalgia. Clin. J. Pain **13:** 189–196.
77. MOUNTZ, J.M., L.A. BRADLEY, J.G. MODELL et al. 1995. Fibromyalgia in women: abnormalities of regional cerebral blood flow in the thalamus and the caudate nucleus are associated with low pain threshold levels. Arthritis Rheum. **38:** 926–938.
78. WELIN, M., B. BRAGEE, F. NYBERG & M. KRISTIANSSON. 1995. Elevated substance P levels are contrasted by a decrease in met-enkephalin-arg-phe levels in CSF from fibromyalgia patients. J. Musculoskeletal Pain **3:** 4.
79. VAEROY, H., R. HELLE, O. FORRE et al. 1988. Elevated CSF levels of substance P and high incidence of Raynaud's phenomenon in patients with fibromyalgia: new features for diagnosis. Pain **32:** 21–26.
80. RUSSELL, I.J., M.D. ORR, B. LITTMAN et al. 1994. Elevated cerebrospinal fluid levels of substance P in patients with the fibromyalgia syndrome. Arthritis Rheum. **37**(11): 1593–1601.
81. BRADLEY, L.A., K.R. ALBERTS, G.S. ALARCON et al. 1996. Abnormal brain regional cerebral blood flow and cerebrospinal fluid levels of substance P in patients and non-patients with fibromyalgia. Arthritis Rheum. **39**(9S): 1109.
82. EVENGARD, B., C.G. NILSSON, G. LINDH et al. 1998. Chronic fatigue syndrome differs from fibromyalgia: no evidence for elevated substance P levels in cerebrospinal fluid of patients with chronic fatigue syndrome. Pain **78:** 153–155.
83. RUSSELL, I.J., H. VAEROY, M. JAVORS & F. NYBERG. 1992. Cerebrospinal fluid biogenic amine metabolites in fibromyalgia/fibrositis syndrome and rheumatoid arthritis [see comments]. Arthritis Rheum. **35:** 550–556.
84. YUNUS, M.B., J.W. DAILEY, J.C. ALDAG et al. 1992. Plasma tryptophan and other amino acids in primary fibromyalgia: a controlled study. J. Rheumatol. **19:** 90–94.
85. CROFFORD, L.J. 1998. Neuroendocrine abnormalities in fibromyalgia and related disorders. Am. J. Med. Sci. **315:** 359–366.
86. VAN DENDEREN, J.C., J.W. BOERSMA, P. ZEINSTRA et al. 1992. Physiological effects of exhaustive physical exercise in primary fibromyalgia syndrome (PFS): is PFS a disorder of neuroendocrine reactivity? Scand. J. Rheumatol. **21:** 35–37.
87. BENNETT, R.M., D.M. COOK, S.R. CLARK et al. 1993. Low somatomedin-C in fibromyalgia patients: an analysis of clinical specificity and pituitary/hepatic responses. Arthritis Rheum. **36**(9S): 62.
88. ELAM, M., G. JOHANSSON & B.G. WALLIN. 1992. Do patients with primary fibromyalgia have an altered muscle sympathetic nerve activity? Pain **48:** 371–375.
89. QIAO, Z.G., H. VAEROY & L. MORKRID. 1991. Electrodermal and microcirculatory activity in patients with fibromyalgia during baseline, acoustic stimulation, and cold pressor tests. J. Rheumatol. **18:** 1383–1389.

90. MAYER, E.A. & H.E. RAYBOULD. 1990. Role of visceral afferent mechanisms in functional bowel disorders. Gastroenterology **99:** 1688–1704.
91. BUZZI, M., M. BONAMINI & R. CERBO. 1993. The anatomy and biochemistry of headache. Funct. Neurol. **8**(6): 395–402.
92. LYNN, R. & L. FRIEDMAN. 1993. Irritable bowel syndrome. N. Engl. J. Med. **329:** 1940–1945.
93. POGACNIK, T., S. SEGA, B. PECNIK & T. KIAUTA. 1993. Autonomic function testing in patients with migraine. Headache **33**(10): 545–550.
94. ROWE, P.C., I. BOU-HOLAIGAH, J.S. KAN & H. CALKINS. 1995. Is neurally mediated hypotension an unrecognised cause of chronic fatigue? Lancet **345:** 623–624.
95. FREEMAN, R. & A.L. KOMAROFF. 1997. Does the chronic fatigue syndrome involve the autonomic nervous system? Am. J. Med. **102:** 357–364.
96. AGGARWAL, A., T.F. CUTTS, T.L. ABELL et al. 1994. Predominant symptoms in irritable bowel syndrome correlate with specific autonomic nervous system abnormalities. Gastroenterology **106:** 945–950.
97. MCALLISTER, C. & J.F. FIELDING. 1988. Patients with pulse rate changes in irritable bowel syndrome: further evidence of altered autonomic function. J. Clin. Gastroenterol. **10:** 273–274.
98. FUKUDO, S. & J. SUZUKI. 1987. Colonic motility, autonomic function, and gastrointestinal hormones under psychological stress on irritable bowel syndrome. Tohoku J. Exp. Med. **151:** 373–385.
99. PAREJA, J.A. 1995. Chronic paroxysmal hemicrania: dissociation of the pain and autonomic features. Headache **35:** 111–113.
100. ZIGELMAN, M., S. APPEL, S. DAVIDOVITCH et al. 1994. The effect of verapamil calcium antagonist on autonomic imbalance in migraine: evaluation by spectral analysis of beat-to-beat heart rate fluctuations. Headache **34:** 569–577.
101. PRUSINSKI, A., S. TRZOS, P. ROZENTRYT et al. 1994. Studies of heart rhythm variability in migraine: preliminary communication. Neurol. Neurochir. Pol. **28:** 23–27.
102. POGACNIK, T., S. SEGA, B. PECNIK & T. KIAUTA. 1993. Autonomic function testing in patients with migraine. Headache **33:** 545–550.
103. APPEL, S., A. KURITZKY, I. ZAHAVI et al. 1992. Evidence for instability of the autonomic nervous system in patients with migraine headache. Headache **32:** 10–17.
104. WHITEHEAD, W.E., B. HOLTKOTTER & P. ENCK. 1990. Tolerance for rectosigmoid distension in irritable bowel syndrome. Gastroenterology **98:** 1187–1192.
105. YUNUS, M.B., T.A. AHLES, J.C. ALDAG & A.T. MASI. 1991. Relationship of clinical features with psychological status in primary fibromyalgia. Arthritis Rheum. **34:** 15–21.
106. AHLES, T.A., S.A. KHAN, M.B. YUNUS et al. 1991. Psychiatric status of patients with primary fibromyalgia, patients with rheumatoid arthritis, and subjects without pain: a blind comparison of DSM-III diagnoses. Am. J. Psychiatry **148:** 1721–1726.
107. BOISSEVAIN, M.D. & G.A. MCCAIN. 1991. Toward an integrated understanding of fibromyalgia syndrome. II. Psychological and phenomenological aspects. Pain **45:** 239–248.
108. WESSELY, S., T. CHALDER, S. HIRSCH et al. 1996. Psychological symptoms, somatic symptoms, and psychiatric disorder in chronic fatigue and chronic fatigue syndrome: a prospective study in the primary care setting. Am. J. Psychiatry **153:** 1050–1059.
109. AARON, L.A., L.A. BRADLEY, G.S. ALARCON et al. 1996. Psychiatric diagnoses in patients with fibromyalgia are related to health care–seeking behavior rather than to illness. Arthritis Rheum. **39:** 436–445.
110. HUDSON, J.I., M.S. HUDSON, L.F. PLINER et al. 1985. Fibromyalgia and major affective disorder: a controlled phenomenology and family history study. Am. J. Psychiatry **142**(4): 441–446.
111. NIH TECHNOLOGY PANEL. 1996. Integration of behavioral and relaxation approaches into the treatment of chronic pain and insomnia. J. Am. Med. Assoc. **276:** 313–318.

Role of Gaseous Neurotransmitters in the Hypothalamic-Pituitary-Adrenal Axis

CATHERINE RIVIER[a]

The Clayton Foundation Laboratories for Peptide Biology, The Salk Institute, La Jolla, California 92037, USA

ABSTRACT: Nitric oxide (NO) is an unstable gas that plays important roles in the brain in general and in neuroendocrine functions in particular. We have shown that NO exerts opposite effects within the median eminence–pituitary axis, where it inhibits ACTH responses to blood-borne signals [such as the systemic injection of proinflammatory cytokines or vasopressin (VP)], and structures protected by the blood-brain barrier, where it stimulates the synthesis of the hypothalamic peptides, corticotropin-releasing factor (CRF) and VP. As a result, when an animal is exposed to stimuli that acutely activate the paraventricular nucleus of the hypothalamus as well as the release of peptides from nerve terminals (such as mild inescapable foot shocks), the net influence of NO on the ACTH response will represent the balance between these two effects. Based on experiments conducted with rats, we propose that, in shocks of low intensity, ACTH release primarily depends, at least in the initial phase, on the interaction between NO and VP (and consequently is augmented by reagents that block NO formation); in shocks of higher intensity, the interaction between NO and the hypothalamus predominates (i.e., it is inhibited by reagents that block NO formation).

NITRIC OXIDE EXERTS OPPOSITE EFFECTS IN THE BRAIN AND THE PERIPHERY

The arrival of nitric oxide (NO) in the field of neuroscience has revolutionized our classical view of the effect and mechanisms of action of brain neurotransmitters since this gas is extremely unstable, does not have a receptor or a reuptake mechanism, and diffuses freely across neurons.[1] Nevertheless, NO is now recognized as an important signal in the central nervous system and this includes a significant influence on the activity of neuroendocrine systems.[2,3] When it became known that NO modulated the effect of cytokines on behavior,[4] we decided to determine whether this gas might also alter the effects of these proteins on the hypothalamic-pituitary-adrenal (HPA) axis. These first experiments provided evidence for an inhibitory influence of NO on the ACTH response to circulating interleukin (IL) 1β, and subsequently other proinflammatory cytokines,[5] and were the starting point for an ongoing project in our laboratory that aims at understanding the pharmacological effects and physiological role played by NO and related entities. As this effect is important for a full understanding of the ability of NO to alter the HPA axis, we

---

[a]Address for correspondence: The Salk Institute, Peptide Biology Laboratory, 10010 North Torrey Pines Road, La Jolla, CA 92037. Voice: 858-453-4100, ext. 1350; fax: 858-552-1546. crivier@salk.edu

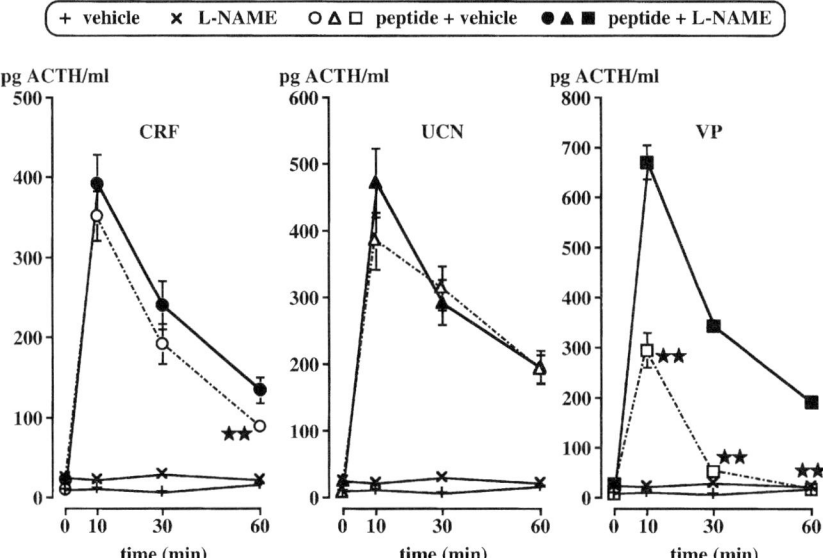

FIGURE 1A. The systemic injection of L-NAME (50 mg/kg, sc, −3 h) significantly augments the ACTH response to VP (0.5 μg/kg), but not to CRF (1 μg/kg) or the related peptide urocortin (UCN, 1 μg/kg). Each point represents the mean ± SEM of 5–6 rats. **$p < 0.01$ vs. vehicle.

illustrate here one of its main aspects, which is to blunt the stimulatory influence of vasopressin [(VP), an important ACTH secretagogue[6]] on corticotrophs activity. This is shown by the fact that blockade of NO formation with the arginine derivative N_ω-nitro-L-arginine-methylester (L-NAME), a compound that inhibits NO synthase (NOS), the enzyme responsible for NOS synthesis,[7] significantly augments VP-induced ACTH release (FIG. 1A). Interestingly, we routinely observe that the ability of the main ACTH secretagogue, corticotropin-releasing factor (CRF), as well as that of the related peptide urocortin, to induce ACTH release is not significantly altered by changes in NO formation. Another intriguing and as yet unexplained finding is that CRF antibodies only partially reduced the ability of L-NAME to increase the ACTH response to VP (FIG. 1B). The effect of VP alone depends on the presence of CRF,[8] a peptide that potentiates the actions of VP on the corticotrophs, as indicated by the virtual lack of ACTH response to VP in rats pretreated with CRF antibodies.[9] However, L-NAME remained capable of enhancing ACTH release due to VP (although less so) despite the lack of CRF. This suggests that interactions between NO and VP depend on factors that may not involve the primary modulator of ACTH release.

In contrast to its inhibitory influence on the median eminence and anterior pituitary, NO markedly stimulates the neuronal activity of the hypothalamic peptides that control ACTH release—an influence that may be exerted on the paraventricular nucleus (PVN) itself and/or its afferents. This is exemplified by the fact that L-

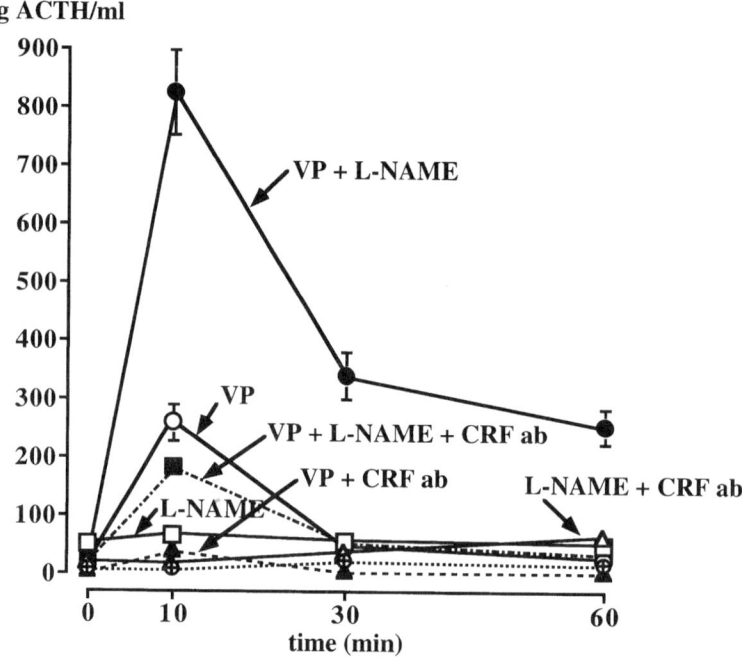

FIGURE 1B. Interaction between L-NAME and CRF antibodies (CRF ab) on the ACTH response to VP. [Statistical levels are not indicated for the sake of clarity. However, responses due to VP, VP + L-NAME, VP + L-NAME + CRF ab, VP + CRF ab, and L-NAME were all different ($p < 0.01$) from that elicited by the vehicle.]

NAME decreases the ACTH response to shocks (FIG. 2) as well as the upregulation of CRF and VP transcripts normally measured in the PVN of the hypothalamus in response to neurogenic stressors,[10–12] and that the intracerebroventricular (icv) injection of the NO donor SIN-1 stimulates PVN CRF and VP cell bodies.[11] Collectively, our work therefore indicates that NO exerts opposite effects in the periphery (where it is inhibitory) and in brain areas protected by the blood-brain barrier (BBB) (where it is stimulatory). This chapter will outline some of our recent studies focused on these brain areas and attempts to shed some light on the way in which the opposite effects of NO interact to modulate the ACTH response to neurogenic stressors.

These types of stressors, which include mild electric foot shocks and restraint, primarily stimulate ACTH secretion by activating neurons in the PVN, in particular those that express CRF and VP [see references 13 and 14]. These peptides are subsequently released from terminals in the median eminence, from which they travel through portal vessels to the pituitary corticotrophs where they activate their specific receptors, thus resulting in ACTH release. Indeed, removal of endogenous CRF and/ or VP, or blockade of their respective receptors, significantly blunts the ACTH response to shocks (FIG. 3). The mechanisms involved in the ACTH response to neurogenic stressors therefore take place at various sites situated in both the brain (PVN neurons and their afferents) and the periphery (median eminence and pituitary).

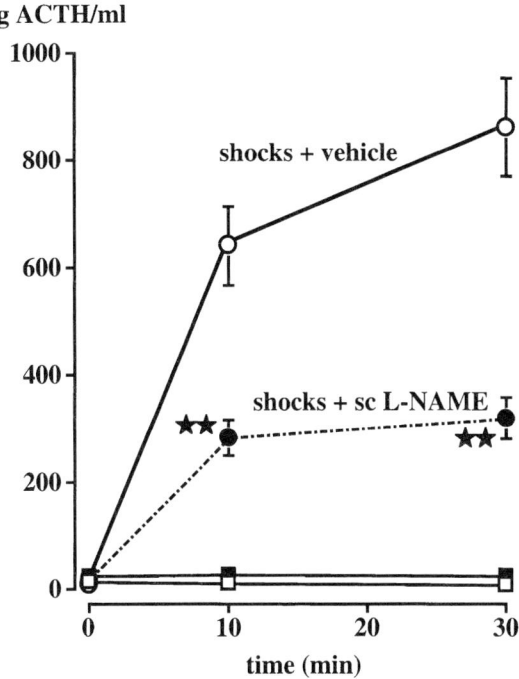

FIGURE 2. The sc injection of L-NAME (50 mg/kg, −3 h) significantly blunts the ACTH response to shocks (1 mA, 1 s duration, 2 shocks/min). Each point represents the mean ± SEM of 6–7 rats. **$p < 0.01$ vs. shocks only.

Consequently, these mechanisms are under both the stimulatory and inhibitory influence of NO. What then determines the net influence of this gas?

WHAT IS THE NET INFLUENCE OF NITRIC OXIDE WHEN A STIMULUS ACTS ON BOTH THE PVN AND THE MEDIAN EMINENCE–PITUITARY AXIS?

As indicated above, studies of the role of NO have classically relied on the use of arginine derivatives that block NOS activity. These reagents readily cross the BBB and are therefore usually injected systemically. While this results in a significant decrease in NO formation in the hypothalamus, it also lowers gas formation in the pituitary (FIG. 4). Consequently, the resulting decrease in shock-induced ACTH secretion (see FIG. 2) represents the combined influence of NO-induced activation of CRF and VP PVN neurons and blunted ability of VP to stimulate the corticotrophs. However, as the net effect of systemically injected L-NAME is to inhibit shock-induced ACTH secretion, it appears that, in this model, the inhibitory effect of NO on PVN neurons prevailed. Is this always the case? First, we reasoned that if we could administer L-NAME directly into the brain, at a dose that did not reach the

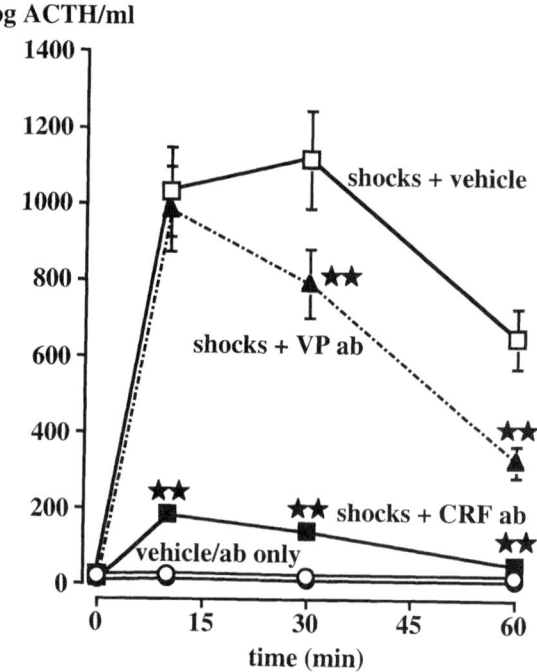

FIGURE 3. Effect of prior (−3 h) iv injection of CRF or VP antibodies (ab) or their vehicle on the ACTH response to shocks (1 mA, 1 s duration, 2 shocks/min). Each point represents the mean ± SEM of 6–7 rats. **$p < 0.01$ vs. shocks only.

pituitary, we could target the hypothalamic site of action of this reagent. We started by determining which dose of the arginine derivative was able to fully inhibit hypothalamic NO formation without altering pituitary NO levels. These studies, which are illustrated in FIGURE 5, indicated that 50 μg, injected icv (into the lateral ventricle), was the dose of choice; 25 μg did not exert a maximum effect on hypothalamic NOS activity and 250 μg leaked to the pituitary, as indicated by a change in enzyme levels. The next step was to examine the influence of the 50-μg dose icv on the ACTH response to shocks: as shown in FIGURE 6, this regimen significantly decreased ACTH release. These results indicated that, as expected, the stimulatory influence of NO on hypothalamic neurons was an important mechanism modulating the HPA axis response to shocks. Then, by comparing the magnitude of the effect of icv and sc L-NAME, we should be able to deduce the participation of the pituitary influence of NO versus its influence in the PVN. However, when we carried out this comparison in the same assay (which is important because the net effect of blocking NO formation can somewhat vary between batches of animals), we found that sc L-NAME decreased the ACTH response to shocks by 43%, while the effect of icv L-NAME was only 36%. While this difference is small, our results would nevertheless argue against a role of an NO/VP interaction at the level of the pituitary. This was somewhat surprising in view of the fact that L-NAME has such a powerful augment-

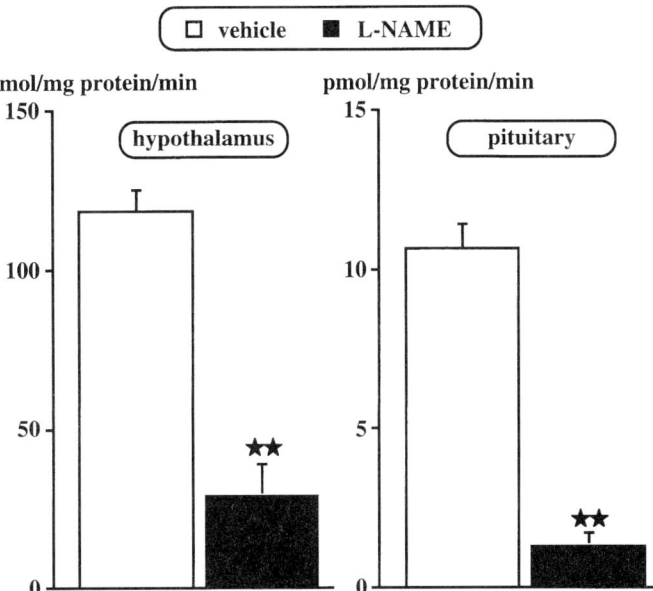

FIGURE 4. The sc injection of L-NAME (50 mg/kg, −3 h) significantly decreases NOS activity in the hypothalamus and pituitary. Each bar represents the mean ± SEM of 5 replicates. **$p < 0.01$ vs. vehicle.

ing influence on even low doses of VP, a peptide that we assume is released during foot shocks because VP antibodies reduced the ACTH response to this stressor.[10]

ROLE OF VP

The second approach that we used was the following: As indicated above, we knew that the ACTH response to shocks depended not only on endogenous CRF, but also on VP. However, we also knew that the contribution of this latter peptide to ACTH released by shocks was delayed, as shown by the fact that VP antibodies decrease the later, not the earlier, phase of shock-induced ACTH release (see FIG. 3). In our earlier studies, we consistently found that blockade of NO formation lowered plasma ACTH levels during the first 30 min of the stressor, which indicated the prevalent influence of central NO on PVN neurons.[10] As can be seen by comparing results obtained in different experiments (see FIGS. 2, 7, and 8), the magnitude of the effect of L-NAME can be somewhat variable. Nevertheless, when we measured pituitary response at later times (30–60 min), we found that L-NAME started to augment the ACTH response of rats exposed to shocks of lower intensities (FIG. 7). This led us to conclude that, in the low-intensity paradigms, the interaction between NO and VP at the pituitary level became functionally more important than that between NO and PVN neurons once VP started to be important for ACTH release. How do we reconcile these results with those obtained by comparing the effect of icv and sc

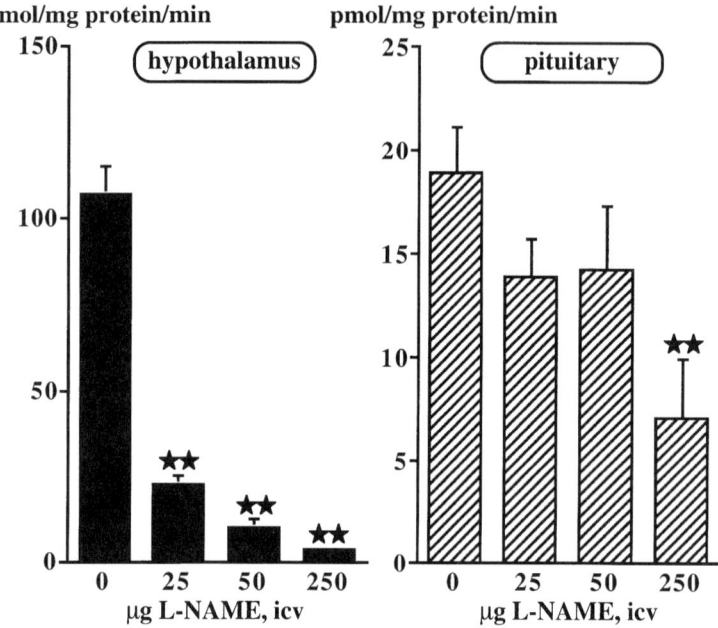

FIGURE 5. Effect of the icv injection of L-NAME on hypothalamic or pituitary NOS activity. Each bar represents the mean ± SEM of 5 replicates. **$p < 0.01$ vs. no L-NAME.

L-NAME? These latter studies were also conducted at a time when we only monitored the first 30 min of the ACTH response to shocks. As we now know that the functional importance of VP and its interaction with NO take place in later phases of this response, the comparison between the two routes of L-NAME administration will have to be repeated with a longer time course.

The final question that we asked was as follows: what would happen to the interaction between shocks and NO in the absence of endogenous VP? If the net influence of sc injected L-NAME represented the sum of its stimulatory effect of NO on CRF/VP neurons and its inhibitory effect on VP-induced ACTH secretion, removing endogenous VP should obliterate this latter inhibitory effect; the augmenting effect of L-NAME on VP-induced ACTH secretion would disappear and the resulting ACTH response to L-NAME should be lower. However, this was not observed. In rats exposed to the 1.0-mA intensity shocks, pretreatment with VP antibodies did not significantly alter the effect of L-NAME alone (FIG. 8). This was not totally unexpected because, in this model, we would expect the influence of the PVN (and, in particular, CRF neurons) to overshadow that of the effect of VP on the pituitary. In contrast, in rats subjected to the low-intensity shocks and injected with VP antibodies prior to L-NAME, the ACTH response was augmented. While this was a surprising finding (see above), the ability of L-NAME itself to significantly enhance the later part of the ACTH response in this particular paradigm may have provided a confounding effect.

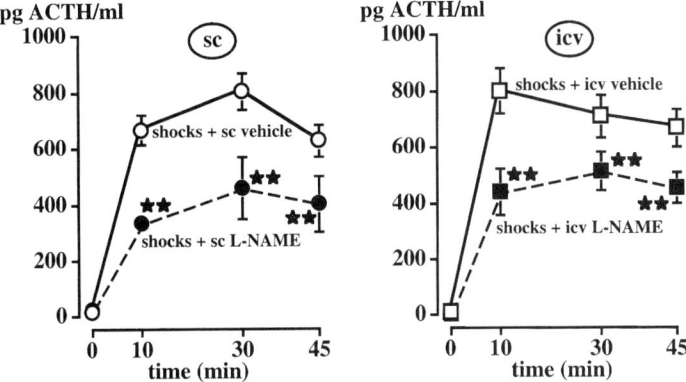

FIGURE 6. Comparison in the same experiment with the effect of sc (50 mg/kg, −3 h) and icv injection of L-NAME (50 μg, −3 h) or its vehicle on the ACTH response to shocks (1 mA, 1 s duration, 2 shocks/min). Each point represents the mean ± SEM of 6–7 rats. Absolute control (abs con) represents animals injected with the vehicle icv, but not exposed to shocks. $**p < 0.01$ vs. icv vehicle.

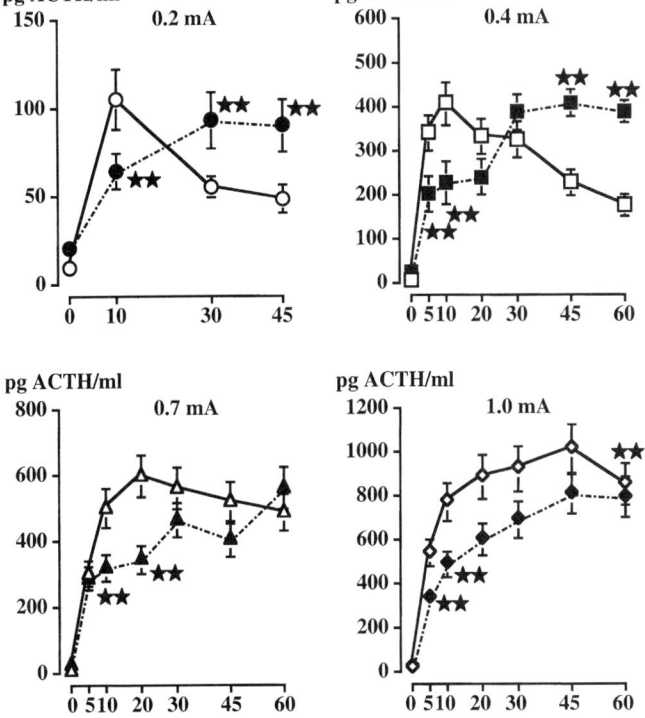

FIGURE 7. Effect of the sc injection of the vehicle (open symbols) or L-NAME (closed symbols; 50 mg/kg, sc, −3 h) on the ACTH response to shocks of four different intensities (all shocks were 1 s duration and delivered at the rate of 2 shocks/min). Each point represents the mean ± SEM of 6–7 rats. $**p < 0.01$ vs. sc vehicle.

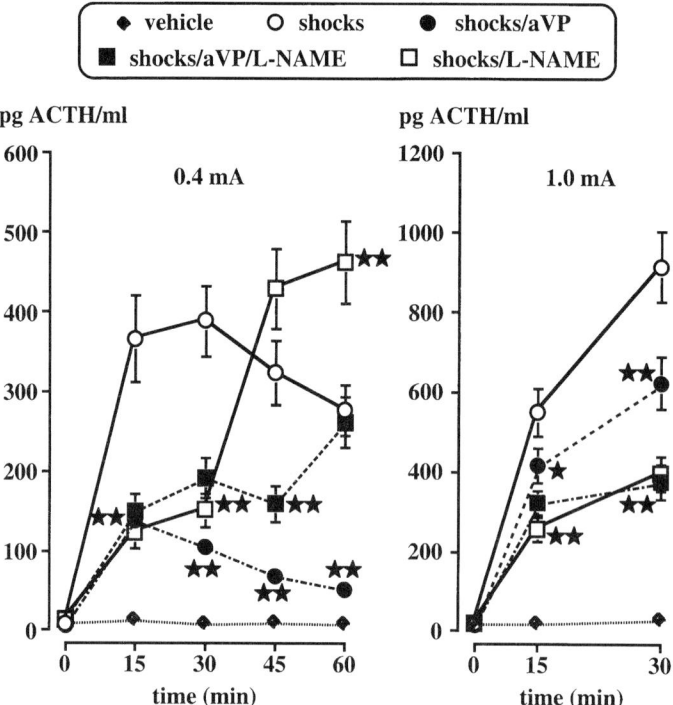

FIGURE 8. Combined effect of VP antibodies (iv, −3 h) and L-NAME (50 mg/kg, sc, −3 h) or their vehicle on the ACTH response to shocks (1 mA, 1 s duration, 2 shocks/min). Each point represents the mean ± SEM of 6–7 rats. $*p < 0.05$ and $**p < 0.01$ vs. shocks only.

CONCLUSIONS

Many stressors release ACTH through mechanisms that depend on both CRF and VP. This means that PVN neurons expressing these peptides are activated and therefore fall under the stimulatory influence of NO and that both peptides act on the pituitary, an influence that in the case of VP is inhibited by NO. The results that we present here provide strong evidence for the importance of these two roles of NO (FIG. 9). However, when we tried to unravel their respective influence in the footshock paradigm, no clear-cut resolution was found. In particular, our recent finding that the interaction between NO and VP on the pituitary may be delayed will require repeating some of our experiments with longer time points.

Finally, as the results illustrated in this chapter were presented in a conference focused on chemical intolerance, it might be useful to speculate on possible interactions between the HPA axis in general, and its modulation by NO in particular, and the host of conditions covered by chemical intolerance.[15] Pathologies such as fibromyalgia and chronic fatigue syndrome have been hypothesized to result from dysregulation of the HPA axis.[16] Many stressors, both inflammatory and noninflammatory, are known to alter NO formation in the brain and, in doing so, the activity

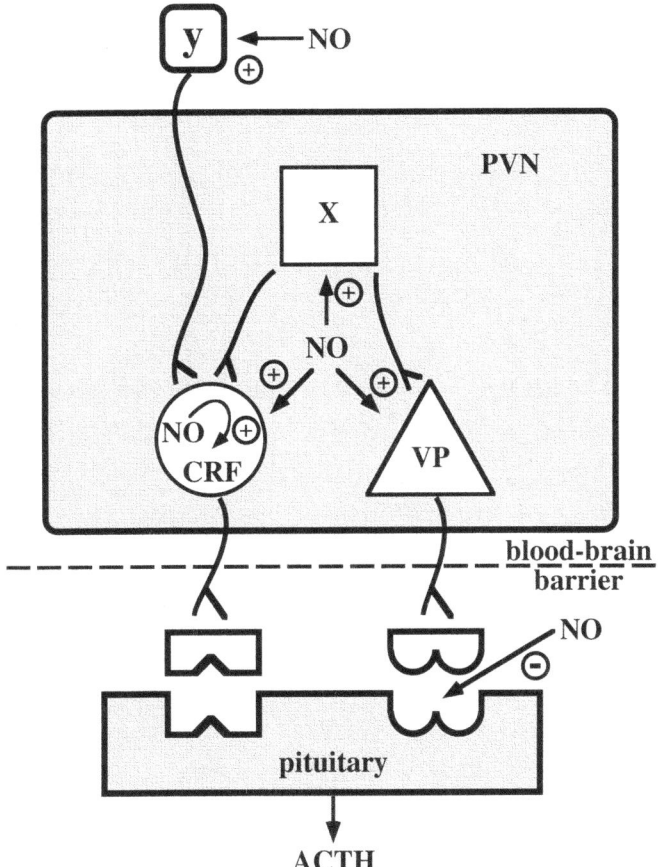

FIGURE 9. Diagram showing the proposed interactions between NO, PVN CRF and VP neurons (illustrated by a circle and a triangle, respectively), and ACTH release as they are presently understood. X (within the PVN) and Y (outside the PVN) designate as yet unidentified neurons and/or glial cells on which NO could act. Placement of the blood-brain barrier is schematized and not meant to be anatomically correct.

of the HPA axis. To our knowledge, very little is known regarding a possible functional link between NO levels and chemical intolerance, but this may represent a fruitful field.

ACKNOWLEDGMENTS

This research was supported by NIH Grant No. MH-51774 and the Foundation for Research. The author is indebted to C. Kwon Kim for his research contribution.

REFERENCES

1. SNYDER, S.H., S.R. JAFFREY & R. ZAKHARY. 1998. Nitric oxide and carbon monoxide: parallel roles as neural messengers. Brain Res. Rev. **26:** 167–175.
2. MANCUSO, C., P. PREZIOSI, A.B. GROSSMAN & P. NAVARRA. 1997. The role of carbon monoxide in the regulation of neuroendocrine function. Neuroimmunomodulation **4:** 225–229.
3. JESSOP, D.S. 1999. Central non-glucocorticoid inhibitors of the hypothalamo-pituitary-adrenal axis. J. Endocrinol. **160:** 169–180.
4. BLUTHÉ, R-M., S. SPARBER & R. DANTZER. 1992. Modulation of the behavioral effects of interleukin-1 in mice by nitric oxide. Neuroendocrinology **3:** 207–209.
5. KIM, C.K. & C. RIVIER. 1998. Influence of nitric oxide synthase inhibitors on the ACTH and cytokine responses to peripheral immune signals. J. Neuroendocrinol. **10:** 353–362.
6. ANTONI, F.A. 1993. Vasopressinergic control of pituitary adrenocorticotropin secretion comes of age. Front. Neuroendocrinol. **14:** 76–122.
7. MASTERS, B.S.S. 1994. Nitric oxide synthases: why so complex? Annu. Rev. Nutr. **14:** 131–145.
8. RIVIER, C. & W. VALE. 1983. Interaction of corticotropin-releasing factor (CRF) and arginine vasopressin (AVP) on ACTH secretion *in vivo*. Endocrinology **113:** 939–942.
9. RIVIER, C., J. RIVIER, P. MORMEDE & W. VALE. 1984. Studies of the nature of the interaction between vasopressin and corticotropin-releasing factor on adrenocorticotropin (ACTH) release in the rat. Endocrinology **115:** 882–886.
10. RIVIER, C. 1994. Endogenous nitric oxide participates in the activation of the hypothalamic-pituitary-adrenal axis by noxious stimuli. Endocr. J. **2:** 367–373.
11. LEE, S., C. KIM & C. RIVIER. 1999. Nitric oxide stimulates ACTH secretion and the transcription of the genes encoding for NGFI-B, corticotropin-releasing factor, corticotropin-releasing factor receptor type 1, and vasopressin in the hypothalamus of the intact rat. J. Neurosci. **19:** 7640–7647.
12. RIVIER, C. 1998. Role of nitric oxide and carbon monoxide in modulating the ACTH response to immune and non-immune signals. Neuroimmunomodulation **5:** 203–213.
13. SAWCHENKO, P.E., E.R. BROWN, R.K.W. CHAN *et al.* 1996. The paraventricular nucleus of the hypothalamus and the functional neuroanatomy of visceromotor responses to stress. *In* Emotional Motor System. Vol. 107, pp. 201–222. Elsevier. Amsterdam/New York.
14. WATTS, A.G. 1996. The impact of physiological stimuli on the expression of corticotropin-releasing hormone (CRH) and other neuropeptide genes. Front. Neuroendocrinol. **17:** 281–326.
15. SORG, B. 1999. Multiple chemical sensitivity: potential role of neural sensitization. Crit. Rev. Neurobiol. **13:** 283–316.
16. CLAUW, D. & G. CHROUSOS. 1997. Chronic pain and fatigue syndromes: overlapping clinical and neuroendocrine features and potential pathogenic mechanisms. Neuroimmunomodulation **4:** 134–153.

Plasticity of the Hippocampus: Adaptation to Chronic Stress and Allostatic Load

BRUCE S. McEWEN[a]

*Laboratory of Neuroendocrinology, The Rockefeller University,
New York, New York 10021, USA*

ABSTRACT: The hippocampus is an important structure for declarative, spatial, and contextual memory and is implicated in the perception of chronic pain. The hippocampal formation is vulnerable to damage from seizures, ischemia, and head trauma and is particularly sensitive to the effects of adrenal glucocorticoids secreted during the diurnal rhythm and chronic stress. Adrenal steroids typically have adaptive effects in the short run, but promote pathophysiology when there is either repeated stress or dysregulation of the HPA axis. The damaging actions of glucocorticoids under such conditions have been termed "allostatic load", referring to the cost to the body of adaptation to adverse conditions. Adrenal steroids display both protective and damaging effects in the hippocampus. They biphasically modulate excitability of hippocampal neurons, and high glucocorticoid levels and severe acute stress impair declarative memory in a reversible manner. The hippocampus also displays structural plasticity, involving ongoing neurogenesis of the dentate gyrus, synaptogenesis under control of estrogens in the CA1 region, and dendritic remodeling caused by repeated stress or elevated levels of exogenous glucocorticoids in the CA3 region. In all three forms of structural plasticity, excitatory amino acids participate along with circulating steroid hormones. Glucocorticoids and stressors suppress neurogenesis in the dentate gyrus. They also potentiate the damage produced by ischemia and seizures. Moreover, the aging rat hippocampus displays elevated and prolonged levels of excitatory amino acids released during acute stress. Our working hypothesis is that structural plasticity in response to repeated stress starts out as an adaptive and protective response, but ends up as damage if the imbalance in the regulation of the key mediators is not resolved. It is likely that morphological rearrangements in the hippocampus brought on by various types of allostatic load alter the manner in which the hippocampus participates in memory functions and it is conceivable that these may also have a role in chronic pain perception.

INTRODUCTION

The hippocampal formation of the brain is involved in episodic, declarative, spatial, and contextual learning and memory and is also a particularly vulnerable and sensitive region of the brain that expresses high levels of receptors for adrenal steroid "stress" hormones.[1–4] Hippocampal neurons are vulnerable to seizures, stroke, and head trauma, as well as responding to stressful experiences.[4–7] At the same time,

---

[a]Address for correspondence: Bruce S. McEwen, Ph.D., The Rockefeller University, Box 165, 1230 York Avenue, New York, NY 10021. Voice: 212-327-8624; fax: 212-327-8634.
mcewen@rockvax.rockefeller.edu

these neurons show remarkable and paradoxical plasticity, involving long-term synaptic potentiation and depression, dendritic remodeling, synaptic turnover, and neurogenesis in the case of the dentate gyrus.[2,8,9]

The hippocampus is also involved in processing of painful stimuli and nociception. Lesions of the dorsal hippocampus in rats increase the vocalization threshold to painful stimuli,[10] whereas electrical stimulation of the hippocampus increases tail-flick latency,[11] and lidocaine injections into the dentate gyrus produce analgesia.[12,13] Electrophysiological recording from the hippocampus has revealed that CA1 pyramidal neurons show prolonged decreases in pyramidal cell activity in response to painful stimuli,[14] and effects of painful stimulation are also evident in the dentate gyrus and CA3 region.[15] Electrical stimulation of the locus coeruleus produces analgesia (see refs. 14 and 16 for citations). The noradrenergic input to the hippocampus is responsive to chronic stress[17,18] and this has been suggested by studies showing that chronic neuropathic pain suppresses hippocampal noradrenergic neurotransmission through elevated local production of the inflammatory cytokine, TNF alpha.[16,19] The fact that the hippocampus shows these changes is consistent with other evidence, reviewed above, that it plays a role in pain perception.

Given the involvement of the hippocampus in the response to stress and in neuropathic pain, it is reasonable to consider its potential involvement in the CNS aspects of chemical intolerance, particularly those aspects that may result from stress and trauma and result in manifestations of chronic pain. This article will discuss the capacity of the hippocampus to change structurally and functionally as a result of chronic restraint and psychosocial stress. Studies of the hippocampus in its response to repeated stress have led to the finding that there are multiple forms of structural and functional plasticity ranging from changes in long-term potentiation to neurogenesis in the dentate gyrus to remodeling of dendrites of CA3 pyramidal neurons.

AN OVERVIEW OF THE STRUCTURAL PLASTICITY OF THE HIPPOCAMPUS

There are three types of plasticity in the hippocampal formation in which adrenal steroids play a role. First, adrenal steroids reversibly and biphasically modulate excitability of hippocampal neurons and influence the magnitude of long-term potentiation, as well as producing long-term depression.[4,7,20,21] These effects on neuronal responses may be involved in biphasic effects of adrenal secretion on excitability and cognitive function and memory during the diurnal rhythm and after stress.[7,22] In particular, acute nonpainful novelty stress inhibits primed-burst potentiation and memory.[23,24] On the other hand, stress involving foot shock and therefore some pain produces an inhibition of hippocampal excitability by a process that is independent of adrenal steroids and, rather, dependent on endogenous opioids.[25,26]

Second, adrenal steroids participate along with excitatory amino acids in regulating neurogenesis of the dentate gyrus granule neuron, in which acute stressful experiences can suppress the ongoing neurogenesis (see ref. 2 for review). Ongoing neurogenesis appears to be a feature of the adult dentate gyrus in species from rodents to humans.[2,27–29] We believe that these effects may be involved in fear-related learning and memory because of the anatomical and functional connections between the dentate gyrus and the amygdala,[30] a brain area important in memory of aversive and fear-producing experiences.[31] Neurogenesis is inhibited by various types of acute and chronic stress.[2] Moreover, during classical (trace) conditioning and spatial maze learning, both involving hippocampal activation, newly formed neurons are protected and differentiate and survive longer as a result of the experience, suggesting that this process may have some role in the memory of the events.[32]

Third, adrenal steroids participate along with excitatory amino acids in a reversible stress-induced remodeling of dendrites in the CA3 region of hippocampus of male rats and tree shrews, a process that affects only the apical dendrites and results in cognitive impairment in the learning of spatial and short-term memory tasks.[2,7] This process is reversible as long as stress is terminated after 21 days[33] and it involves the coordinated activity of adrenal steroids and excitatory amino acids working in concert to produce the shortening and debranching of the apical dendrites of CA3 pyramidal neurons.[2] Pharmaceutical treatment with phenytoin, an antiepileptic drug, and an NMDA receptor blocker prevents the remodeling, and glucocorticoid administration can mimic the effects of stress to cause remodeling by a process that is also blocked by phenytoin (see ref. 2 for review).

The ability of repeated stress to produce structural changes in hippocampus is an example of allostatic load, as will be described below. The wear and tear, produced by repeated stress and/or dysregulation of the HPA axis and of excitatory amino acids, that results in adaptive plasticity of hippocampal nerve cells also leads to conditions that may result in permanent damage to the hippocampus, as will be discussed in the next section.

ALLOSTASIS AND ALLOSTATIC LOAD IN THE BRAIN

Allostasis is the process of adaptation to challenge that maintains stability, or homeostasis, through an active process that may change the operating set points or range of systems that participate in adaptation,[34] and allostatic load is the wear and tear produced by the repeated activation of allostatic, or adaptive, mechanisms.[35,36] Four types of allostatic load have been identified. These consist of (1) repeated challenges, for example, chronic stress, (2) failure to habituate with repeated challenges, (3) failure to shut off the response after the challenge is past, and (4) failure to mount an adequate response. (See ref. 35.) In the hippocampus, we can recognize at least two types of allostatic load involving excitatory amino acid release, namely, the potential to cause damage with repeated stressful challenges and the failure in aging rats to shut off glutamate release after stress.

Under restraint stress, rats show increased extracellular levels of glutamate in hippocampus, as determined by microdialysis, and adrenalectomy markedly attenuates this elevation.[37] Glucocorticoids appear to be involved in potentiating the increased extracellular levels of excitatory amino acids under stress.[38] Similar results have been reported using lactography, a method that is based upon the stimulation of glucose metabolism by increased neuronal activity.[39,40] The consequences of this increased level of glutamate extracellularly will be discussed below in terms of hippocampal dendritic remodeling, which is an example of type 1 allostatic load. In aging rats, hippocampal release of excitatory amino acids during restraint stress is markedly potentiated[41] and this constitutes an example of type 3 allostatic load in the brain, that is, the failure to shut off the production and/or removal of a mediator of neuronal activation.

Free radical formation is a by-product of excitatory amino acid release and a consequence of the activation of second messenger systems.[42,43] A key factor in regulating production of free radicals is the maintenance of homeostasis of calcium ions.[44] When excitatory amino acid neurotransmitters are released, calcium ions are mobilized via activation of NMDA and AMPA receptors, and second messenger systems are activated, leading to a cascade of effects including the long-term potentiation and long-term depression that are believed to be related to information storage mechanisms.[45,46]

The reuptake and rebuffering of calcium ions constitute an active process.[44,47] If the calcium ions are not removed and put back into intracellular stores rapidly and efficiently, the cascade of events is potentiated and can result in the increased accumulation of free radicals and free-radical induced by-products of lipid peroxidation that can produce an allostatic load on brain and cardiovascular cells.[42,44]

There is a link between stressful events and the production of the free radicals, namely, that acute stress increases the production of free radicals in the brain and other organs.[48] However, the role of glucocorticoids in this process is not known. Glucocorticoids may play a role in the process by facilitating the activity of NMDA receptors,[49,50] by impairing glucose uptake and reducing intracellular energy supplies,[6,43] and by increasing calcium currents (see above), and individual differences in glucocorticoid secretion over the life course may thus make a contribution. What is the basis of these individual differences?

DEVELOPMENTAL DETERMINANTS OF INDIVIDUAL DIFFERENCES IN ALLOSTATIC LOAD

The vulnerability of many systems of the body to stress is influenced by experiences early in life. In animal models, unpredictable prenatal stress causes increased emotionality and increased reactivity of the HPA axis and autonomic nervous system and these effects last throughout the life span.[51] Postnatal handling in rats, a mild stress involving brief daily separation from the mother, counteracts the effects of prenatal stress and results in reduced emotionality and reduced reactivity of the HPA axis and autonomic nervous system.[52–54]

For prenatal stress and postnatal handling, once the emotionality and the reactivity of the adrenocortical system are established by events early in life, it is the subsequent actions of the hypothalamo-pituitary-adrenal (HPA) axis in adult life, as discussed above, that are likely to contribute to the rate of brain and body aging. Rats with increased HPA reactivity show early decline of cognitive functions associated with the hippocampus[55] as well as increased propensity to self-administer drugs such as amphetamine and cocaine.[56,57] In contrast, rats with a lower HPA reactivity as a result of neonatal handling have a slower rate of cognitive aging and a reduced loss of hippocampal function.[58–60] Thus, lifelong patterns of adrenocortical function, determined by early experience, contribute to rates of brain aging, at least in experimental animals.

Evidence for a human counterpart to the story of individual differences in rat HPA activity and hippocampal aging is very limited. Individual differences in human brain aging that are correlated with cortisol levels have been recognized in otherwise healthy individuals that are followed over a number of years.[61-63] In the most extensive investigation, healthy elderly subjects were followed over a 4-year period and those who showed a significant and progressive increase in cortisol levels, during yearly exams, over the 4 years, and had high basal cortisol levels in year 4, showed deficits on tasks measuring explicit memory as well as selective attention, compared to subjects with either decreasing cortisol levels over 4 years or subjects with increasing basal cortisol, but moderate current cortisol levels.[61] Using MRI, they also showed a hippocampus that was 14% smaller than age-matched controls who did not show progressive cortisol increases and were not cognitively impaired.[62]

NATURE OF BRAIN CHANGES CAUSED BY CHRONIC STRESS

In order to emphasize the role of allostatic load produced by chronic stress in changing brain structure and function, the effects of two types of repeated stress will be summarized below before considering changes in hippocampus and other brain structures in a number of human conditions.

Multiple Cumulative Effects of Restraint Stress

Restraint stress does not appear on the surface to be a major stress for rats. Upon placing them into a plastic or wire-mesh restrainer for the first time, there is some struggling and a large elevation of glucocorticoids in the blood. With repetition of restraint stress over days, there is a progressive habituation of the HPA response to stress, characterized by an initial peak of corticosterone that is turned off earlier and earlier on subsequent days of stress.[64-66] In spite of this apparent habituation, rats do not show dendritic remodeling until day 21 of repeated restraint, at which time they also show impairment of hippocampal-dependent learning.[67,68] The 21 days of restraint stress also leads to a suppression of neurogenesis in the dentate gyrus, which is not evident after a single restraint stress session.[69] Moreover, in spite of the HPA habituation, administration of adrenal steroid synthesis blockers during 21 days of restraint prevents dendritic remodeling.[66]

After 21 days of repeated restraint stress, rats show increased fear in an open field and increased fear conditioning to both tone and context.[33] They also show enhanced aggressive behavior towards cage mates, which increases over the course of the 3 weeks of repeated restraint (G. Wood, unpublished observations). Thus, the picture that emerges from chronic restraint stress is of a series of behavioral compensations that manifest themselves as increased fear and aggressivity in spite of habituated HPA function in response to the same stressor.

Multiple Cumulative Effects of Psychosocial Stress

Psychosocial stress by conspecifics constitutes an even more powerful stressful experience than restraint stress. In the Visible Burrow System[70] (VBS), five males placed with two females establish a dominance hierarchy in which some of the subordinate rats die within the several weeks they are living together. Among the survivors, the most severely affected subordinates (nonresponding subordinates or NRS) show very low testosterone levels and an impaired HPA response to restraint stress and other stressors, and they have low hypothalamic CRF mRNA levels.[71,72] Both NRS and subordinates that show HPA responses have elevated amygdala CRF levels compared to dominants and cage controls,[72] and both types of subordinates have elevated locus coeruleus tyrosine hydroxylase mRNA and protein levels that point to elevated noradrenergic tone throughout the forebrain.[73] The big surprise is that it is the dominants that show the greatest degree of remodeling of dendrites on CA3 pyramidal neurons in the hippocampus.[74] Not only that, dominants show the greatest downregulation of serotonin transporters in the CA3 region, which points to a role for increased serotonin in the dendritic remodeling.[74] Interestingly, an atypical antidepressant, tianeptine, which increases serotonin reuptake, prevents dendritic remodeling caused by stress and by elevated glucocorticoids.[75,76] Besides 5HT transporters, two other VBS-sensitive serotonergic parameters are the 5HT2 receptors labeled with iodoketanserin and the 5HT1A receptors labeled with 8-OH DPAT.[71] In parietal cerebral cortex, 5HT2 receptor binding was increased in subordinates more so than in dominants. On the other hand, 5HT1A receptor binding was decreased in both dominants and subordinates in many regions of the hippocampus. It should be noted that deletion of the 5HT1A receptor in mice is associated with increased anxiety.[77,78]

Subordinate rats also show dendritic remodeling in the VBS, and another situation in which stress causes dendritic remodeling is seen in the resident-intruder model with tree shrews. In this model, 28 days of residence next to a dominant tree shrew causes dendritic remodeling of apical dendrites of CA3 pyramidal neurons, very much like what is seen after restraint stress in rats.[79] As in rats, remodeling is prevented by phenytoin administration during chronic stress and this treatment does not reduce either glucocorticoid or catecholamine elevations caused by the psychosocial stress.[79] Thus, actions of excitatory amino acids are involved in causing the dendritic remodeling in the tree shrew as well as in the rat. No information is available about the status of dendrites in the dominant tree shrews because they are too precious to sacrifice.

The resident-intruder studies on tree shrews also revealed that neurogenesis is reduced by 28 days of chronic stress.[80] Thus, in both the tree shrew and rat restraint stress models, repeated stress causes dendritic remodeling of CA3 pyramidal neurons and suppresses neurogenesis in the dentate gyrus. Acute psychosocial stress in marmosets also causes a suppression of neurogenesis in the dentate gyrus.[81]

HIPPOCAMPAL STRUCTURAL CHANGES IN DEPRESSIVE ILLNESS AND PTSD

The human hippocampus is capable of dynamic changes in volume. London taxicab drivers are reported to have a larger ventral hippocampus and a smaller dorsal hippocampus, and hippocampal volume is related to length of service on the job.[82] Moreover, as noted above, there are individual differences in human hippocampal aging, with some individuals who show progressively elevated glucocorticoids over 5 years showing a smaller hippocampus than age-matched controls who do not show increased cortisol levels.

In addition, the human brain shows signs of atrophy as a result of elevated glucocorticoids and severe, traumatic stress (e.g., Holocaust survivors; see ref. 6). Advances in brain imaging techniques have allowed for a regional analysis of the atrophy of various brain structures. Recent evidence indicates that the human hippocampus is particularly sensitive in this respect and tends to show greater changes than other brain areas, in particular in Cushing's syndrome, recurrent depressive illness, posttraumatic stress disorder (PTSD), schizophrenia, and aging prior to overt dementia.[83-89]

The diversity of conditions in which atrophy occurs raises two questions, namely, whether there is a common mechanism and whether the atrophy is permanent or reversible. Based upon what is summarized above, the atrophy might be due to one of at least four different processes: (1) a reduced volume of Ammon's horn or dentate gyrus due to reduced dendritic branching; (2) a reduction in dentate gyrus neuron number due to a suppression of neurogenesis; (3) a decreased rate of neuron survival; (4) permanent neuron loss. In addition, it is noteworthy that atrophy of other brain regions has been reported in depressive illness—for example, prefrontal cortex[90] and amygdala.[91] Moreover, new evidence suggests that glial cell depletion may contribute to atrophy of brain regions like the prefrontal cortex and amygdala[91-94] and the contribution of glial cell changes must now be considered for the hippocampus.

Because of the high density of intracellular receptors for adrenal steroids in hippocampus, it is tempting to attribute the occurrence of hippocampal atrophy solely to the actions of glucocorticoids. As summarized above, the hippocampus shows influences of adrenal steroids on plasticity as well as on the loss and damage to hippocampal neurons in conditions like ischemia and aging (see refs. 5–7 and 95 for reviews). However, adrenal steroids produce their effects on plasticity (see earlier discussion) and on damage in ischemia and aging (see above references) by acting in concert with neuromodulators and neurotransmitters, in particular the endogenous excitatory amino acids. Nevertheless, the role of glucocorticoids should not be ignored. Glucocorticoids are elevated in Cushing's syndrome and may also be somewhat elevated in depressive illness, but this is probably not the case for PTSD, at least at the time the PTSD subjects are studied, except as there are elevations in glucocorticoids associated with the diurnal rhythm and stressful experiences that take place on a daily basis.

In this connection, it is important to emphasize that sustained stress levels, or Cushing's-like elevations, of adrenal steroids are not required to produce structural changes in hippocampus. For example, in animal models of stress-induced remodeling of CA3 apical dendrites, periodic adrenocortical stress responses over 21 days are all that are needed, and even those responses tend to habituate and show an earlier shutoff with the repetition of the daily stressor.[7] With regard to human hippocampal atrophy, individual differences in stress responsiveness may play a role in making some people more vulnerable to their own stress hormones: for example, some individuals who are exposed to repeated psychosocial stress (e.g., public speaking) fail to habituate their cortisol elevation and these individuals lack self-esteem and self-confidence.[96] Therefore, one could imagine that individuals with a more reactive stress hormone profile will expose themselves to more cortisol and experience more stress-elevated neural activity than other people who can more easily habituate to psychosocial challenges.

In this regard, events related to the course of illness in recurrent depressive illness may involve very distinct pathways of selective and repeated elevations of glucocorticoid hormones in relation to the individual experiences and reactivities. We are largely ignorant of the history of the depressed individual with regard to endocrine function and neurochemical activity, as well as responses to stressful life experiences. In both disorders, a long-term pattern of increased neurochemical, autonomic, and HPA reactivity to experiences may underlie a progression of neuronal structural changes, involving atrophy that might lead to permanent damage, including neuronal loss. Regarding the neurochemical aspects, there is need to measure the activity of excitatory amino acids in the brain during recurrent depressive illness since neural activity is likely to be a major factor in the long-term atrophy of key brain regions such as hippocampus, amygdala, and prefrontal cortex.

Regarding reversibility or irreversibility of these structural changes, treatment with drugs like phenytoin or tianeptine, both of which block stress-induced atrophy in the model of CA3 dendritic remodeling,[2] is a potential means of both testing the mechanism and at the same time demonstrating the reversibility of human hippocampal atrophy. There is already some indication that hippocampal atrophy in Cushing's syndrome is reversible.[97] On the other hand, there may be irreversible loss of hippocampal neurons, and some of the evidence in the MRI of recurrent depressive illness is consistent with this possibility.[84] Insofar as atrophy of the hippocampus and accompanying cognitive impairment are signs of reversible neuronal remodeling, they may be treatable with agents that block the neuronal remodeling in animal models. On the other hand, where atrophy involves neuronal loss, treatment strategies should focus on the earlier traumatic or recurrent events, and it may be possible to devise strategies to reduce or prevent neuronal damage.

CONCLUSIONS

The hippocampus, amygdala, and prefrontal cortex are three brain areas that show morphological changes as a result of stress-related disorders such as depression and PTSD. Based upon animal models of repeated psychosocial and restraint stress, and studies of underlying cellular changes, there are multiple mechanisms for changes in volume of brain structure ranging from neuronal damage to glial cell loss to dendritic remodeling and reduced dentate gyrus granule cell number. The HPA axis appears to play a significant role in mediated changes in the hippocampus, along with excitatory amino acid neurotransmitters and free radicals. Other types of animal model studies have revealed that experiences early in life, centering around stress and maternal care of infants, play a powerful role in determining patterns of lifelong reactivity of the systems that lead to atrophy of hippocampus and other brain structures. Thus, the role of early experience and a childhood history of abuse and neglect (e.g., see ref. 98) should also be considered in relation to chronic pain and increased chemical sensitivities.

The functional consequences of the changes in brain structure include impairment of declarative memory and it is also likely that the morphological changes within these brain structures also contribute to other symptoms of the disorders. Much less is known about chronic pain and virtually nothing is known about increased chemical sensitivities, as far as structural and functional changes in the hippocampus and other brain regions are concerned. However, because the hippocampus is implicated in the perception of pain (see INTRODUCTION), it is likely that alterations in hippocampal structure and function, such as described in this article, lead to changes in pain perception. This is a possibility that can be tested in animal models. An additional and most intriguing question for future study is whether chronic pain itself leads to alterations in brain structure and function.

ACKNOWLEDGMENTS

Research support for studies described in this paper was obtained from MH 41256, Center Grant P50 MH 58911, Servier (France), and The Health Foundation (New York).

REFERENCES

1. MCEWEN, B.S., J. WEISS & L. SCHWARTZ. 1968. Selective retention of corticosterone by limbic structures in rat brain. Nature **220:** 911–912.
2. MCEWEN, B.S. 1999. Stress and hippocampal plasticity. Annu. Rev. Neurosci. **22:** 105–122.
3. EICHENBAUM, H. 1997. How does the brain organize memories? Science **277:** 330–332.
4. DEKLOET, E.R., E. VREUGDENHIL, M.S. OITZL & M. JOELS. 1998. Brain corticosteroid receptor balance in health and disease. Endocr. Rev. **19:** 269–301.
5. SAPOLSKY, R., L. KREY & B.S. MCEWEN. 1986. The neuroendocrinology of stress and aging: the glucocorticoid cascade hypothesis. Endocr. Rev. **7:** 284–301.
6. SAPOLSKY, R. 1992. Stress, the Aging Brain, and the Mechanisms of Neuron Death. Volume 1, pp. 423. MIT Press. Cambridge, MA.
7. MCEWEN, B.S., D. ALBECK, H. CAMERON *et al.* 1995. Stress and the Brain: A Paradoxical Role for Adrenal Steroids. *In* Vitamins and Hormones, pp. 371–402. Academic Press. New York.
8. CAMERON, H.A. & E. GOULD. 1996. The Control of Neuronal Birth and Survival. *In* Receptor Dynamics in Neural Development, pp. 141–157. CRC Press. New York.
9. MCEWEN, B.S. & S.H. ALVES. 1999. Estrogen actions in the central nervous system. Endocr. Rev. **20:** 279–307.
10. BLANCHARD, R.J. & R.A. FIAL. 1968. Effects of limbic lesions on passive avoidance and reactivity to shock. J. Comp. Physiol. Psychol. **66:** 606–612.
11. PRADO, W.A.R.M.H.T. 1985. An assessment of the antinociceptive and aversive effects of stimulating identified sites in the rat brain. Brain Res. **340:** 219–228.
12. MCKENNA, J.E. & R. MELZACK. 1992. Analgesia produced by lidocaine microinjection into the dentate gyrus. Pain **49:** 105–112.
13. YEUNG, J.C., T.L. YAKSH & T.A. RUDY. 1977. Concurrent mapping of brain sites for sensitivity to the direct application of morphine and focal electrical stimulation in the production of antinociception in the rat. Pain **4:** 23–40.
14. KHANNA, S. & J.G. SINCLAIR. 1989. Noxious stimuli produce prolonged changes in the CA1 region of the rat hippocampus. Pain **39:** 337–343.
15. BRANKACK, J. & G. BUZSAKI. 1986. Hippocampal responses evoked by tooth pulp and acoustic stimulation: depth profiles and effect of behavior. Brain Res. **378:** 303–314.
16. IGNATOWSKI, T.A., W.C. COVEY, P.R. KNIGHT *et al.* 1999. Brain-derived TNF mediates neuropathic pain. Brain Res. **841:** 70–77.
17. ABERCROMBIE, E.D., R.W. KELLER, JR. & M.J. ZIGMOND. 1988. Characterization of hippocampal norepinephrine release as measured by microdialysis perfusion: pharmacological and behavioral studies. Neuroscience **27:** 897–904.

18. NISENBAUM, L., M. ZIGMOND, A. SVED & E. ABERCROMBIE. 1991. Prior exposure to chronic stress results in enhanced synthesis and release of hippocampal norepinephrine in response to a novel stressor. J. Neurosci. **11:** 1478–1484.
19. COVEY, W.C., T.A. IGNATOWSKI, P.R. KNIGHT & R.N. SPENGLER. 2000. Brain-derived TNF: involvement in neuroplastic changes implicated in the conscious perception of persistent pain. Brain Res. **859:** 113–122.
20. PAVLIDES, C., S. OGAWA, A. KIMURA & B.S. MCEWEN. 1996. Role of adrenal steroid mineralocorticoid and glucocorticoid receptors in long-term potentiation in the CA1 field of hippocampal slices. Brain Res. **738:** 229–235.
21. KERR, D.S., A.M. HUGGETT & W.C. ABRAHAM. 1994. Modulation of hippocampal long-term potentiation and long-term depression by corticosteroid receptor activation. Psychobiology **22:** 123–133.
22. BARNES, C., B. MCNAUGHTON, G. GODDARD et al. 1977. Circadian rhythm of synaptic excitability in rat and monkey central nervous system. Science **197:** 91–92.
23. DIAMOND, D.M., M. FLESHNER & G.M. ROSE. 1994. Psychological stress repeatedly blocks hippocampal primed burst potentiation in behaving rats. Behav. Brain Res. **62:** 1–9.
24. DIAMOND, D.M., M. FLESHNER, N. INGERSOLL & G.M. ROSE. 1996. Psychological stress impairs spatial working memory: relevance to electrophysiological studies of hippocampal function. Behav. Neurosci. **110:** 661–672.
25. SHORS, T., T. SEIB, S. LEVINE & R. THOMPSON. 1989. Inescapable versus escapable shock modulates long-term potentiation in the rat hippocampus. Science **244:** 224–226.
26. SHORS, T., S. LEVINE & R. THOMPSON. 1990. Effect of adrenalectomy and demedullation on the stress-induced impairment of long-term potentiation. Neuroendocrinology **51:** 70–75.
27. GOULD, E., P. TANAPAT, T. RYDEL & N. HASTINGS. 2000. Regulation of hippocampal neurogenesis in adulthood. Biol. Psychiatry. In press.
28. CAMERON, H.A. & D.G. MCKAY. 1999. Restoring production of hippocampal neurons in old age. Nat. Neurosci. **2:** 849–858.
29. KEMPERMANN, G. & F.H. GAGE. 1999. New nerve cells for the adult brain. Sci. Am. **280:** 48–53.
30. IKEGAYA, Y., H. SAITO & K. ABE. 1997. The basomedial and basolateral amygdaloid nuclei contribute to the induction of long-term potentiation in the dentate gyrus *in vivo*. Eur. J. Neurosci. **8:** 1833–1839.
31. LEDOUX, J.E. 1995. In search of an emotional system in the brain: leaping from fear to emotion and consciousness. *In* The Cognitive Neurosciences, pp. 1049–1061. MIT Press. Cambridge, MA.
32. GOULD, E., A. BEYLIN, P. TANAPAT et al. 1999. Learning enhances adult neurogenesis in the hippocampal formation. Nat. Neurosci. **2:** 260–265.
33. CONRAD, C.D., A.M. MAGARINOS, J.E. LEDOUX & B.S. MCEWEN. 1999. Repeated restraint stress facilitates fear conditioning independently of causing hippocampal CA3 dendritic atrophy. Behav. Neurosci. **113:** 902–913.
34. STERLING, P. & J. EYER. 1988. Allostasis: a new paradigm to explain arousal pathology. *In* Handbook of Life Stress, Cognition, and Health, pp. 629–649. Wiley. New York.
35. MCEWEN, B.S. 1998. Protective and damaging effects of stress mediators. N. Engl. J. Med. **338:** 171–179.
36. MCEWEN, B.S. & E. STELLAR. 1993. Stress and the individual: mechanisms leading to disease. Arch. Intern. Med. **153:** 2093–2101.
37. LOWY, M.T., L. GAULT & B.K. YAMAMOTO. 1993. Adrenalectomy attenuates stress-induced elevations in extracellular glutamate concentrations in the hippocampus. J. Neurochem. **61:** 1957–1960.
38. MOGHADDAM, B., M.L. BOLIANO, B. STEIN-BEHRENS & R. SAPOLSKY. 1994. Glucocorticoids mediate the stress-induced extracellular accumulation of glutamate. Brain Res. **655:** 251–254.
39. SCHAASFOORT, E., L. DEBRIN & J. KORF. 1988. Mild stress stimulates rat hippocampal glucose utilization transiently via NMDA receptors as assessed by lactography. Brain Res. **575:** 58–63.

40. DE BRUIN, L.A., M.C. SCHASFOORT, A.B. STEFENS & J. KORF. 1994. Effects of stress and exercise on rat hippocampus and striatum extracellular lactate. Am. J. Physiol. **259:** R773–R779.
41. LOWY, M.T., L. WITTENBERG & B.K. YAMAMOTO. 1995. Effect of acute stress on hippocampal glutamate levels and spectrin proteolysis in young and aged rats. J. Neurochem. **65:** 268–274.
42. MCCORD, J. 1985. Oxygen-derived free radicals in postischemic tissue injury. N. Engl. J. Med. **312:** 159–163.
43. REAGAN, L.P. & B.S. MCEWEN. 1997. Controversies surrounding glucocorticoid-mediated cell death in the hippocampus. J. Chem. Neuroanat. **13:** 149–167.
44. KELLER, J.N. & M.P. MATTSON. 1998. Roles of lipid peroxidation in modulation of cellular signaling pathways, cell dysfunction, and death in the nervous system. Rev. Neurosci. **9:** 105–116.
45. MAREN, S. 1999. Long-term potentiation in the amygdala: a mechanism for emotional learning and memory. TINS **22:** 561–567.
46. BLISS, T.V.P. & G.L. COLLINGRIDGE. 1993. A synaptic model of memory: long-term potentiation in the hippocampus. Nature **361:** 31–39.
47. CHOI, D. 1988. Calcium-mediated neurotoxicity: relationship to specific channel types and role in ischemic damage. TINS **11:** 465–469.
48. LIU, J., A. FISCHER, N. AMIRI *et al.* 1998. Stress-induced oxidative damage in the brain: stress hormones enhance, but an antistress hormone (DHEA) inhibits, oxidative damage and beta-amyloid production in cell culture. Oxygen Society Meeting poster [abstract].
49. WEILAND, N.G., M. ORCHINIK & P. TANAPAT. 1997. Chronic corticosterone treatment induces parallel changes in N-methyl-D-aspartate receptor subunit messenger RNA levels and antagonist binding sites in the hippocampus. Neuroscience **78:** 653–662.
50. BARTANUSZ, V., J.M. AUBRY, S. PAGLIUSI *et al.* 1995. Stress-induced changes in messenger RNA levels of N-methyl-D-aspartate and AMPA receptor subunits in selected regions of the rat hippocampus and hypothalamus. Neuroscience **66:** 247–252.
51. WEINSTOCK, M., T. POLTYREV, D. SCHORER-APELBAUM *et al.* 1998. Effect of prenatal stress on plasma corticosterone and catecholamines in response to foot shock in rats. Physiol. Behav. **64:** 439–444.
52. ADER, R. 1968. Effects of early experiences on emotional and physiological reactivity in the rat. J. Comp. Physiol. Psychol. **66:** 264–268.
53. HESS, J.L., V.H. DENENBERG, M.X. ZARROW & W.D. PFEIFER. 1968. Modification of the corticosterone response curve as a function of handling in infancy. Physiol. Behav. **4:** 109–111.
54. LEVINE, S., G. HALTMEYER, G. KARA & V. DENENBERG. 1967. Physiological and behavioral effects of infantile stimulation. Physiol. Behav. **2:** 55–59.
55. DELLU, F., W. MAYO, M. VALLEE *et al.* 1994. Reactivity to novelty during youth as a predictive factor of cognitive impairment in the elderly: a longitudinal study in rats. Brain Res. **653:** 51–56.
56. PIAZZA, P.V., M. MARINELLI, C. JODOGNE *et al.* 1994. Inhibition of corticosterone synthesis by metrapone decreases cocaine-induced locomotion and relapse of cocaine self-administration. Brain Res. **658:** 259–264.
57. DEROCHE, V., P.V. PIAZZA, M. LEMOAL & H. SIMON. 1993. Individual differences in the psychomotor effects of morphine are predicted by reactivity to novelty and influenced by corticosterone secretion. Brain Res. **623:** 341–344.
58. MEANEY, M., D. AITKEN, H. BERKEL *et al.* 1988. Effect of neonatal handlng of age-related impairments associated with the hippocampus. Science **239:** 766–768.
59. CATALANI, A., M. MARINELLI, S. SCACCIANOCE *et al.* 1993. Progeny of mothers drinking corticosterone during lactation has lower stress-induced corticosterone secretion and better cognitive performance. Brain Res. **624:** 209–215.
60. MEANEY, M.J., B. TANNENBAUM, D. FRANCIS *et al.* 1994. Early environmental programming hypothalamic-pituitary-adrenal responses to stress. Semin. Neurosci. **6:** 247–259.
61. LUPIEN, S., A.R. LECOURS, I. LUSSIER *et al.* 1994. Basal cortisol levels and cognitive deficits in human aging. J. Neurosci. **14:** 2893–2903.

62. LUPIEN, S.J., M.J. DELEON, S. DE SANTI et al. 1998. Cortisol levels during human aging predict hippocampal atrophy and memory deficits. Nat. Neurosci. **1:** 69–73.
63. SEEMAN, T.E., B.S. MCEWEN, B.H. SINGER et al. 1997. Increase in urinary cortisol excretion and memory declines: MacArthur studies of successful aging. J. Clin. Endocrinol. Metab. **82:** 2458–2465.
64. WATANABE, Y., E. GOULD & B.S. MCEWEN. 1992. Stress induces atrophy of apical dendrites of hippocampus CA3 pyramidal neurons. Brain Res. **588:** 341–344.
65. MAGARINOS, A.M. & B.S. MCEWEN. 1995. Stress-induced atrophy of apical dendrites of hippocampal CA3c neurons: comparison of stressors. Neuroscience **69:** 83–88.
66. MAGARINOS, A.M. & B.S. MCEWEN. 1995. Stress-induced atrophy of apical dendrites of hippocampal CA3c neurons: involvement of glucocorticoid secretion and excitatory amino acid receptors. Neuroscience **69:** 89–98.
67. LUINE, V., M. VILLEGAS, C. MARTINEZ & B.S. MCEWEN. 1994. Repeated stress causes reversible impairments of spatial memory performance. Brain Res. **639:** 167–170.
68. CONRAD, C.D., L.A.M. GALEA, Y. KURODA & B.S. MCEWEN. 1996. Chronic stress impairs rat spatial memory on the Y-maze and this effect is blocked by tianeptine pre-treatment. Behav. Neurosci. **110:** 1321–1334.
69. PHAM, K., J. NACHER, P.R. HOF & B.S. MCEWEN. 2000. Repeated, but not acute, restraint stress suppresses proliferation of neural precursor cells and increases PSA-NCAM expression in the adult rat dentate gyrus. J. Neurosci. In press.
70. BLANCHARD, R.J., M. HEBERT, R.R. SAKAI et al. 1998. Chronic social stress: changes in behavioral and physiological indices of emotion. Aggressive Behav. **24:** 307–321.
71. MCKITTRICK, C.R., D.C. BLANCHARD, R.J. BLANCHARD et al. 1995. Serotonin receptor binding in a colony model of chronic social stress. Biol. Psychiatry **37:** 383–393.
72. ALBECK, D.S., C.R. MCKITTRICK, D.C. BLANCHARD et al. 1997. Chronic social stress alters levels of corticotropin-releasing factor and arginine vasopressin mRNA in rat brain. J. Neurosci. **17:** 4895–4903.
73. WATANABE, Y., C.R. MCKITTRICK, D.C. BLANCHARD et al. 1995. Effects of chronic social stress on tyrosine hydroxylase mRNA and protein levels. Mol. Brain Res. **32:** 176–180.
74. MCKITTRICK, C.R., A.M. MAGARINOS, D.C. BLANCHARD et al. 2000. Chronic social stress reduces dendritic arbors in CA3 of hippocampus and decreases binding to serotonin transporter sites. Synapse **36:** 85–94.
75. WATANABE, Y., E. GOULD, D. DANIELS et al. 1992. Tianeptine attenuates stress-induced morphological changes in the hippocampus. Eur. J. Pharmacol. **222:** 157–162.
76. MAGARINOS, A.M., A. DESLANDES & B.S. MCEWEN. 1999. Effects of antidepressants and benzodiazepine treatments on the dendritic structure of CA3 pyramidal neurons after chronic stress. Eur. J. Pharmacol. **371:** 113–122.
77. RAMBOZ, S., R. OOSTING, D. AIT AMARA et al. 1998. Serotonin receptor 1A knockout: an animal model of anxiety-related disorder. Proc. Natl. Acad. Sci. U.S.A. **95:** 14476–14481.
78. SIBILLE, E., C. PAVLIDES, D. BENKE & M. TOTH. 2000. Genetic inactivation of the serotonin$_{1A}$ receptor in mice results in downregulation of major GABA$_A$ receptor subunits, reduction of GABA$_A$ receptor binding, and benzodiazepine-resistant anxiety. J. Neurosci. **20:** 2758–2765.
79. MAGARINOS, A.M., B.S. MCEWEN, G. FLUGGE & E. FUCHS. 1996. Chronic psychosocial stress causes apical dendritic atrophy of hippocampal CA3 pyramidal neurons in subordinate tree shrews. J. Neurosci. **16:** 3534–3540.
80. GOULD, E., B.S. MCEWEN, P. TANAPAT et al. 1997. Neurogenesis in the dentate gyrus of the adult tree shrew is regulated by psychosocial stress and NMDA receptor activation. J. Neurosci. **17:** 2492–2498.
81. GOULD, E., P. TANAPAT, B.S. MCEWEN et al. 1998. Proliferation of granule cell precursors in the dentate gyrus of adult monkeys is diminished by stress. Proc. Natl. Acad. Sci. U.S.A. **95:** 3168–3171.
82. MAGUIRE, E.A., D.G. GADIAN, I.S. JOHNSRUDE et al. 2000. Navigation-related structural change in the hippocampi of taxi drivers. Proc. Natl. Acad. Sci. U.S.A. In press.
83. STARKMAN, M., S. GEBARSKI, S. BERENT & D. SCHTEINGART. 1992. Hippocampal formation volume, memory dysfunction, and cortisol levels in patients with Cushing's syndrome. Biol. Psychiatry **32:** 756–765.

84. SHELINE, Y.I., P.W. WANG, M.H. GADO et al. 1996. Hippocampal atrophy in recurrent major depression. Proc. Natl. Acad. Sci. U.S.A. **93:** 3908–3913.
85. BREMNER, D.J., P. RANDALL, T.M. SCOTT et al. 1995. MRI-based measurement of hippocampal volume in patients with combat-related posttraumatic stress disorder. Am. J. Psychiatry **152:** 973–981.
86. GURVITS, T.V., M.E. SHENTON, H. HOKAMA et al. 1996. Magnetic resonance imaging study of hippocampal volume in chronic, combat-related posttraumatic stress disorder. Biol. Psychiatry **40:** 1091–1099.
87. BOGERTS, B., J.A. LIEBERMAN, M. ASHTAIR et al. 1993. Hippocampus-amygdala volumes and psychopathology in chronic schizophrenia. Biol. Psychiatry **33:** 236–246.
88. FUKUZAKO, H., T. FUKUZAKO, T. HASHIGUCHI et al. 1996. Reduction in hippocampal formation volume is caused mainly by its shortening in chronic schizophrenia: assessment by MRI. Biol. Psychiatry **39:** 938–945.
89. SHELINE, Y.I., M. SANGHAVI, M.A. MINTUN & M.H. GADO. 1999. Depression duration, but not age predicts hippocampal volume loss in medically healthy women with recurrent major depression. J. Neurosci. **19:** 5034–5043.
90. DREVETS, W.C., J.L. PRICE, J.R. SIMPSON, JR. et al. 1997. Subgenual prefrontal cortex abnormalities in mood disorders. Nature **386:** 824–827.
91. SHELINE, Y.I., M.H. GADO & J.L. PRICE. 1998. Amygdala core nuclei volumes are decreased in recurrent major depression. NeuroReport **9:** 2023–2028.
92. DREVETS, W.C., D. ONGUR & J.L. PRICE. 1998. Neuroimaging abnormalities in the subgenual prefrontal cortex: implications for the pathophysiology of familial mood disorders. Mol. Psychiatry **3:** 220–226.
93. RAJKOWSKA, G., J.J. MIGUEL-HIDALGO, J. WEI et al. 1999. Morphometric evidence for neuronal and glial prefrontal cell pathology in major depression. Biol. Psychiatry **45:** 1085–1098.
94. ONGUR, D., W.C. DREVETS & J.L. PRICE. 1998. Glial loss in the subgenual prefrontal cortex in familial mood disorders. Abstr. Soc. Neurosci. **24:** 990 (no. 386.13).
95. LANDFIELD, P.W. & J.C. ELDRIDGE. 1994. Evolving aspects of the glucocorticoid hypothesis of brain aging: hormonal modulation of neuronal calcium homeostasis. Neurobiol. Aging **15:** 579–588.
96. KIRSCHBAUM, C., J.C. PRUSSNER, A.A. STONE et al. 1995. Persistent high cortisol responses to repeated psychological stress in a subpopulation of healthy men. Psychosom. Med. **57:** 468–474.
97. STARKMAN, M.N., B. GIORDANI, S.S. GEBRSKI et al. 1999. Decrease in cortisol reverses human hippocampal atrophy following treatment of Cushing's disease. Biol. Psychiatry **46:** 1595–1602.
98. FELITTI, V.J., R.F. ANDA, D. NORDENBERG et al. 1998. Relationship of childhood abuse and household dysfunction to many of the leading causes of death in adults: the adverse childhood experiences (ACE) study. Am. J. Prev. Med. **14:** 245–258.

Acquiring Symptoms in Response to Odors: A Learning Perspective on Multiple Chemical Sensitivity

OMER VAN DEN BERGH,[a,b] STEPHAN DEVRIESE,[b] WINNIE WINTERS,[b] HENDRIK VEULEMANS,[c] BENOIT NEMERY,[c] PAUL EELEN,[b] AND KAREL P. VAN DE WOESTIJNE[c]

[b]*Department of Psychology,* [c]*Faculty of Medicine, University of Leuven, Belgium*

ABSTRACT: In this chapter, a learning account is discussed as a potential explanation for the symptoms in multiple chemical sensitivity. Clinical evidence is scarce and anecdotal. A laboratory model provides more convincing results. After a few breathing trials containing CO_2-enriched air as an unconditioned stimulus in a compound with harmless odor substances as conditioned stimuli, subjective symptoms are elicited and respiratory behavior is altered by the odors only. Also, mental images can become conditioned stimuli to trigger subjective symptoms. The learning effects cannot be explained by a response bias or by conditioned arousal, and they appear to involve basic associative processes that do not overlap with aware cognition of the relationship between the odors and the CO_2 inhalation. Learned symptoms generalize to new odors and they can be eliminated in a Pavlovian extinction procedure. In accordance with clinical findings, neurotic subjects and psychiatric cases are more vulnerable to learning subjective symptoms in response to odors. Consistent with a learning account, cognitive-behavioral treatment techniques appear to produce beneficial results in clinical cases. Several criticisms and unresolved questions regarding the potential role of learning mechanisms are discussed.

INTRODUCTION

Several excellent reviews on multiple chemical sensitivity (MCS; or idiopathic environmental intolerance, IEI)[1–4] and special issues of journals[d] document its symptoms, prevalence, prognostic course, and possible pathogenic mechanisms. Two major features characterize this syndrome: (1) the presence of a wide variety of nonspecific subjective symptoms, such as fatigue and weakness, cognitive difficulties (concentration and memory), dizziness, pounding heart, shortness of breath, anxiety, headache, and muscle tension;[5,e] and (2) a spatiotemporal relationship between the symptoms and the presence of (often odorous) chemical substances that are often structurally unrelated and at doses below those known to cause harmful

---

[a]Address for correspondence: Omer Van den Bergh, Department of Psychology, University of Leuven, Tiensestraat 102, B-3000 Leuven, Belgium. Voice: +32 16 32.60.58; fax: +32 16 32.60.55.
omer.vandenbergh@psy.kuleuven.ac.be

[d]See, for example: *Toxicol. Ind. Health*, 1994, **10**(4,5); *Environ. Health Perspect.*, 1997, **105**; and *Occup. Med.*, 2000, **15**(3).

[e]The symptoms also occur, for example, in chronic fatigue syndrome,[5] fibromyalgia,[5] panic disorder,[6,7] posttraumatic stress disorder,[8] and hyperventilation syndrome.[9]

effects in the population.[10] Thus, the basic questions regarding MCS are as follows: what is the origin of these symptoms and how can the link with chemical substances be explained?

In the present chapter, we will discuss the evidence for one potential explanation, namely Pavlovian conditioning. The evidence will not be discussed in the context of an antithesis between psychologic and biologic explanations. Such an antithesis is, we believe, counterproductive. First, the subjective symptoms of MCS are by definition the result of psychologic processes. Part of their input may come from biologic dysregulation and part may come from mental processes, but perceptual-cognitive processes of symptom perception and interpretation are the final route to all subjective symptoms. Second, Pavlovian conditioning should be regarded as an adaptive psychobiologic process. The salivation of Pavlov's dog is a biologic response, and the mental processes that trigger it have a biologic substrate. The difference between a psychologic and a biologic explanation is therefore mainly a matter of level of description. Nevertheless, these different levels may suggest quite different approaches to treatment. In this chapter, we will argue that evidence for a Pavlovian conditioning hypothesis is accumulating, that it has great explanatory power, and that it offers interesting treatment options.

THE PAVLOVIAN CONDITIONING HYPOTHESIS OF MCS

In its simplest form, Pavlovian conditioning relies on the co-occurrence of two events. An unconditional stimulus (US; e.g., a toxic exposure or another traumatic event) may trigger an unconditional response (UR; e.g., an array of bodily responses and subjective symptoms). The occurrence of this US in a spatiotemporal relationship with a neutral^f stimulus (a conditioned stimulus, CS; e.g., an odor or harmless chemical) may endow the CS with the capacity to elicit UR-like responses that, at that moment, become conditioned responses (CRs) (see FIG. 1).

We translated this simple Pavlovian schema into a laboratory model in order to test whether subjective symptoms induced by a physiological challenge in association with a harmless odoring chemical could be elicited by presenting the latter stimulus only. The basic model implied the administration of a number of breathing trials of two minutes each (see FIG. 2). Air enriched with 7.5% CO_2 served as a respiratory US and two odors as CSs, for example, dilute ammonia and niaouli (a mixture containing mainly eucalyptus oil). In the learning phase, subjects breathed one odor mixed with CO_2 (called the CS+ trial) and the other odor mixed with room air (called the CS− trial).

In the test phase, the breathing trials contained the odors only, that is, there was no CO_2. Respiratory frequency, tidal volume, end-tidal fractional concentration of CO_2, and heart rate were measured throughout the experiment and subjective symptoms were registered after each trial. Often, conscious awareness of the contingency relationship between the CS+ odor and the experienced symptoms during the acquisition phase was also registered.

---

^{f}A CS is not necessarily neutral in an absolute way, but in a relative way in that it does not elicit the same URs as the US by itself.

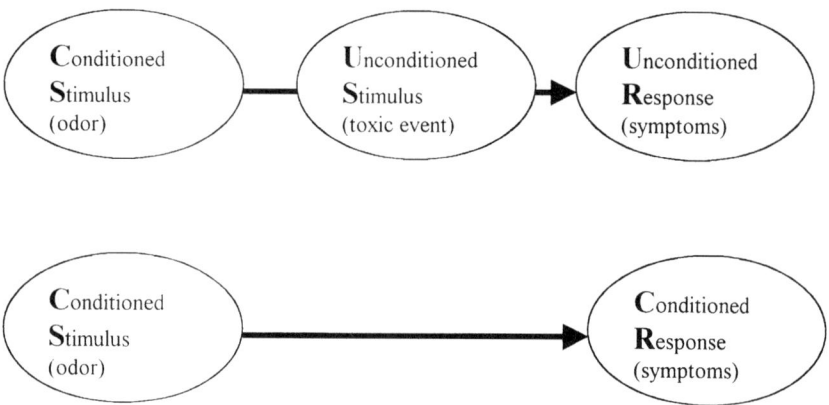

FIGURE 1. Traditional Pavlovian schema (applied to MCS).

This experimental model replicates important features of MCS: (1) it involves human subjects; (2) the major dependent variable consists of a variety of subjective symptoms; (3) CO_2 inhalation may represent a conceptual analogue for a toxic exposure; and (4) harmless odoring chemicals are introduced to serve as elicitors of the symptoms.

In addition, both bodily responses and subjective symptoms are measured, allowing investigation of the concordance/divergence among the two sets of responses. An important methodological advantage is also that the conditioning effect can be tested both within subject and within odor, meaning that the subject and the odor serve as their own controls. The following results were obtained in a series of experiments:

(1) After a few pairings of the CS+ odor with CO_2, presenting the CS+ odor alone altered respiratory behavior and induced elevated levels of somatic symptoms "as if the subjects were still breathing CO_2".[11–15]

(2) The learning effect was selective: conditioning effects only occurred to foul-smelling ammonia as CS+ odor and not to neutral/pleasant-smelling niaouli as CS+ (see FIG. 2). When both CS odors were foul smelling (irritant ammonia and nonirritant butyric acid), learned symptoms emerged to both, suggesting that affective valence of the odors was the critical variable for the selective association effect.[11–14]

(3) The learning effect was specific: no conditioning effects appeared for symptoms usually not provoked by CO_2 ("dummy symptoms") and the effects could not be explained by conditioned arousal/anxiety only. We never observed a conditioned heart rate increase, and the effects were largest for the subset of symptoms that are typically elicited by CO_2.[12–14]

(4) Conscious awareness of the relationship between the odor and CO_2-induced symptoms was not critical for the effects to occur. For all odors used as CS+, the participants were roughly equally aware of the experimentally induced contingencies, yet they only showed conditioning effects to foul-smelling CSs. This suggests that more basic learning processes than those reflected by conscious awareness are involved.[12–14]

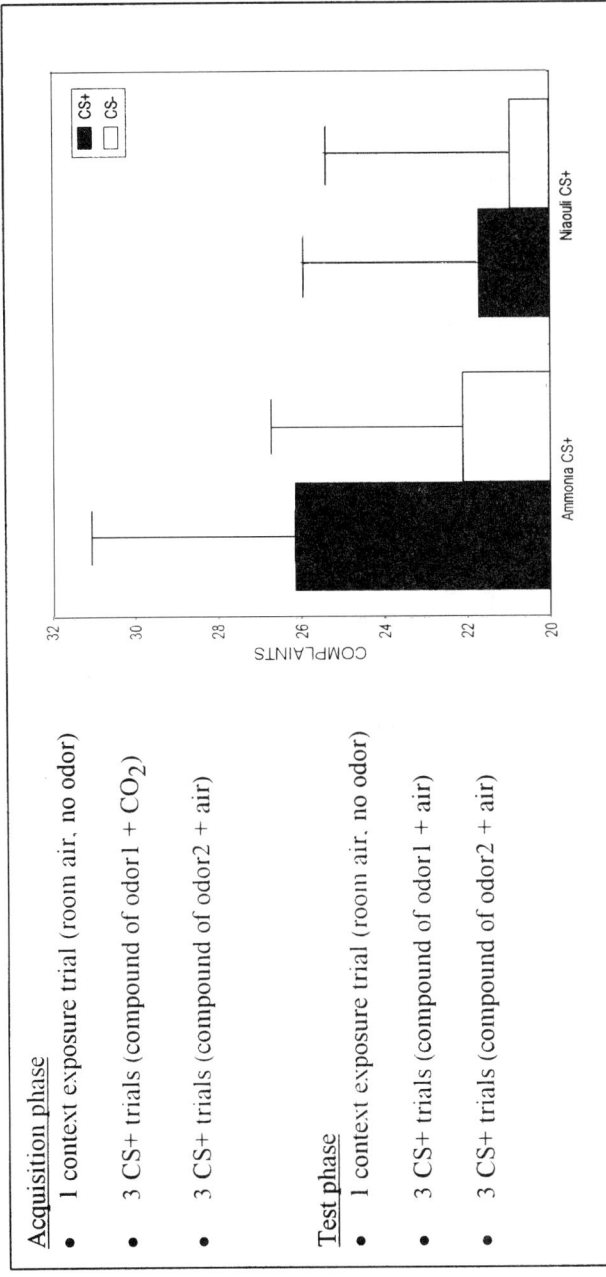

FIGURE 2. Schema of a respiratory conditioning paradigm and a typical result (means ± SEM).[12] The specific odor used as CS+ or CS− is counterbalanced across subjects and presented in low concentrations to avoid US effects of the odors themselves. The three CS+ and three CS− trials are presented in a semirandomized order. Both phases are preceded by a baseline trial: the participant breathes through the system, but no odor or CO_2 is added.

(5) A straightforward extinction procedure, involving a series of unreinforced CS exposures, readily reduced the learned symptoms.[14]

(6) Once symptoms to one odor were learned, they generalized to newly presented odors provided that they had a negative affective valence (i.e., were foul smelling). For example, subjects conditioned to have symptoms to ammonia showed elevated symptoms also to (first time presented) foul-smelling butyric acid and acetic acid, but not to fresh-smelling citric aroma.[15]

(7) Mental cues and images can also serve as CSs: Merely evoking an image of a situation that was previously paired with the experience of CO_2-induced symptoms elicited those symptoms and altered respiratory behavior. Again, negative emotional valence of the images appeared to be an important modulator: learning effects only showed up when the imagined situations were stressful.[16]

(8) Although both (respiratory) symptoms and altered respiratory behavior were learned, the symptoms in the test phase were not a reflection of the actual (learned) physiologic responses. Rather, the symptoms were relying on an activated memory representation of the symptoms experienced in the acquisition phase. This activation process was automatic in that it required little or no conscious mental resources.[13]

(9) Important individual differences occurred:

(a) The level of neuroticism or negative affectivity (NA) in normals modulated the conditioning effects: Learned symptoms and their generalization to new odors were, overall, more elevated in a group of subjects scoring high on negative affectivity.[13,15]

(b) The learning effects on symptoms were overall stronger in a group of "psychosomatic" patients. This suggests that psychopathological groups are more vulnerable to learning symptoms.[12]

The latter findings are strikingly similar with the fact that neuroticism or NA is a risk factor for developing MCS[17] and that psychiatric populations are more likely to develop MCS. Especially high rates of MCS are found in patients suffering from medically unexplained symptoms such as chronic fatigue syndrome and fibromyalgia.[18]

Overall, this set of experimental data provides strong evidence for the plausibility of a learning explanation for MCS. In general, our effects were highly reliable, although they were limited in magnitude and well below clinical levels. However, learning theory implies that much stronger USs produce stronger learning effects, reduce the likelihood of extinction, and enhance generalization. For obvious reasons, stronger USs are difficult to apply in humans for experimental purposes.

MCS WITHIN A CONTEMPORARY VIEW ON PAVLOVIAN CONDITIONING

Although the experimental model sketched above apparently represents a straightforward application of Pavlov's classical procedure, this does not mean that Pavlov's original mechanistic theoretical framework applies to explain the results. Contemporary views heavily rely on an information processing framework (see

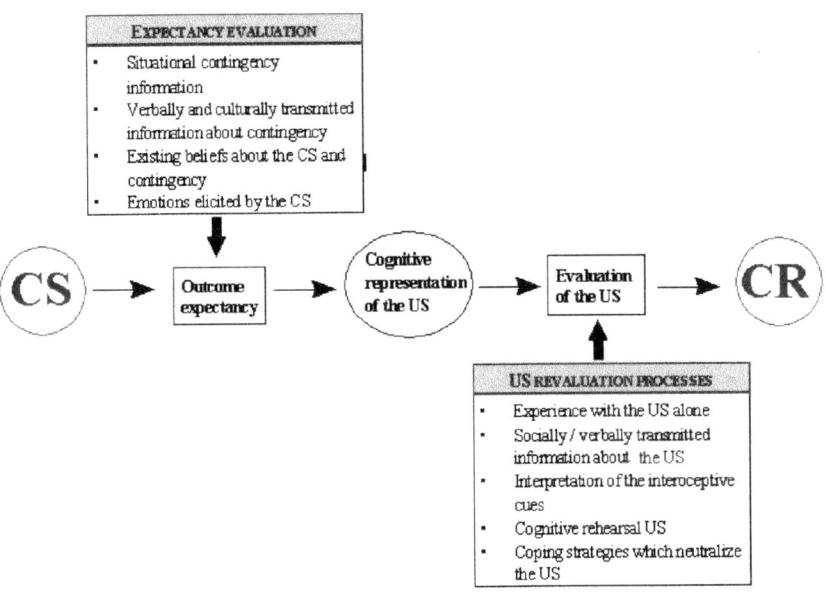

FIGURE 3. A contemporary schema of Pavlovian conditioning. From reference 20.

FIG. 3), linking Pavlovian conditioning even to forms of causal reasoning.[18] An extensive discussion of these more liberal theoretical views is beyond the scope of this chapter. Only a few aspects will be mentioned here and their potential implications for MCS will be discussed in the next section.

If a CS is co-occurring in some regular manner with a US, an associative link with a certain strength is formed between the memory representations of the two events. A CS allows for the prediction of an upcoming US, implying the activation of the memory representation of the US, which in turn may elicit (adaptive) conditioned CRs. The associative link does not depend on actual pairings of the CS and US only, but on the informational value of other relevant events as well (see, e.g., phenomena such as blocking, latent inhibition, etc.).[19] In animals, actual events are the main source of information, but humans also possess other sources that may modulate their expectancy once a CS occurred. Davey[20] (see FIG. 3), for example, lists situational, verbally and culturally transmitted information, existing beliefs, and emotions elicited by the CS.

An activated memory representation of a US does not directly translate into a response either. Learning and performance appear quite distinct phenomena: a learned association may remain behaviorally silent in some conditions and suddenly show up in other conditions. Conditioning effects may also be modulated by postconditioning manipulations. For example, when an organism has learned a tone-shock relationship, subsequent presentations of a much stronger shock alone may induce a reevaluation of the US in memory and inflate later CRs to the CS.[19] In Davey's model,[20] reevaluation of acquired associations in humans may occur through verbally transmitted information, interpretations given to interoceptive cues, cognitive rehearsal, and coping strategies (see FIG. 3). In summary, several processes may modulate the formation of associative links and their translation into behavioral output.

Some reviews and editorials about MCS give only brief consideration to associative learning, if at all, and subsequently dismiss it as being inadequate. Often, this is based upon an impoverished view on conditioning processes. We will elaborate on some criticisms within a contemporary view on associative learning.

CRITICISMS AND UNRESOLVED QUESTIONS

What Is the US in MCS?

The conditioning hypothesis is often rejected on the grounds that, very often, no previous toxic exposure is found in the history of an MCS patient. Referring to Pavlov's prototypical dog, Staudenmayer[21] phrased this as "where is the meat?". In other words, there would be no US. We suggest that, for instance, regular stress-induced hyperventilation episodes in a "chemical context" may act as a US in the same way as shown in our experiments with CO_2-induced hyperventilation. However, because learning processes may loosen the link between symptoms and their physiological correlates (see above), a one-to-one relationship between hypocapnia and the presence of symptoms should not be considered critical for this hypothesis.[22] This view may explain a number of observations: (1) the origin of MCS appears in some cases to be linked to episodes of stress and not to toxic exposures;[23] (2) a substantial overlap exists among the symptoms of MCS and those of hyperventilation, such as intermittent flares of fatigue and weakness, dizziness or light-headedness, cognitive difficulties (concentration and memory), shortness of breath, sore throat, dry mouth, palpitations and "racing heart", gastrointestinal problems, and feelings of anxiety or depression;[4,9,11,24] (3) the exposure of MCS patients to their chemical trigger induced hyperventilation in 73% of them.[25] In some cases, both hyperventilation and toxic exposures may be involved. For example, a toxic exposure may be a primary US, causing conditioned symptoms and anxiety to odoring substances or specific "contaminated" environments. Subsequent exposures to the CS may induce hyperventilation as part of anticipatory anxiety, and in this way become a secondary US.

What Is the CS?

The likelihood for a given cue (CS) to become associated with a US is determined by a number of variables. One is its salience, which may in turn be influenced by culturally transmitted information, preexisting beliefs, and/or emotional reactions to available cues (see FIG. 3). For example, the belief that the air is chemically polluted may facilitate associating symptoms to perceived chemicals. Even thoughts and mental images may function as CSs for learned symptoms, as was shown in one of our studies[16] (see above). The images in that study were selected as being relevant for panic, but it would be interesting to investigate mental images relevant for MCS as well. For example, imagining being in polluted places may potentially come to serve as mental CSs. As a consequence, tangible or measurable CSs may not always be present in the environment or perceivable to an outside observer.

This may explain why the incidence and prevalence of MCS appear to vary between geographical areas. Although epidemiological data are scarce, MCS appears to be very much an American disease and much less a European disease. Within Europe, the distribution is likely to vary depending on the level of awareness of environmental pollution and the salience of cues.

Why Do Not All Toxic Exposures Lead to MCS?

A similar question has been dealt with extensively in the context of conditioning models of fear and anxiety: why is it that severe traumatic events produce PTSD in only 30% of the cases?[26] The probability of MCS following a US (toxic exposure or hyperventilation) may be determined by aspects of the US, the CS, characteristics of the individual, and/or their interaction. Actually, this was typically shown in a recent experiment:[15] learning effects only occurred in subjects scoring high on negative affectivity (NA) who had a foul-smelling odor (ammonia) as CS. Subjects with the same number and intensity of USs, but having had a neutral/fresh odor as CS and/or not scoring high on NA, did not show effects.

NA in MCS patients may contribute in several ways to the development of MCS. First, a toxic exposure or a hyperventilation episode may impact stronger upon persons with NA and produce stronger autonomic responses as internal responses (URs). Second, persons high on NA may interpret these URs as more threatening, thus affecting the experienced intensity. Third, NA may bias persons to link negative events (US) to negative cues in their environment (CS). Fourth, such subjects may comparatively be more affected by culturally transmitted information about the presence and toxicity of environmental chemicals and hence form more explicit preexisting beliefs in this regard. Fifth, persons with NA may be more vulnerable to postconditioning cognitive processes: worrying and catastrophical interpretations after a toxic or hyperventilatory event may increase the CRs (see below).

Why Is There No Spontaneous Extinction?

Repeated nonreinforced exposures to conditioned odors should produce extinction of the learned responses. Because most patients cannot avoid being exposed to odorous substances, the question is why do symptoms not extinguish in patients. A selection bias may operate here because only patients present themselves to doctors and hospitals, and little is known about the course of events in those subjects whose symptoms do gradually decline after a toxic accident. Also, the persistence of the symptoms may be due to extensive avoidance behavior, preventing exposure to critical cues for a duration sufficiently long to allow extinction. More importantly, however, is recent evidence showing that Pavlovian extinction does not produce unlearning.[27,28] Rather, additional knowledge is acquired in such a procedure, implying that, in some contexts or at some moments in time, the learned CS-US relation does not hold. Conditioning, therefore, is like learning *a rule* (CS predicts US) and extinction is like learning contextually dependent *exceptions-to-the-rule* (CS predicts US, but not now/here[28]). Thus, what is extinguished in one context may still emerge in another.

Several processes modulating conditioning can also retard or prevent extinction, such as very intense USs in subjects high on neuroticism[29] and postconditioning processes (mental rumination, worrying, catastrophic thinking acting as reevaluations of the US; see above). To the extent that hyperventilation is involved, each new episode potentially induced by anticipatory stress will reinforce the existing association and prevent effective extinction as well.

Range of Stimuli Amenable to Generalization

Devriese et al.[15] demonstrated that learned symptoms generalized from the CS odor to newly presented odors, following stimulus valence as a generalization gradient (i.e., generalization occurred to foul-smelling odors, but not to neutral or positively valent ones). However, patients often show symptoms to perfumes, fresh odors, and even tastes and foods. Again, stronger USs than we used in our experiments may broaden the range of stimuli amenable to generalization.[30] In addition, several variables promoting blurring or forgetting about the attributes of the CS (duration, context shifts) may substantially broaden the generalization gradient.[31] Also, existing cognitive schemata may play a role. For example, the conviction that perfumes also contain certain chemicals or that both air quality and foods are contaminated by similar chemical substances may turn these items into negative ones and broaden the generalization gradient. Furthermore, the a priori conviction that a confrontation with some chemical may be dangerous may evoke anticipatory anxiety and hyperventilation, causing new conditioning experiences and establishing self-fulfilling prophecies.

What Is the Actual UR/CR?

In our experiments, we applied CO_2 inhalation as a US and we registered subjective symptoms, breathing behavior, and (sometimes) heart rate as URs. In reality, a toxic exposure or other negative event as US may trigger a wide variety of URs in both mental and bodily systems, including the autonomic, immune, and endocrine responses. Up to now, little is known about the causal role of these systems to explain the symptoms of MCS patients. Indeed, observed differences in autonomic responses to odors or other stimuli between patients and normals may be a result rather than a cause of patient status or simply be correlates of higher neuroticism. Even less is known about the potential role of conditioned modulation of autonomic, immune, and endocrine responses in MCS to explain the symptoms of MCS (see Siegel and Kreutzer[32] for interesting suggestions).

It should be noted that co-occurring variations in conditioned physiological and subjective responses should not readily be interpreted as a causal path from the former to the latter. Each dependent variable may be controlled by different mechanisms, as we demonstrated in one experiment.[13] Learned respiratory symptoms still showed up when a manipulation (a reaction time task) overruled the conditioned alterations of respiratory behavior and prevented them to occur. This suggests that acquired symptoms are depending on learned perceptual-cognitive processes underlying symptom perception and not on the presence of altered respiratory behavior.

More detailed analyses of these perceptual-cognitive mechanisms in MCS patients are needed: Do MCS patients have an attentional bias towards odors and symptoms? Do they have a negative interpretation bias? Do they ruminate and/or catastrophize about causes and consequences of their illness? How do they attribute symptoms to causes? All these processes have been shown to have an important impact upon somatic symptoms and to contribute to a self-perpetuating cycle in many ways.[33]

Conditioning and (Neural) Sensitization

Neural sensitization refers to an increasing intensity of responses to stimuli, such as drugs, as a result of repeated intermittent exposure. In MCS, it is hypothesized that olfactory, limbic, mesolimbic, and related pathways of the CNS are involved.[34,35] Sensitization effects are more likely with stronger stimuli and in conditions of physical and psychological stress. A special case is time-dependent sensitization (TDS),[36] which specifies that the increase in the response is not just a matter of repeated exposures, but also of the time interval between initial and later exposures.

Neural sensitization has been contrasted with conditioning as a potential model for MCS.[2,34,37] Both basic forms of learning are often distinguished as nonassociative (implying one stimulus) and associative learning (implying two stimuli becoming associated), respectively. Despite some apparent procedural differences, Ramsay and Woods[38] in an astute analysis of conditioning cogently argued that also sensitization to drugs represents a form of associative learning, provided that the proper analysis is made of what actually constitutes the US, UR, CS, and CR.[g] In this view, contrasting sensitization and conditioning regarding the processes involved may not be fruitful. One important difference at the procedural level, however, is that a sensitization paradigm requires a reactivity to an initial exposure of a stimulus, whereas a conditioning paradigm does not (see table 1 in Bell et al.[40]). Given the wide variety of potential triggers of MCS symptoms, many of which are completely harmless and never before elicited even the slightest symptom, it appears reasonable to assume that a new response was learned toward a chemical rather than that a preexisting one was sensitized. In addition, for many of the hypothesized neurobiological processes in (often animal) sensitization studies, it remains to be seen how they actually relate to subjective symptoms in humans triggered by harmless chemicals.

Implications for Treatment

One of the important implications from our perspective as opposed to a toxicological view concerns the treatment options. For example, a learning perspective suggests a cognitive-behavioral approach implying exposure to the symptom-provoking stimulus, whereas toxicological or immunological reasoning may actually advise avoidance behavior. Consistent with our perspective is that systematic desensitization (SD), a behavioral treatment technique relying on extinction and counterconditioning principles, has been shown to produce positive treatment results.[41–43] Because the efficacy of a treatment is no proof of the correctness of its rationale,[37] controlled large-scale treatment studies are needed to corroborate the efficacy of cognitive-behavioral treatment for MCS. They should also assess whether the effects mainly involve reduction of associated avoidance behavior, of associated autonomic arousal, or also of the very symptoms of MCS. In addition, because extinction effects

---

[g]Interoceptive cues, associated with the presence of the drug in the body, may serve as CSs.[39] Those situations may erroneously appear as nonassociative.

appear highly sensitive to contextual conditions (see above), care should be taken to enhance the generalization of extinction effects in order to improve its effectiveness.[44]

CONCLUDING REMARKS

Our laboratory experiments have convincingly documented the plausibility of an associative learning model for MCS: odor stimuli that have been associated with a physiologic challenge inducing symptoms may subsequently elicit comparable symptoms by themselves. It should be noted, however, that a Pavlovian paradigm mainly refers to a procedure stimulating the formation of associative connections, which in turn can initiate and modulate different perceptual-cognitive and physiologic processes underlying the experience of symptoms. In addition, because several external, cognitive, and emotional factors may modulate both the probability of association formation and their expression into observable effects (see above),[20] Pavlovian conditioning should not be regarded as a specific explanation, but as an open framework stimulating the search for critical processes underlying MCS symptoms.

Although the account sketched above offers testable predictions for further investigations, it implies tough challenges for the scientific community. Indeed, it has been suggested that CSs need not necessarily be observable to an outside observer; that hyperventilation may be involved as an important mechanism, but should not be present during every symptom episode; and that several hard to measure mental processes may play a critical role. However, the involvement of processes that are difficult to measure may actually be the very reason why MCS is still poorly understood.

ACKNOWLEDGMENTS

This work was supported by Grant No. G.0399.98 N (Fund for Scientific Research, Flanders, Belgium) and Grant No. OT-97/16 (Research Council of the University of Leuven).

REFERENCES

1. FIEDLER, N. & H. KIPEN. 1997. Chemical sensitivity: the scientific literature. Environ. Health Perspect. **105:** 409–415.
2. SORG, B.A. 1999. Multiple chemical sensitivity: potential role for neural sensitization. Crit. Rev. Neurobiol. **13:** 283–316.
3. GRAVELING, R.A., A. PILKINGTON, J.P.K. GEORGE *et al.* 1999. A review of multiple chemical sensitivity. Occup. Environ. Med. **56:** 73–85.
4. SHUSTERMAN, D.J. 1992. Critical review: the health significance of environmental odor pollution. Arch. Environ. Health **47:** 76–87.
5. FIEDLER, N., H.M. KIPEN, J. DELUCA *et al.* 1996. A controlled comparison of multiple chemical sensitivities and chronic fatigue syndrome. Psychosom. Med. **58:** 38–49.
6. MILLER, C.S. 1994. Chemical sensitivity: history and phenomenology. Toxicol. Ind. Health **10:** 253–276.
7. KURT, T.L. 1995. Multiple chemical sensitivities: a syndrome of pseudotoxicity manifest as exposure perceived symptoms. Clin. Toxicol. **33:** 101–105.

8. BINKLEY, K.E. & S.K. KUTCHER. 1997. Panic response to sodium lactate infusion in patients with multiple chemical sensitivity syndrome. J. Allergy Clin. Immunol. **99:** 570–574.
9. LEHRER, P.M. 1997. Psychophysiological hypotheses regarding multiple chemical sensitivity syndrome. Environ. Health Perspect. **105:** 479–483.
10. DAGER, S.R., J.P. HOLLAND, D.S. COWLEY et al. 1987. Panic disorder precipitated by exposure to organic solvents in the workplace. Am. J. Psychiatry **144:** 1056–1058.
11. VAN DEN BERGH, O., P.J. KEMPYNCK, K.P. VAN DE WOESTIJNE et al. 1995. Respiratory learning and somatic complaints: a conditioning approach using CO_2-enriched air inhalation. Behav. Res. Ther. **33:** 517–527.
12. VAN DEN BERGH, O., K. STEGEN & K.P. VAN DE WOESTIJNE. 1997. Learning to have psychosomatic complaints: conditioning of respiratory behavior and somatic complaints in psychosomatic patients. Psychosom. Med. **59:** 13–23.
13. VAN DEN BERGH, O., K. STEGEN & K.P. VAN DE WOESTIJNE. 1998. Memory effects on symptom reporting in a respiratory learning paradigm. Health Psychol. **17:** 241–248.
14. VAN DEN BERGH, O., K. STEGEN, I. VAN DIEST et al. 1999. Acquisition and extinction of somatic symptoms in response to odors: a Pavlovian paradigm relevant to multiple chemical sensitivity. Occup. Environ. Med. **56:** 295–301.
15. DEVRIESE, S., W. WINTERS, K. STEGEN et al. 2000. Generalization of acquired somatic symptoms in response to odors: a Pavlovian perspective on multiple chemical sensitivity. Psychosom. Med. **62:** 751–759.
16. STEGEN, K., K. DE BRUYNE, W. RASSCHAERT et al. 1999. Fear-relevant images as conditioned stimuli for somatic complaints, respiratory behavior, and reduced end-tidal pCO_2. J. Abnorm. Psychol. **108:** 143–152.
17. PENNEBAKER, J.W. 1994. Psychological bases of symptom reporting: perceptual and emotional aspects of chemical sensitivity. Toxicol. Ind. Health **10:** 497–509.
18. SHANKS, D.R., D. CHARLES, R.J. DARBY et al. 1998. Configural processes in human associative learning. J. Exp. Psychol. Learn. Mem. Cogn. **24:** 1353–1378.
19. DOMJAN, M. 1993. The Principles of Learning and Behavior. Brooks/Cole Pub. Pacific Grove, CA.
20. DAVEY, G.C.L. 1997. A conditioning model of phobias. In Phobias: A Handbook of Theory, Research, and Treatment, pp. 301–322. Wiley. New York/Chichester.
21. STAUDENMAYER, H. 1997. Multiple chemical sensitivities or idiopathic environmental intolerances: psychophysiologic foundation of knowledge for a psychogenic explanation. J. Allergy Clin. Immunol. **99:** 434–437.
22. HORNSVELD, H.K., B. GARSSEN, M.J. DOP et al. 1996. Double-blind placebo-controlled study of the hyperventilation provocation test and the validity of the hyperventilation syndrome. Lancet **348:** 154–158.
23. SCHOTTENFELD, R.S. 1987. Workers with multiple chemical sensitivities: a psychiatric approach to diagnosis and treatment. Occup. Med. State Art Rev. **2:** 739–753.
24. PEARSON, D.J. 1988. Psychologic and somatic interrelationships in allergy and pseudoallergy. J. Allergy Clin. Immunol. **81:** 351–361.
25. LEZNOFF, A. 1997. Provocative challenges in patients with multiple chemical sensitivity. J. Allergy Clin. Immunol. **99:** 434–437.
26. TOMB, D.A. 1994. The phenomenology of post-traumatic stress disorder. Psychiatr. Clin. N. Am. **17:** 237–250.
27. BAEYENS, F., P. EELEN & G. CROMBEZ. 1995. Pavlovian associations are forever: on classical conditioning and extinction. J. Psychophysiol. **9:** 127–141.
28. BOUTON, M.E. 1994. Conditioning, remembering, and forgetting. J. Exp. Psychol. Anim. Behav. Processes **20:** 219–231.
29. EYSENCK, H.J. 1979. The conditioning model of neurosis. Behav. Brain Sci. **2:** 155–199.
30. BOUTON, M.E., J.B. NELSON & J.M. ROSAS. 1999. Stimulus generalization, context change, and forgetting. Psychol. Bull. **125:** 171–186.
31. RICCIO, D.C., V.C. RABINOWITZ & S. AXELROD. 1994. Memory: when less is more. Am. Psychol. **49:** 917–926.
32. SIEGEL, S. & R. KREUTZER. 1997. Pavlovian conditioning and multiple chemical sensitivity. Environ. Health Perspect. **105:** 521–526.
33. BARSKY, A.J. & J.F. BORUS. 1999. Functional somatic syndromes. Ann. Intern. Med. **1:** 910–921.

34. BELL, I.R., J. ROSSI, M.E. GILBERT et al. 1997. Testing the neural sensitization and kindling hypothesis for illness from low levels of environmental chemicals. Environ. Health Perspect. **105:** 539–547.
35. SORG, B.A. & T. HOCHSTATTER. 1999. Behavioral sensitization after repeated formaldehyde exposure in rats. Toxicol. Ind. Health **15:** 346–355.
36. ANTELMAN, S.M. 1994. Time-dependent sensitization in animals: a possible model of multiple chemical sensitivity in humans. Toxicol. Ind. Health **10:** 335–342.
37. BELL, I.R., C.M. BALDWIN, M. FERNANDEZ & G.E. SCHWARTZ. 1999. Neural sensitization model for multiple chemical sensitivity: overview of theory and empirical evidence. Toxicol. Ind. Health **15:** 295–304.
38. RAMSAY, D.S. & S.C. WOODS. 1997. Biological consequences of drug administration: implications for acute and chronic tolerance. Psychol. Rev. **104:** 170–193.
39. GREELEY, J., D.A. LÊ & C.X. POULOS. 1984. Alcohol is an effective cue in the conditional control of tolerance to alcohol. Psychopharmacology **83:** 159–162.
40. BELL, I.R., G.E. SCHWARTZ, C.M. BALDWIN et al. 1997. Individual differences in neural sensitization and the role of context in illness from low-level environmental chemical exposures. Environ. Health Perspect. **105:** 457–466.
41. SPYKER, D.A. 1995. Multiple chemical sensitivities: syndrome and solution. Clin. Toxicol. **33:** 95–99.
42. GUGLIELMI, R.S., D.J. COX & D.A. SPYKER. 1994. Behavioral treatment of phobic avoidance in multiple chemical sensitivity. J. Behav. Ther. Exp. Psychiatry **25:** 197–209.
43. STENN, P. & K. BINKLEY. 1998. Successful outcome in a patient with chemical sensitivity. Psychosomatics **39:** 547–550.
44. MINEKA, S., J.L. MYSTKOWSKI, D. HLADEK et al. 1999. The effects of changing context on return of fear following exposure therapy for spider phobia. J. Consult. Clin. Psychol. **67:** 599–604.

Pavlovian Conditioning of Emotional Responses to Olfactory and Contextual Stimuli

A Potential Model for the Development and Expression of Chemical Intolerance

TIM OTTO[a,b] AND NICHOLAS D. GIARDINO[c]

[b]*Program in Biopsychology and Behavioral Neuroscience,*
[c]*Program in Clinical Psychology, Department of Psychology, Rutgers University, Piscataway, New Jersey 08854, USA*

ABSTRACT: Chemical intolerance (CI) in humans is a poorly understood phenomenon of uncertain etiology, seemingly influenced by multiple factors both within and between affected individuals. Several authors have suggested that the development of CI in some individuals may be due, at least in part, to Pavlovian conditioning processes in which the expression of overt symptoms to certain substances reflects classically conditioned responses to previously neutral olfactory and contextual stimuli. In this paper, we describe the potential relationship between olfactory and contextual conditioning in experimental animals and the development and expression of CI in humans. Furthermore, as significant advances have been made in delineating the brain areas that underlie these learned responses, we also review recent research on the contributions of the amygdala and perirhinal cortical region to olfactory and contextual fear conditioning.

Chemical intolerance (CI) in humans is a poorly understood phenomenon of uncertain etiology, seemingly influenced by multiple factors both within and between affected individuals. Given the lack of consensus on the etiology and maintenance of CI, as well as the lack of agreement on effective treatment for the syndrome, it seems prudent to continue to evaluate scientifically plausible explanations for this condition, especially those grounded by empirical research.

Pavlovian conditioning (also called classical conditioning) is one such well-studied mechanism that may play a role in the development of CI. As discussed below in more detail, several features of CI are consistent with known conditioning principles. In addition, certain medical and psychological phenomena that appear to share significant overlap with CI are widely agreed to be mediated by Pavlovian conditioning. Thus, a review of conditioning principles and their possible relevance to CI may assist attempts to better understand and treat this condition.

Several authors have suggested that one possible means by which CI may develop in some individuals is via a process similar to that of Pavlovian, or "classical", con-

---

[a]Voice: 732-445-0719; fax: 732-445-2263.
totto@rci.rutgers.edu

ditioning.[1–6] Briefly, this hypothesis suggests that the overt symptoms of CI in some individuals likely reflect conditioned behavioral and physiological responses to chemical stimuli due to previous pairings of these stimuli with natural, biological responses to aversive stimuli. In this paper, we will critically review the data supporting this hypothesis. Because most cases of CI involve physiological responses to odorous chemicals or to discrete spatial locations, and because recent data suggest that olfactory and contextual cues can be particularly robust stimuli in classical conditioning studies, we will focus mainly on experiments examining olfactory and contextual conditioning in experimental animals. Furthermore, as significant advances have been made in delineating brain areas that underlie these learned responses, we also review recent research on the contributions of three brain areas implicated in the acquisition and expression of conditioned emotional responses: the amygdala, perirhinal cortex, and hippocampus.

OLFACTORY AND CONTEXTUAL FEAR CONDITIONING: BEHAVIORAL STUDIES

As described above, the primary focus of this paper is to review the data examining olfactory and contextual conditioning in experimental animals. Among the many successful approaches used to explore the acquisition of conditioned emotional, autonomic, and overt behavioral responses has been an examination of the acquisition, expression, and retention of Pavlovian "fear" conditioning in rats.[7–11] In these studies, an initially neutral stimulus (the conditioned stimulus [CS]; for example, a tone, light, or odor) and an aversive unconditioned stimulus ([US]; for example, foot shock) are typically paired in a forward manner. Following several pairings, subsequent reexposure to the CS or to the context in which CS-US pairing took place elicits in rats a variety of behavioral and physiological responses, including increased heart rate and blood pressure, increased defecation and urination, and freezing behavior, collectively thought to reflect an internal state of fear (see refs. 7 and 11 for reviews).

We have recently found that an olfactory stimulus can serve effectively as a CS in fear conditioning paradigms and that the basic principles governing the acquisition of emotional responses conditioned to auditory and visual CSs can be extended to the olfactory system.[12] In the first experiment of this series, male Sprague-Dawley rats were assigned to one of three groups. One group (FOR) received 6 forward pairings of a 20-s odorant CS (15% pyridine) and a 2-s, 0.8-mA foot shock; the CS and US coterminated, and successive CS-US pairings were separated by a 4-min intertrial interval (ITI). A second group (BAC) was treated similarly, but delivery of the US preceded CS onset by 30 s. A third group (CS-ONLY) received 6 presentations of the CS alone.

Twenty-four hours after training, conditioned fear was assessed in a 6-min session by examining freezing behavior to re-presentations of the odorant CS in a novel chamber. During the first minute of testing, no odorant was present; the CS was then presented throughout each of the following 5 min of testing. Freezing behavior, characterized by a crouching posture and an absence of visible movement except that due to breathing,[13] was assessed by an experimenter who was blind to the animals' treatment condition.

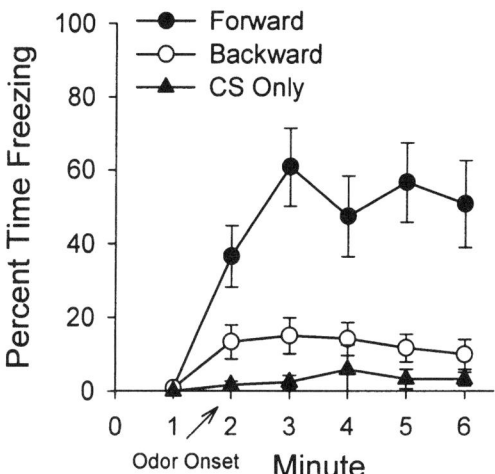

FIGURE 1. Freezing responses of separate groups of animals presented with an olfactory CS in a novel context 24 h after training with either forward (FOR) or backward (BAC) pairings of the CS and foot shock, or presentations of the olfactory CS only. Plotted values represent the mean ± 1 SEM.

As illustrated in FIGURE 1, none of the groups exhibited freezing behavior during the first minute of testing, suggesting that subjects did not generalize the training and testing contexts. Only those animals previously receiving forward pairings of the CS and US exhibited significant levels of freezing behavior during minutes 2–6. Furthermore, the fact that neither the BAC nor the CS-ONLY group froze significantly more during the period of CS exposure (minutes 2–6) than during the period prior to exposure (minute 1) suggests that the robust freezing behavior of the FOR subjects is likely not due to an increased tendency to freeze to simple reexposures of an odorant in a novel context. Finally, the BAC subjects were no more likely to freeze during the period of CS reexposure than were the CS-ONLY subjects, suggesting that backward pairings of the odorant and shock did not result in the acquisition of conditioned fear. Collectively, these data suggest that the increased tendency of the FOR subjects to freeze in the presence of the CS likely reflects a learned CS-US association.

With respect to fear conditioned to discrete contexts, there is now a wealth of data suggesting that simply receiving mild foot shocks in a novel, distinct spatial context results in a robust expression of conditioned fear when the animal is reintroduced into that context (reviewed in ref. 14). Consistent with this general pattern of results, recent findings in our laboratory indicate that simply returning an animal to the chamber in which it had previously received forward pairings of odor and foot shock results in a robust freezing response in the absence of the olfactory CS, suggesting the animal has formed an association between the previously neutral uni- and multimodal sensory cues comprising the training context and the aversive foot shock US.

In addition to examining the acquisition of olfactory and contextual fear conditioning, we have also examined whether rats exhibit latent inhibition when preexposed to the olfactory CS prior to conditioning. Latent inhibition, a phenomenon in which unreinforced exposure to a stimulus attenuates conditioning when that stimulus is later paired with a US,[15] has been an important tool in exploring the relative role of various neural systems in attentional and mnemonic processes.[16] With this in mind, a recent study in our laboratory examined the extent to which rats demonstrate latent inhibition of odor-guided conditioned fear following preexposure to the CS.[12]

Male Sprague-Dawley rats were assigned to one of two experimental groups. Subjects in one group received a total of 30 preexposures to the odorant CS in the training chamber over 3 consecutive days prior to training; subjects in a second group were placed into the same behavioral training chamber, but were not presented with the odorant CS. All subjects then received 6 forward pairings of the odorant CS and foot shock US as described above. Testing for fear conditioned to the CS was conducted 24 h after training in a novel chamber. As illustrated in FIGURE 2, no subjects displayed freezing behavior during the first minute of testing prior to odor onset. Similarly, those subjects that received exposure to the olfactory CS prior to conditioning failed to exhibit significant levels of freezing behavior in the presence of the olfactory CS. In contrast, those subjects that did not receive CS preexposure exhibited significant freezing behavior during the period of odor presentation. Thus, these data suggest that preexposure to the odorant CS prior to training results in a robust latent inhibition of odor-guided fear conditioning. It should be noted that the level of freezing observed in animals that did not receive preexposure to the olfactory CS was significantly lower than that observed in the animals receiving forward odor-shock pairings presented in FIGURE 1. This attenuation of freezing is likely due to the extended handling animals received during preexposure.

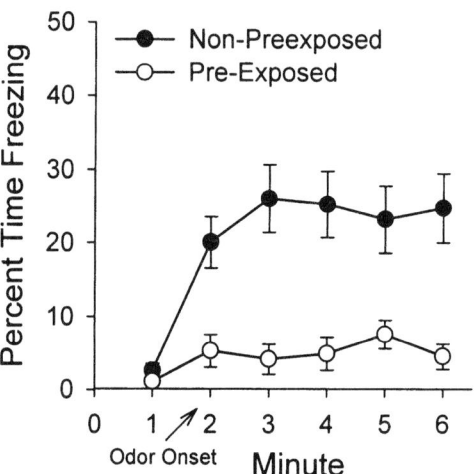

FIGURE 2. Latent inhibition in the olfactory fear conditioning paradigm. Animals preexposed to the olfactory CS prior to conditioning failed to exhibit freezing responses when re-presented with the CS 24 h following training. Plotted values represent the mean ± 1 SEM.

It has been demonstrated repeatedly that subjects preexposed to a CS in one context and subsequently presented with CS-US pairings in a different context typically fail to exhibit latent inhibition.[17] This "contextual specificity" of latent inhibition has been a particularly useful means of identifying the neural substrates of contextual information processing (e.g., see ref. 18). With this in mind, a final study in this series examined the extent to which the latent inhibition of odor-guided fear conditioning was sensitive to variations in the preexposure and training contexts.

Male Sprague-Dawley rats were assigned to one of two conditions. All subjects received preexposure and training in the same conditioning chamber per se, but contexts were differentiated by their auditory and visual attributes: one context was brightly illuminated and quiet; the other context was dark and a 3.5-kHz, 80-dB tone sounded continuously. Subjects in one condition received 30 preexposures to the odorant CS in the same context as subsequent CS-US pairing; subjects in a second condition received CS preexposure in a context different from that used during subsequent CS-US pairing. Conditioned freezing to re-presentations of the odorant CS was assessed 24 h after CS-US pairing in a separate chamber.

As illustrated in FIGURE 3, only those subjects receiving preexposure and training in different contexts exhibited significant conditioned freezing behavior to subsequent re-presentations of the odorant CS. These data suggest that the latent inhibition of odor-guided fear conditioning is context-specific: only those subjects preexposed and trained in the same context exhibited attenuated freezing behavior during re-presentation of the olfactory CS. Thus, it appears that simple alterations in the visual and auditory attributes of the training context are sufficient to exert substantial contextual control over conditioning.

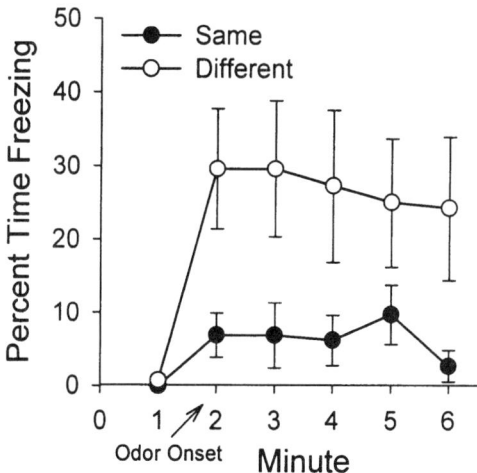

FIGURE 3. Contextual specificity of latent inhibition in the olfactory fear conditioning paradigm. Only those animals preexposed to the CS and trained in the same context exhibited latent inhibition. Plotted values represent the mean ± 1 SEM.

OLFACTORY AND CONTEXTUAL FEAR CONDITIONING: POTENTIAL RELATIONSHIP TO CI

As described above, olfactory fear conditioning is a robust phenomenon. Although the behavioral aspects of this type of learning have been well delineated in nonhuman animal research, it is, as always, wise to be cautious in generalizing these findings to human behavior and particularly to poorly understood conditions such as CI. Nonetheless, there are several reasons to believe that olfactory fear conditioning as demonstrated in animal research does occur similarly in humans and, more importantly, may contribute to at least some aspects of CI in some individuals.

First, symptom-provoking chemicals in CI are rarely odorless. Given this fact, it is at least possible that Pavlovian conditioning may play some role in odor-related symptom presentations. For example, an odor present at the time of a toxin or toxicant exposure or other symptom-inducing event (whether or not the odor is constituently related to the noxious compound) may serve as a CS to elicit the same or similar symptoms in the absence of the original stimulus.

In an elegant series of experimental studies, Van den Bergh and colleagues have demonstrated that harmless odors can serve as potent conditioned stimuli in human subjects, triggering somatic symptoms similar to those produced by a noxious US with which that odor had previously been paired.[6,19–21] These studies, described in more detail elsewhere in this volume, suggest that Pavlovian conditioning may play a role in at least some cases of CI.

Several clinical and experimental reports of CI cases and groups with CI are also consistent with a potential involvement of Pavlovian odor-guided conditioning. Shusterman, Balmes, and Cone reported cases of CI in which odors linked to an acute overexposure to a chemical subsequently triggered hyperventilation symptoms, including chest pain, dizziness, perspiration, dyspnea, and resting tremors in patients.[22] Bolla-Wilson and colleagues also described several cases of patients with multiple chemical sensitivities that, according to the authors, may most simply be explained by odor conditioning.[23] Still others have reported case and controlled studies in which desensitization through repeated exposures to untolerated, but nontoxic chemicals greatly reduced or extinguished illness responses to odors in patients with CI. Finally, Staudenmayer, Selner, and Buhr conducted double-blind exposures of CI subjects to multiple chemicals to which they reported sensitivity and found that, when the odor of each compound was masked by a nonoffensive odor (e.g., peppermint), subjects could not reliably distinguish tolerated from untolerated chemicals.[24]

CONTEXTUAL CONDITIONING AND SICK-BUILDING SYNDROME

The principles of Pavlovian contextual conditioning described briefly above may also be relevant to some types of CI. One particularly relevant class of CI-related symptoms is known as "sick-building" syndrome.[25] Sick-building syndrome is typically characterized by CI-like symptoms occurring in a particular building or section of a building, often at the workplace, that diminish after leaving the premises. In the presence of a noxious chemical, these symptoms are very likely unconditioned responses to that substance; it is also likely that subsequent exposures to that spatial context (the building) in the absence of the offending chemical reflect conditioned responses similar in nature to contextual conditioning. Thus, after one or several pairings of a noxious chemical and a particular spatial context, subsequent symptom expression in that same context may occur in the absence of the chemical due to Pavlovian contextual conditioning.

PAVLOVIAN CONDITIONING AND INDIVIDUAL DIFFERENCES IN CI

A Pavlovian conditioning perspective on CI as presented thus far, however, suffers from at least one apparent flaw. If CI can be induced by Pavlovian conditioning processes as we have suggested, then why does not everyone develop CI? After all, most people are exposed to many of the same substances that are untolerated by those with CI syndromes. However, although chemical odor intolerance in mild form is fairly common, occurring in 15–30% of adults,[26,27] clinical CI occurs in less than 5% of the general population.[28] Even in the case of industrial chemical spills and other documented toxic exposures, many exposed individuals do not manifest odor-related illness symptoms. One plausible explanation is that individuals naturally vary in their sensitivity to certain chemicals. While this is a distinct and likely possibility in most cases, there exist several well-documented means by which conditioning-related phenomena may help to explain individual differences in susceptibility to CI.

As described above, latent inhibition of olfactory conditioning in experimental animals is a robust and replicable effect of preexposure to a substance that is subsequently paired with a noxious US. Strong latent inhibition effects have also been observed in humans.[29,30] Latent inhibition effects may contribute to individual differences in the development of CI. For example, individuals who have previously been exposed to an odor prior to a noxious conditioning event might be less susceptible to developing conditioned aversions to that (or a very similar) odor. In addition, while latent inhibition in itself may serve to explain some of the variability in the acquisition of conditioned CI, there are also stable individual differences in the extent to which latent inhibition (LI) occurs. For example, individuals who score high on questionnaire measures of psychosis-proneness and disinhibition, as well as high achievers who report openness to experience, tend to exhibit reduced LI.[31–33]

Individual differences in the acquisition of learned associations in general have been observed since the earliest days of conditioning research. Pavlov noted that significant individual differences existed between animals in their conditioning performance.[34] Since that time, several factors have been identified that predict the rate at which individuals differentially acquire associations and suggest mechanisms by which these differences occur. For example, on a neurobiological level, recent evidence suggests that one likely mechanism underlying individual differences in learning is an innate difference between organisms in their basal level of synaptic efficacy, or the strength of synaptic communication.[35] Moreover, in humans, anxiety is often associated with enhanced conditioning to aversive events, while impulsivity is associated with greater conditioning to appetitive stimuli.[36] Consistent with these personality correlates, individuals with greater autonomic (e.g., heart rate, skin conductance) reactivity demonstrate better acquisition of conditional responses to aversive stimuli.[37]

A concrete example of the relationship between autonomic reactivity and conditioning can be observed in cancer patients undergoing chemotherapy. Approximately 60–70% of patients who receive highly emetic anticancer drugs develop nausea or vomiting in *anticipation* of chemotherapy sessions after their first two or three treatments.[38] This anticipatory reaction is believed to be caused by Pavlovian conditioning in which the sight, smell, or sound associated with drug administration triggers a conditioned response in patients similar to that induced by the chemotherapy drug itself. In one study, investigators tested patients on a benign conditioning task before their first chemotherapy session and found that those who went on to develop anticipatory nausea and vomiting exhibited greater cardiovascular reactivity and conditioning to an auditory CS than those who did not develop symptoms.[39]

There is also some evidence that certain individuals may be more susceptible to the effects of odor conditioning per se. In one recent study, subjects answered questions assessing the impact of odor on their liking for people, places, foods, and health and beauty products. The investigators reported that the level of affective importance that subjects gave to odors strongly predicted performance on a subsequent odor-guided Pavlovian conditioning task. Those who were highly odor-oriented showed greater aversive responses to previously neutral visual stimuli that had been paired with disliked odors.[40]

A CAVEAT

A point that has been made often, but is worth reinforcing, is that although conditioning processes may in some cases contribute to CI, we are not suggesting that CI is "all in the head" or, worse still, that CI is best explained as a psychiatric disorder. Advocates of an exclusively neurotoxicological explanation of CI, for example, have used the plethora of abnormal clinical test results reported in patients as evidence against a psychological origin of CI (e.g., see ref. 41). However, contemporary Western medical science both accepts and embraces the notion that psychological processes—Pavlovian conditioning in particular—play a role in even well-established medical diseases, including arthritis, cancer, asthma, and diabetes. Consistent with this notion, we suggest that Pavlovian conditioning processes should be considered a plausible mechanism contributing to some aspects of CI as well.

NEURAL SUBSTRATES OF OLFACTORY AND CONTEXTUAL FEAR CONDITIONING

A full appreciation for the potential ramifications of the Pavlovian conditioning model for the development and expression of some aspects of CI necessarily includes an understanding of the brain mechanisms underlying the acquisition of these conditioned responses. Recent study has focused on the contributions of several brain areas to the acquisition and maintenance of Pavlovian fear conditioning. Because this review has focused primarily on olfactory and contextual fear conditioning in rats, the following sections will summarize recent work examining the neural substrates of conditioning in these paradigms.

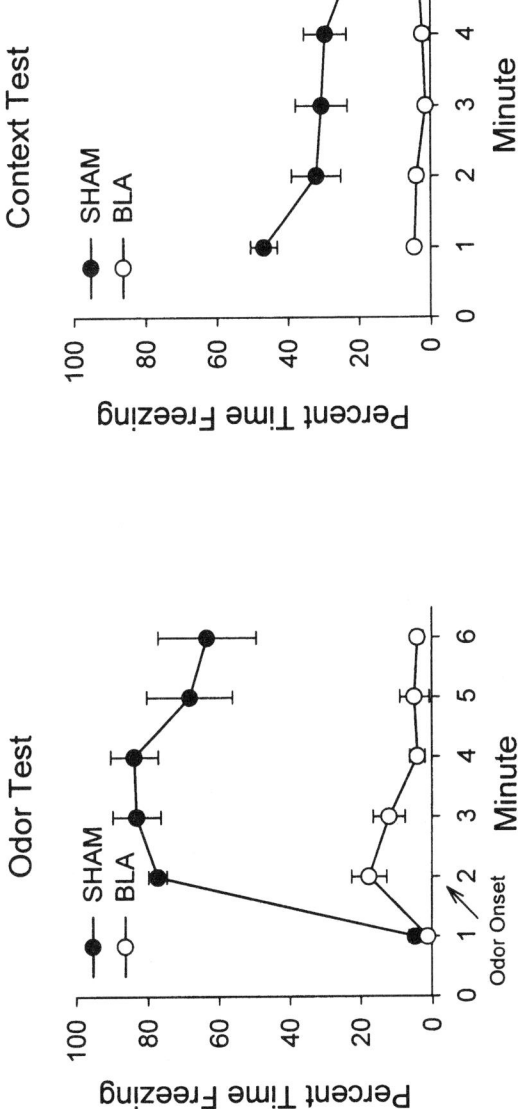

FIGURE 4. Freezing behavior of animals receiving either pretraining control surgical procedures (SHAM) or pretraining excitotoxic lesions of the basolateral amygdala (BLA). (**Left**) Freezing behavior during a 6-min CS reexposure session at 24 h after conditioning. Odor was presented during minutes 2–6 only. (**Right**) Freezing behavior during a 5-min context reexposure session at 48 h after conditioning. Plotted values represent the mean ± 1 SEM.

As reviewed elsewhere,[42] primary olfactory structures establish particularly dense and immediate connections to the amygdala and the perirhinal cortex (PRH), two brain areas implicated in many forms of learning. We have recently examined in detail the contributions of both of these areas to olfactory and contextual fear conditioning; these studies are described below.

Amygdala

With respect to the brain areas mediating the acquisition and expression of conditioned fear, a substantial body of neuroanatomical, neuropsychological, and electrophysiological data suggests that the amygdala plays a critical role in the development of learned associations between emotionally neutral sensory stimuli and aversive unconditioned stimuli. Specifically, lesions of the amygdala that include the lateral nucleus (LA) have been found to disrupt the acquisition and expression of fear conditioned *both* to auditory and visual CSs and to the context in which CS-US pairing occurred.[43–45]

We have recently shown that the amygdala participates critically in olfactory fear conditioning as well.[46] In our initial experiment, subjects received either excitotoxic (NMDA) lesions of the basolateral amygdaloid nucleus (BLA) or sham surgery prior to a single conditioning session consisting of 6 discrete forward pairings of odor and mild foot shock. Freezing behavior during reexposure to the odorant CS and to the training context was examined separately. Control subjects exhibited high levels of freezing upon reexposure to the olfactory CS and to the training context. In contrast, subjects with excitotoxic lesions of the BLA did not exhibit freezing behavior during either test period (see FIG. 4). Control experiments indicated that the two groups of subjects did not differ in basal locomotor activity or in acquisition of a successive-cue odor discrimination task, suggesting that deficits in freezing behavior exhibited by subjects with BLA lesions were due neither to a general enhancement of locomotor activity nor to an impairment in primary aspects of olfaction.

In a second experiment in this series, subjects received NMDA lesions of the BLA or sham surgery either 1 day or 15 days after olfactory fear conditioning, and conditioned freezing responses during reexposure to the odor and to the training context were examined 7–8 days after surgery. While operated control subjects exhibited robust freezing behavior upon reexposure to the odor CS and to the training context, subjects with lesions of the BLA did not, regardless of the training-to-lesion interval; these data are illustrated in FIGURE 5.

Collectively, these results suggest that, as for auditory and visual stimuli, the BLA participates critically and in an enduring manner in the expression of fear conditioned to olfactory CSs. With respect to auditory stimuli, previous work has demonstrated that the LA, in particular, likely plays a prominent role in the acquisition and expression of CS-US associations.[47,48] These data are consistent with anatomical findings indicating that the LA is the primary amygdalar target for fibers originating in both the auditory thalamus and the secondary and tertiary auditory cortical areas.[49–53] Relative to auditory projections, however, projections from primary olfactory regions to the BLA are considerably less dense. Thus, if associative learning in fear conditioning paradigms is subserved, at least in part, by a convergence within the BLA of pathways encoding the sensory properties of the CS and US, the source of projections coding for the CS in olfactory fear conditioning remains a question.

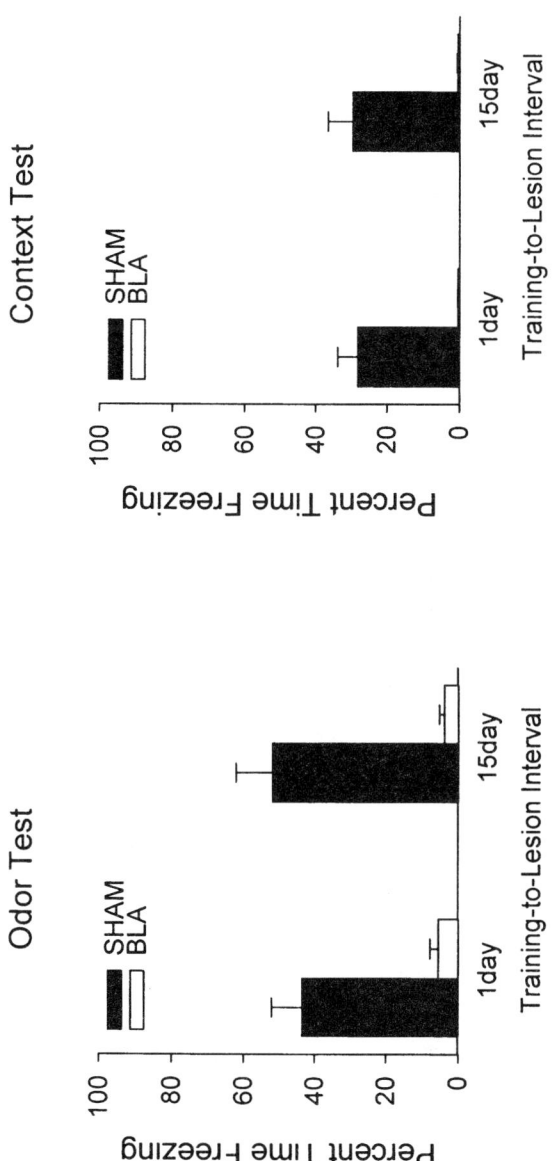

FIGURE 5. Freezing behavior of animals receiving control surgical procedures (SHAM) or excitotoxic lesions of the basolateral amygdala (BLA) at either 1 or 15 days after conditioning. (**Left**) Freezing responses during CS reexposure in a novel context. (**Right**) Freezing responses during reexposure to the training context. Plotted values represent the mean ± 1 SEM.

Anatomical and neuropsychological evidence suggests that the critical olfactory information *may* project to the BLA via anterior PRH. As described previously, the anterior PRH receives monosynaptic input from the olfactory bulb and piriform cortex, and in turn projects to several subnuclei of the BLA, most prominently the LA. Thus, it is possible that CS-US associations during olfactory fear conditioning result from a convergence within the BLA of fibers originating in part from anterior PRH with those coding for the somatosensory aspects of the US. The results of several studies exploring this possibility are described in the following section.

Perirhinal Cortex

A number of previous neuropsychological studies have demonstrated the importance of the PRH to memory in a variety of learning paradigms. For example, lesions restricted to PRH or of the entire rhinal cortical region have been found to impair recognition memory in both primates and rats[54–57] and also typically disrupt learning guided by extramaze spatial cues in rats.[58–61] Thus, it is possible that, as with other forms of learning and memory, the PRH contributes actively to associative memory processes in some forms of Pavlovian fear conditioning.

In order to examine the involvement of anterior PRH in fear conditioned to an explicit olfactory CS and to the context in which CS-US pairing takes place, we examined the effect of small aspirative[8] or excitotoxic[9] lesions of this area on olfactory and contextual fear conditioning. One group served as sham-operated control subjects and a second group received small lesions of anterior PRH. Following recovery, all subjects received 6 forward pairings of the olfactory CS and foot shock US as described previously. Conditioned freezing to re-presentations of the odorant CS was examined 24 h after training. Conditioned freezing to the training context was examined in a single 5-min session 48 h following training.

Both aspirative and excitotoxic lesions of PRH severely attenuated fear conditioned to the olfactory CS, but, interestingly, *not* to the training context; the effects of excitotoxic lesions on fear conditioning are illustrated in FIGURE 6. It should be noted that the observed deficits in conditioning to the explicit CS are likely not due to a lesion-induced deficit in olfactory perceptual processes; previous studies examining the effects of much larger rhinal cortical lesions (that typically included the area examined in this study) on olfactory learning have demonstrated that lesioned animals are fully capable of accurately performing other odor-guided learning tasks.[56,62]

It is at present unclear whether the deficits in conditioning to the explicit CS observed in the present study are secondary to elimination of the relevant afferents to amygdala or rather reflect a more general role of the PRH in associative learning. Furthermore, it remains to be determined whether these behavioral deficits reflect impaired acquisition, retention, retrieval, and/or expression of conditioned fear. The fact that all trained PRH-lesioned animals displayed normal contextual conditioning, however, strongly suggests that conditioning deficits to the explicit CS were not merely due to an inability to express a fear response.

Hippocampus

The data reviewed above suggest that the amygdala contributes to both olfactory and contextual fear conditioning, while the anterior PRH contributes to olfactory

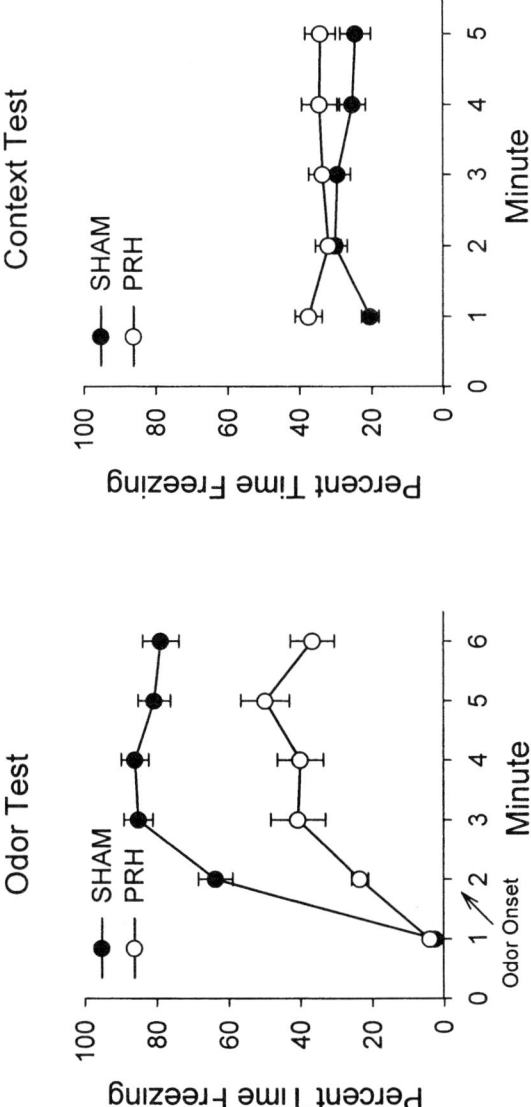

FIGURE 6. Freezing behavior of animals receiving either pretraining control surgical procedures (SHAM) or pretraining excitotoxic lesions of the anterior perirhinal cortex (PRH). **(Left)** Freezing behavior during a 6-min CS reexposure session in a novel context 24 h after conditioning. Odor was presented during minutes 2–6 only. **(Right)** Freezing behavior during a 5-min context reexposure session 48 h after conditioning. Plotted values represent the mean ± 1 SEM.

conditioning only. Recent work has suggested that contextual conditioning may depend upon interactions between the amygdala and a second limbic structure implicated in a variety of forms of learning, the hippocampus.

The role of the hippocampal formation in fear conditioning is currently the topic of considerable interest and debate. The results of a number of both early and more recent studies indicate that, although both pre- and posttraining lesions of the hippocampus have no effect on fear conditioned to an explicit CS,[10,63,64] they profoundly impair contextual fear conditioning.[64–66] These data, which are largely compatible with the effects of hippocampal lesions on contextual conditioning in appetitively motivated tasks,[67–69] were viewed as consistent with the well-established role of the hippocampus in memory for the complex spatial relationships among multiple unimodal and polymodal stimuli continuously present within the training apparatus (i.e., "spatial" memory). The once-widely accepted proposition that the hippocampus participates critically in the acquisition of fear conditioned to contextual stimuli, but not explicit CSs, however, has recently been called into question for several reasons. First, McNish et al.[70] have recently reported that, consistent with many previous studies, posttraining electrolytic lesions of dorsal hippocampus impaired the freezing response typically observed in unoperated animals during re-presentations of the training context; these lesions failed, however, to impair fear-potentiated startle. This effect was interpreted as evidence supporting the notion that hippocampal lesions disrupt the freezing response typically used as an index of "fear", but do not affect contextual conditioning per se. While this interpretation may be, in part, correct (see below), other data suggest the following: although electrolytic lesions of hippocampus often result in the generation of a competing response (i.e., hyperactivity), this competing response likely does not interact significantly with conditioned freezing measures. For example, as shown by Maren et al.,[71] there is no correlation between activity levels and contextual freezing in rats with hippocampal lesions. Also, whereas electrolytic lesions of dorsal hippocampus that are produced 1 day following training attenuate freezing elicited by the training context, they have no effect when made 28 days after training.[10] Finally, as described briefly above, electrolytic lesions of hippocampus typically have no effect on freezing responses to re-presentations of the explicit CS previously paired with foot shock.[10,63,64] Thus, while the hyperactivity often observed following electrolytic lesions of the hippocampus may result in a subtle modulation or masking of the freezing response, this effect appears not to interact significantly enough with the freezing response so as to render this response an unreliable index of conditioned fear.

A second finding calling into question the notion that hippocampus is critically involved in contextual fear conditioning is that while hippocampal lesions typically impair conditioning to the training context when an explicit CS is, within that context, paired with a US (i.e., the context was a background stimulus), this effect is absent when no CS is presented (i.e., the context was a foreground cue).[66] McNish et al.[70] argue that the competing response of hyperactivity may interact with weak versus strong conditioned associations such that weak associations (context as a background stimulus) are more vulnerable to disruption than are strong associations (context as a foreground stimulus).

A final study calling into question the role of the hippocampus in contextual fear conditioning concerns the effect of excitotoxic hippocampal lesions on contextual fear conditioning. Specifically, Maren, Aharonov, and Fanselow[72] found that pretraining lesions of the dorsal hippocampus produced by intracerebral injection of the excitotoxin N-methyl-D-aspartate (NMDA) had no effect on fear conditioned to the conditioning context, independent of whether the context was a foreground or background cue. The failure of pretraining excitotoxic lesions of hippocampus to disrupt contextual fear conditioning is especially noteworthy because of the nature of the lesion: excitotoxic lesions have become the preferred method of producing discrete brain damage because this method destroys only neurons at or near the injection site, while leaving fibers coursing through the lesioned region intact.[73] It should be noted that in the Maren *et al.*[72] study described here, and consistent with the effects of posttraining electrolytic lesions of hippocampus, posttraining excitotoxic hippocampal lesions produced soon after training impaired contextual conditioning. Interestingly, and in contrast to the effect typically observed following electrolytic lesions, however, excitotoxic hippocampal lesions impaired fear conditioned to the explicit auditory CS as well. Thus, while the contribution of the hippocampus to contextual conditioning appeared for some time to be fairly straightforward, the effects of excitotoxic hippocampal damage described here suggest that the issue deserves considerable reevaluation and continued study.

NEURAL SUBSTRATES OF CONDITIONING IN HUMANS?

Controlled studies examining the contribution of various brain areas to human behavior are, of course, much more difficult to carry out. Nonetheless, a growing number of studies employing contemporary brain imaging techniques support the notion that homologous brain structures are involved in Pavlovian conditioning in humans and nonhumans. Earlier reports of amygdala activation during exposure to a feared stimulus in phobia patients[74,75] have recently been extended to show involvement of this and related brain areas in the acquisition of conditioned emotional responses in healthy human subjects as well. For example, Buchel and colleagues[76] paired pictures of neutral faces (CS) with an aversive tone (US). Using functional magnetic resonance imaging (fMRI), they observed differential evoked responses in the anterior cingulate and anterior insular cortical regions, as well as a time-dependent response in the amygdalae, during subsequent presentation of the CS alone. LaBar *et al.*,[77] also using fMRI, observed a temporally graded amygdala response during conditioned fear acquisition and extinction in healthy human subjects. Finally, Schneider *et al.*[78] paired a noxious (but nontoxic) or neutral odor to pictures of neutral faces in subjects with social phobia and matched healthy control subjects. Again, using fMRI, they found increased activation in the amygdala and hippocampus of phobic subjects only during presentation of the CS associated with the negative odor. Thus, although not as conclusive as the findings from animal studies, research conducted with humans nonetheless supports the idea that the same areas that underlie odor-guided aversive conditioning in rats do so in humans as well.

SUMMARY AND CONCLUSIONS

While many, if not most, cases of CI likely reflect innate responses of sensitive individuals to biologically noxious compounds, it is likely that Pavlovian conditioning plays an important role in the development of symptoms in at least some individuals. Of particular relevance in this regard are recent data indicating that many species, including humans and experimental animals (rats), can develop conditioned responses to odorous substances and to spatial contexts that had previously been paired with a noxious stimulus. Thus, by this account, aversive reactions to odorous compounds or to particular buildings or places may, in some individuals, reflect conditioned responses resulting from prior exposure to that odor or place paired with exposure to a nonodorous noxious chemical or other aversive stimulus. Moreover, individual differences in development of CI might result from a process similar or identical to that of latent inhibition. Finally, studies examining the neural substrates of Pavlovian "fear" conditioning in rats suggest that the amygdala, perirhinal cortex, and hippocampus contribute to the acquisition and maintenance of conditioned responses; it remains to be determined whether these brain areas contribute to the acquisition and expression of CI in humans.

ACKNOWLEDGMENTS

This research was supported by NSF Grant Nos. IBN9514526 and IBN9817145, and a grant from the Charles and Johanna Busch Biomedical Research Fund. We would like to thank Graham Cousens and Christopher Herzog, who participated in many of the studies described here.

REFERENCES

1. BOLLA-WILSON, K., R. WILSON & M.L. BLEEKER. 1988. Conditioning of physical symptoms after neurotoxic exposure. J. Occup. Med. 30: 684–686.
2. GIARDINO, N.D. & P.M. LEHRER. 2000. Behavioral conditioning and idiopathic environmental intolerances. In Occupational Medicine: State of the Art Reviews. Vol. 15: Idiopathic Environmental Intolerances. Hanley & Belfus. Philadelphia.
3. SIEGEL, S. & R. KREUTZER. 1997. Pavlovian conditioning and multiple chemical sensitivity. Environ. Health Perspect. 105: S521–S526.
4. SHUSTERMAN, D.J. 1992. Critical review: the health significance of environmental odor pollution. Arch. Environ. Health 47: 76–87.
5. SPARKS, P.J., W. DANIELL, D.W. BLACK et al. 1994. Multiple chemical sensitivity syndrome: a clinical perspective. II. Evaluation, diagnostic testing, treatment, and social considerations. J. Occup. Med. 36: 731–737.
6. VAN DEN BERGH, O., K. STEGEN, I. VAN DIEST et al. 1999. Acquisition and extinction of somatic symptoms in response to odors: a Pavlovian paradigm relevant to multiple chemical sensitivity. Occup. Environ. Med. 56: 295–301.
7. DAVIS, M. 1992. The role of the amygdala in fear and anxiety. Annu. Rev. Neurosci. 15: 353–375.
8. HERZOG, C.D. & T. OTTO. 1997. Odor-guided fear conditioning. II. Lesions of anterior perirhinal cortex disrupt fear conditioned to the explicit CS, but not to the training context. Behav. Neurosci. 111: 1265–1274.
9. HERZOG, C.D. & T. OTTO. 1998. Contributions of anterior perirhinal cortex to olfactory and contextual fear conditioning. Neuroreport 9: 1855–1859.
10. KIM, J.J. & M.S. FANSELOW. 1992. Modality-specific retrograde amnesia of fear. Science 256: 675–677.
11. LEDOUX, J.E. 1995. Emotion: clues from the brain. Annu. Rev. Neurosci. 46: 209–235.
12. OTTO, T., G. COUSENS & K. RAJEWSKI. 1997. Odor-guided fear conditioning. I. Acquisition, retention, and latent inhibition. Behav. Neurosci. 111: 1257–1264.

13. FANSELOW, M.S. 1986. Associative vs. topographic accounts of the immediate shock-freezing deficit in rats: implications for the response selection rules governing species-specific defensive reactions. Learn. Motiv. **17:** 16–39.
14. FANSELOW, M.S. 2000. Contextual fear, gestalt memories, and the hippocampus. Behav. Brain Res. **110:** 73–81.
15. LUBOW, R.E. & A.U. MOORE. 1959. Latent inhibition: the effect of nonreinforced preexposure to the conditioned stimulus. J. Comp. Physiol. Psychol. **52:** 415–419.
16. WEINER, I. 1990. Neural substrates of latent inhibition: the switching model. Psychol. Bull. **108:** 442–461.
17. BOUTON, M.E. 1990. Context and retrieval in extinction and in other examples of interference in simple associative learning. *In* Current Topics in Animal Learning: Brain, Emotion, and Cognition, pp. 25–53. Erlbaum. Hillsdale, NJ.
18. HONEY, R.C. & M. GOOD. 1993. Selective hippocampal lesions abolish the contextual specificity of latent inhibition and conditioning. Behav. Neurosci. **107:** 23–33.
19. VAN DEN BERGH, O., P.J. KEMPYNCK, K.P. VAN DE WOESTIJNE *et al.* 1995. Respiratory learning and somatic complaints: a conditioning approach using CO_2-enriched air inhalation. Behav. Res. Ther. **33:** 517–527.
20. VAN DEN BERGH, O., K. STEGEN & K.P. VAN DE WOESTIJNE. 1997. Learning to have psychosomatic complaints: conditioning of respiratory behavior and somatic complaints in psychosomatic patients. Psychosom. Med. **59:** 13–23.
21. VAN DEN BERGH, O., K. STEGEN & K.P. VAN DE WOESTIJNE. 1998. Memory effects on symptom reporting in a respiratory learning paradigm. Health Psychol. **17:** 241–248.
22. SHUSTERMAN, D., J. BALMES & J. CONE. 1988. Behavioral sensitization to irritants/odorants after acute overexposure. J. Occup. Med. **30:** 565–567.
23. BOLLA-WILSON, K., R. WILSON & M.L. BLEEKER. 1988. Conditioning of physical symptoms after neurotoxic exposure. J. Occup. Med. **30:** 684–686.
24. STAUDENMAYER, H., J.C. SELNER & M.P. BUHR. 1993. Double-blind provocation chamber challenges in 20 patients presenting with "multiple chemical sensitivity". Regul. Toxicol. Pharmacol. **18:** 44–53.
25. MENZIES, D. & J. BOURBEAU. 1997. Building-related illnesses. N. Engl. J. Med. **337:** 1524–1531.
26. BELL, I.R., G.E. SCHWARTZ, J.M. PETERSON & D. AMEND. 1993. Self-reported illness from chemical odors in young adults without clinical syndromes or occupational exposures. Arch. Environ. Health **48:** 6–13.
27. BELL, I.R., G.E. SCHWARTZ, J.M. PETERSON *et al.* 1993. Possible time-dependent sensitization to xenobiotics: self-reported illness from chemical odors, foods, and opiate drugs in an older adult population. Arch. Environ. Health **48:** 315–327.
28. MEGGS, W.J., K.A. DUNN, R.M. BLOCH *et al.* 1996. Prevalence and nature of allergy and chemical sensitivity in a general population. Arch. Environ. Health **51:** 275–282.
29. LUBOW, R.E. 1973. Latent inhibition. Psychol. Bull. **79:** 398–407.
30. VAITL, D. & O.V. LIPP. 1997. Latent inhibition and autonomic responses: a psychophysiological approach. Behav. Brain Res. **88:** 85–93.
31. GIBBONS, H. & T.H. RAMMSAYER. 1997. Differential effects of personality traits related to the P ImpUSS dimension on latent inhibition in healthy female subjects. Pers. Individ. Differ. **27:** 1157–1166.
32. LUBOW, R.E., Y. INGBERG-SACHS, N. ZALSTEIN-ORDA & J.C. GEWIRTZ. 1992. Latent inhibition in low and high "psychotic-prone" normal subjects. Pers. Individ. Differ. **13:** 563–572.
33. PETERSON, J. & S. CARSON. 2000. Latent inhibition and openness to experience in a high-achieving student population. Pers. Individ. Differ. **28:** 323–332.
34. PAVLOV, I.P. 1920. Conditioned Reflexes. Oxford University Press. London/New York.
35. MATZEL, L.D., C.C. GANDHI & I.A. MUZZIO. 2000. Synaptic efficacy is commonly regulated within a nervous system and predicts individual differences in learning. Neuroreport **27:** 1253–1258.
36. ZINBARG, R.E. & J. MOHLMAN. 1998. Individual differences in the acquisition of affectively valenced associations. J. Pers. Soc. Psychol. **74:** 1024–1040.

37. ÖHMAN, A. & G. BOHLIN. 1973. The relationship between spontaneous and stimulus-correlated electrodermal responses in simple and discriminative conditioning paradigms. Psychophysiology **10:** 589–600.
38. MORROW, G.R. 1988. Anticipatory nausea and vomiting in cancer patients undergoing chemotherapy: prevalence, etiology, and behavioral interventions. Clin. Psychol. Rev. **8:** 517–556.
39. KVALE, G., C. PSYCHOL & K. HUGDAHL. 1994. Cardiovascular conditioning and anticipatory nausea and vomiting in cancer patients. Behav. Med. **20:** 78–83.
40. WRZESNIEWSKI, A., C. MCCAULEY & P. ROZIN. 1999. Odor and affect: individual differences in the impact of odor on liking for places, things, and people. Chem. Senses **24:** 713–721.
41. ZIEM, G. & J. MCTAMNEY. 1997. Profile of patients with chemical injury and sensitivity. Environ. Health Perspect. **105:** S417–S436.
42. OTTO, T., G. COUSENS & C. HERZOG. 2000. Behavioral and neuropsychological foundations of olfactory fear conditioning. Behav. Brain Res. **110:** 119–128.
43. CAMPEAU, S. & M. DAVIS. 1995. Involvement of the central nucleus and basolateral complex of the amygdala in fear conditioning measured with fear-potentiated startle in rats trained concurrently with auditory and visual conditioning. J. Neurosci. **15:** 2301–2311.
44. MAREN, S., G. AHARONOV & M.S. FANSELOW. 1996. Retrograde abolition of conditional fear after excitotoxic lesions in the basolateral amygdala of rats: absence of a temporal gradient. Behav. Neurosci. **110:** 718–726.
45. ROMANSKI, L.M., M.C. CLUGNET, F. BORDI & J.E. LEDOUX. 1993. Somatosensory and auditory convergence in the lateral nucleus of the amygdala. Behav. Neurosci. **107:** 444–450.
46. COUSENS, G. & T. OTTO. 1998. Both pre- and post-training lesions of the basolateral amygdala abolish the expression of olfactory and contextual fear conditioning. Behav. Neurosci. **112:** 1092–1103.
47. LEDOUX, J.E., P. CICCHETTI, A. XAGORARIS & L.M. ROMANSKI. 1990. The lateral amygdaloid nucleus: sensory interface of the amygdala in fear conditioning. J. Neurosci. **10:** 1062–1069.
48. QUIRK, G.J., J.C. REPA & J.E. LEDOUX. 1995. Fear conditioning enhances short-latency auditory responses of lateral amygdala neurons: parallel recordings in the freely behaving rat. Neuron **15:** 1029–1039.
49. LEDOUX, J.E., C.R. FARB & L.M. ROMANSKI. 1991. Overlapping projections to the amygdala and striatum from auditory processing areas of the thalamus and cortex. Neurosci. Lett. **134:** 139–144.
50. MASCAGNI, F., A.J. MACDONALD & J.R. COLEMAN. 1993. Corticoamygdaloid and corticocortical projections of the rat temporal cortex: a *Phaseolus vulgaris* leucoagglutinin study. Neuroscience **52:** 697–715.
51. OTTERSON, O.P. 1982. Connections of the amygdala in the rat. IV. Corticoamygdaloid and intra-amygdaloid connections as studied with axonal transport of HRP. J. Comp. Neurol. **205:** 30–48.
52. ROMANSKI, L.M. & J.E. LEDOUX. 1993. Information cascade from primary auditory cortex to the amygdala: corticocortical and corticoamygdaloid projections of temporal cortex in the rat. Cereb. Cortex **3:** 515–532.
53. TURNER, B.H. & M. HERKENHAM. 1981. An autoradiographic study of the thalamo-amygdaloid connections in the rat. Anat. Rec. **199:** 260A.
54. GAFFAN, D. 1994. Dissociated effects of perirhinal cortex ablation, fornix transection, and amygdalectomy: evidence for multiple memory systems in the primate temporal lobe. Exp. Brain Res. **99:** 411–422.
55. MEUNIER, M., J. BACHEVALIER, M. MISHKIN & E.A. MURRAY. 1993. Effects on visual recognition of combined and separate ablations of the entorhinal and perirhinal cortex in rhesus monkeys. J. Neurosci. **13:** 5418–5432.
56. OTTO, T. & H. EICHENBAUM. 1992. Complementary roles of orbital prefrontal cortex and the perirhinal/entorhinal cortices in an odor-guided delayed non-matching to sample task. Behav. Neurosci. **106:** 763–775.

57. ZOLA-MORGAN, S., L.R. SQUIRE, D.G. AMARAL & W.A. SUZUKI. 1989. Lesions of perirhinal and parahippocampal cortex that spare the amygdala and hippocampal formation produce severe memory impairment. J. Neurosci. **9:** 4355–4370.
58. HUNT, M.E., R.B. KESNER & R.B. EVANS. 1994. Memory for spatial location: functional dissociation of entorhinal cortex and hippocampus. Psychobiology **22:** 186–194.
59. NAGAHARA, A.H., T. OTTO & M. GALLAGHER. 1995. Entorhinal lesions impair performance in two versions of place learning in the Morris water maze. Behav. Neurosci. **109:** 3–9.
60. OTTO, T., D. WOLF & T. WALSH. 1997. Combined lesions of perirhinal and entorhinal cortex impair rats' performance in two versions of the spatially guided radial arm maze. Neurobiol. Learn. Mem. **68:** 21–31.
61. WIIG, K.A. & D.K. BILKEY. 1994. Perirhinal cortex lesions in rats disrupt performance in a spatial DNMS task. Neuroreport **5:** 1405–1408.
62. OTTO, T., F. SCHOTTLER, U. STAUBLI et al. 1991. The hippocampus and olfactory discrimination learning: effects of entorhinal cortex lesions on odor memory in a successive-cue, go, no-go task. Behav. Neurosci. **105:** 111–119.
63. PHILLIPS, R.G. & J.E. LEDOUX. 1992. Differential contribution of amygdala and hippocampus to cued and contextual fear conditioning. Behav. Neurosci. **106:** 274–285.
64. SELDEN, N.R.W., B.J. EVERITT, L.E. JARRARD & T.W. ROBBINS. 1991. Complementary roles for the amygdala and hippocampus in aversive conditioning to explicit and contextual cues. Neuroscience **42:** 335–350.
65. MAREN, S. & M.S. FANSELOW. 1997. Electrolytic lesions of the fimbria/fornix, dorsal hippocampus, or entorhinal cortex produce anterograde deficits in contextual fear conditioning in rats. Neurobiol. Learn. Mem. **67:** 142–149.
66. PHILLIPS, R.G. & J.E. LEDOUX. 1994. Lesions of the dorsal hippocampal formation interfere with background, but not foreground contextual fear conditioning. Learn. Mem. **1:** 34–44.
67. HONEY, R.C. & M. GOOD. 1993. Selective hippocampal lesions abolish the contextual specificity of latent inhibition and conditioning. Behav. Neurosci. **107:** 23–33.
68. GOOD, M. & D. BANNERMAN. 1997. Differential effects of ibotenic acid lesions of the hippocampus and blockade of N-methyl-D-aspartate receptor-dependent long-term potentiation on contextual processing in rats. Behav. Neurosci. **111:** 1171–1183.
69. HALL, G., D. PURVES & C. BONARDI. 1996. Contextual control of conditioned responding in rats with dorsal hippocampal lesions. Behav. Neurosci. **110:** 933–945.
70. MCNISH, K.A., J.C. GEWIRTZ & M. DAVIS. 1997. Evidence of contextual fear after lesions of the hippocampus: a disruption of freezing, but not fear-potentiated startle. J. Neurosci. **17:** 9353–9360.
71. MAREN, S., S.G. ANAGNOSTARAS & M.S. FANSELOW. 1998. The startled sea horse: is the hippocampus necessary for contextual fear conditioning? Trends Cognit. Sci. **2:** 39–42.
72. MAREN, S., G. AHARONOV & M.S. FANSELOW. 1997. Neurotoxic lesions of the dorsal hippocampus and Pavlovian fear conditioning in rats. Behav. Brain Res. **88:** 261–274.
73. JARRARD, L.E. 1989. On the use of ibotenic acid to lesion selectively different components of the hippocampal formation. J. Neurosci. Methods **29:** 251–259.
74. FREDRIKSON, M., G. WIK, P. ANNAS et al. 1995. Functional neuroanatomy of visually elicited simple phobic fear: additional data and theoretical analysis. Psychophysiology **32:** 43–48.
75. FURMARK, T., H. FISCHER, G. WIK et al. 1997. The amygdala and individual differences in human fear conditioning. Neuroreport **8:** 3957–3960.
76. BUCHEL, C., J. MORRIS, R.J. DOLAN & K.J. FRISTON. 1998. Brain systems mediating aversive conditioning: an event-related fMRI study. Neuron **20:** 947–957.
77. LABAR, K.S., J.C. GATENBY, J.C. GORE et al. 1998. Human amygdala activation during conditioned fear acquisition and extinction: a mixed-trial fMRI study. Neuron **20:** 937–945.
78. SCHNEIDER, F., U. WEISS, C. KESSLER et al. 1999. Subcortical correlates of differential classical conditioning of aversive emotional reactions in social phobia. Biol. Psychiatry **45:** 863–871.

Central Nervous System Effects from a Peripherally Acting Cholinesterase Inhibiting Agent: Interaction with Stress or Genetics

KEVIN D. BECK,[a] GUANPING ZHU,[b] DAWN BELDOWICZ,[a]
FRANCIS X. BRENNAN,[a] JOHN E. OTTENWELLER,[a,b] ROBERTA L. MOLDOW,[c]
AND RICHARD J. SERVATIUS[a,b,d]

[a]*Neurobehavioral Unit, Veterans Affairs New Jersey Health Care System, East Orange, New Jersey 07018, USA*

[b]*Department of Neuroscience, New Jersey Medical School–UMDNJ, Newark, New Jersey 07103, USA*

[c]*Department of Biology, Seton Hall University, South Orange, New Jersey 07079, USA*

Many pharmacological agents are developed to have specific loci of action. However, these loci may have different distributions due to individual differences in physiology (genetics) or because of significant changes in physiology due to environmental conditions (i.e., increased chemical sensitivity). Pyridostigmine bromide (PB), a peripheral cholinesterase inhibitor, has been implicated as a compound that has different loci of effect based on these conditions (genetics and environment). Epidemiological research suggests that some individuals, who experienced lasting effects from ingesting PB during Gulf War operations, may have a genetic disposition that equates into an oversensitive cholinesterase phenotype when challenged with PB.[1] Other research suggests environmental conditions, causing a stress state, and leading to physiological changes both acutely and persistently that altered the distribution of drug action. Basic research into the malleability of PB's loci of effect suggests it may be altered if ingested while the individual is in a stress state.[2] The following is a brief review of a series of studies that examined these two hypotheses (individual differences and role of environmental stressors) in relation to PB's actions on behavior and physiology.

INDIVIDUAL DIFFERENCES

Using Sprague-Dawley (SD) and Wistar-Kyoto (WKY) rats, we modeled individual differences in chemical sensitivity. The SD is a commonly used strain for behavior and physiology modeling, whereas the WKY strain was developed as a control for hypertensive rats and is considered a stress-sensitive strain that models depression.[3] The WKY rat also differs in its normal circulating butyrylcholinesterase

---

[d]Address for correspondence: Richard J. Servatius, Neurobehavioral Unit (127A), Veterans Affairs New Jersey Health Care System, East Orange, NJ 07018. Voice: 973-676-1000, ×3678; fax: 973-395-7111.

rjs@njneuromed.org

TABLE 1. Acoustic startle responses (arbitrary units) following a week of PB administration (mean response magnitude ± SEM)

	Posttreatment day 1	Posttreatment day 7	Posttreatment day 14
Individual differences			
WKY			
Water (8)	1.30 ± 0.06	1.65 ± 0.06	1.46 ± 0.08
Water + PB (7)	1.36 ± 0.05	1.58 ± 0.04	1.92 ± 0.11*
SD			
Water (8)	1.38 ± 0.07	1.49 ± 0.08	1.60 ± 0.04
Water + PB (7)	1.54 ± 0.06	1.59 ± 0.06	1.58 ± 0.07
Environmental stressors			
SD			
Water-NS (14)	1.06 ± 0.17	1.18 ± 0.17	1.09 ± 0.19
PB-NS (14)	1.40 ± 0.17*	1.19 ± 0.18	1.10 ± 0.15
Water-stress (14)	1.60 ± 0.34*	1.21 ± 0.16	0.98 ± 0.12
PB-stress (14)	1.11 ± 0.15	1.15 ± 0.19	1.04 ± 0.12

NOTE: An asterisk (*) denotes a significant difference from same-strain water or water-NS groups ($p < 0.05$).

(BuChE) activity.[4] We sought to determine if chronic PB ingestion would lead to the development of a persistent or emergent change in behavior.[4] Two weeks following the end of PB treatment via the drinking water (0.045 mg/mL over 7 days, producing a modest 20–25% reduction in plasma BuChE activity), acoustic startle responses were exaggerated in WKY rats, but not in SD rats (TABLE 1). This behavioral effect was dose-dependent and could be reinstated 7 weeks later following a second week of administration. The most parsimonious explanation for this occurrence is the phenotype of the WKY rat. Even without any experimental manipulation, WKY rats exhibit less open field activity and quicker paw-lick latencies when compared to SD rats[4] and develop ulcers more readily than other strains when stressed.[3] These characteristics suggest that WKY rats are more sensitive to both environmental (novelty) and physiological (interoceptive) stimuli. PB's acute physiological effects (muscle tremors, decreased salivation, etc.) may serve as an internal stressor to the WKY rat. In this regard, the WKY rat may serve as a model for somatoform disorders.

ROLE OF ENVIRONMENTAL STRESSORS

An individual's physiological response to pharmacological agents could be influenced by the presence of environmental stressors. By chronically stressing SD rats (1-hour supine restraint) on 7 PB treatment days (0.045 mg/mL in drinking water), we examined whether changes in startle responding would develop posttreatment (as in the WKY model). Despite stress-induced decreases in plasma BuChE, behavioral differences did not occur.[5] PB-treated SD rats showed an exaggerated startle on the last day of treatment and on the first day posttreatment (acute effect), but not at 7 or

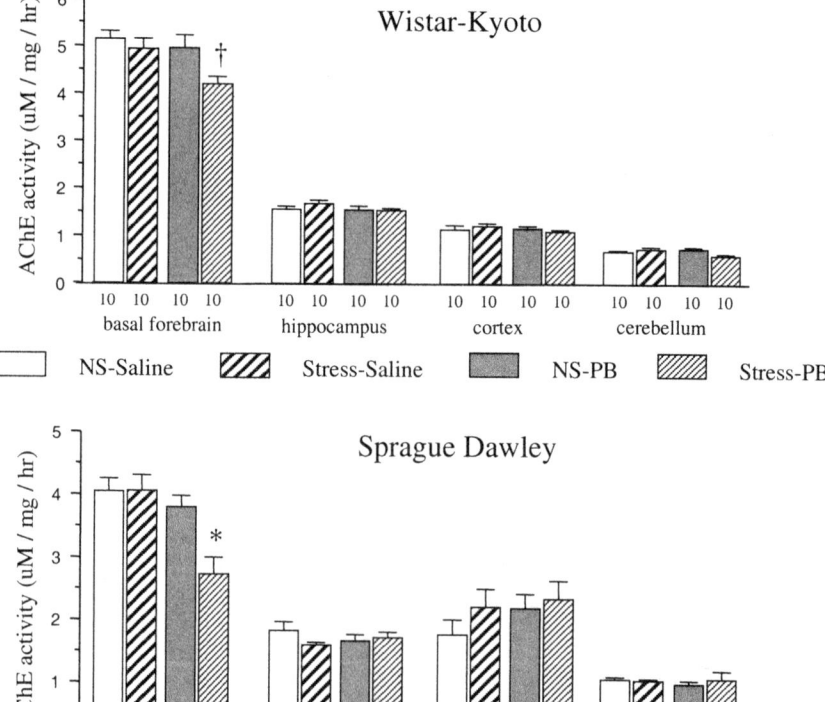

FIGURE 1. AChE activity (RIA) in the brain after 1-hour tail shock stress and PB injection (2 mg/kg ip). An asterisk (*) represents differences from all other groups and a cross (†) denotes a difference from naive-saline subjects ($p < 0.05$, Bonferroni multiple comparison).

14 days later (TABLE 1). Stressed PB-treated SD rats did not show an exaggerated startle on any of the testing days. Thus, combining stress with PB ingestion in a standard strain did not result in the same delayed-onset behavioral effects as in the highly sensitive WKY strain.

INDIVIDUAL DIFFERENCES, ENVIRONMENTAL STRESSORS, AND PB CENTRAL ACTION

We questioned how PB was mediating the behavioral changes. PB should not affect brain cholinesterase activity and we have found this to be true acutely. However, when we analyzed the brains of SD and WKY rats at 24 hours after the end of a week-long PB treatment (drinking water), with and without concomitant restraint stress, we observed changes in AChE activity in the basal forebrain/basal ganglia area of the brain (data not shown). In SD rats, stress (regardless of PB treatment) increased AChE above that of naive-saline rats. In contrast, the same procedures in WKY rats produced a PB-dependent increase in AChE (regardless of stress). These unexpected central AChE changes following chronic treatment led us to test whether an acute dose of PB could affect AChE in the brain. Using both the standard (SD) and stress-sensitive (WKY) rats, we administered PB (2 mg/kg ip) in nonstressed or stressed subjects. We used a more severe stress (1-hour tail shock) because other labs using less intense stressors have reported discrepant results.[2,6] Regardless of strain, the interaction of stress with PB treatment resulted in lower brain AChE activity, an effect localized in the basal forebrain/basal ganglia (see FIG. 1). Why AChE is inhibited only in the basal forebrain/basal ganglia following stress and PB administration is not clear at this juncture. Interestingly, a recent report also suggests the basal ganglia may be morphologically different in some veterans reporting symptoms associated with Gulf War syndrome.[7] Still, the evidence regarding PB CNS effects comprises indirect measures and no lab has presented direct evidence that PB (or its metabolites) crosses the blood-brain barrier.

CONCLUSIONS

Our research exemplifies the complexity of the interaction between genetics, the environment, and reactivity to pharmacological agents. Our work with PB and the WKY rat may apply to unexplained illnesses, such as Gulf War syndrome or somatoform disorders (DSM IV). On the other hand, environmental stressors can lead to different behavioral and physiological changes since the type of stress and model species used are critical in this interaction. Therefore, selecting specific animal strains and testing under different environmental conditions can provide more information about sensitivity changes that can occur when exposed to any particular chemical agent.

ACKNOWLEDGMENTS

This work was supported by funding from the Center for Environmental Hazards Research and DVA Medical Research to R. J. Servatius.

REFERENCES

1. HALEY, R.W., S. BILLECKE & B.N. LA DU. 1998. Association of low PON1 type Q (type A) arylesterase activity with neurologic symptom complexes in Gulf War veterans. Toxicol. Appl. Pharmacol. **157:** 227–233.
2. FRIEDMAN, A., D. KAUFER, J. SHEMER *et al.* 1996. Pyridostigmine brain penetration under stress enhances neuronal excitability and induces early immediate transcriptional response. Nat. Med. **2:** 1382–1385.
3. PARÉ, W.P. 1989. Stress ulcer susceptibility and depression in Wistar Kyoto (WKY) rats. Physiol. Behav. **46:** 993–998.
4. SERVATIUS, R.J., J.E. OTTENWELLER, D. BELDOWICZ *et al.* 1998. Persistently exaggerated startle responses in rats treated with pyridostigmine bromide. J. Pharmacol. Exp. Ther. **287:** 1020–1028.

5. SERVATIUS, R.J., J.E. OTTENWELLER, W. GUO et al. 2000. Effects of inescapable stress and treatment with pyridostigmine bromide on plasma butyrylcholinesterase and the acoustic startle response in rats. Physiol. Behav. **69:** 239–246.
6. LALLEMENT, G., A. FOQUIN, D. BAUBICHON et al. 1998. Heat stress, even extreme, does not induce penetration of pyridostigmine into the brain of guinea pigs. Neurotoxicology **19:** 759–766.
7. HALEY, R.W., W.W. MARSHALL, G.G. MCDONALD et al. 2000. Brain abnormalities in Gulf War syndrome: evaluation with ^{1}H MR spectroscopy. Radiology **215:** 807–817.

Symptom Learning in Response to Odors in a Single Odor Respiratory Learning Paradigm

WINNIE WINTERS,[a] STEPHAN DEVRIESE,[a] PAUL EELEN,[a]
HENDRIK VEULEMANS,[b] BENOIT NEMERY,[b] AND OMER VAN DEN BERGH[a]

[a]*Faculty of Psychology, Center for Ergonomics and Health Psychology,*
[b]*Faculty of Medicine, University of Leuven, B-3000 Leuven, Belgium*

Among the many different explanations given for multiple chemical sensitivity (MCS), classical conditioning has often been suggested and experimental evidence consistent with such an explanation is accumulating.[1] Most of this experimental evidence was acquired using a differential respiratory conditioning paradigm with odors as conditioned stimuli (CS) and CO_2-enriched air (e.g., 7.5%) as the unconditioned stimulus (US). This operationalization may mimic the effects of a toxic exposure or occasional (stress-induced) hyperventilation (US) in an odorous context (CS). The differential paradigm uses two distinct innocuous odors, implying two types of breathing trials for each subject: one containing an odor mixed with CO_2-enriched air and the other mixed with room air (the combination of the specific odor with CO_2 or air is counterbalanced between subjects). In the test phase, breathing trials are administered without CO_2 and symptoms to the odors alone are registered. This paradigm typically showed elevated symptoms to the odor that was previously mixed with CO_2. However, the effect only occurred when the conditioned odor was unpleasant (ammonia or butyric acid) and not when it was neutral/pleasant (niaouli).[2–4] Since a differential paradigm induces a form of discrimination learning, we wanted to extend our findings to a standard conditioning paradigm, pairing one single odor with the aversive event (CO_2 inhalation) during the acquisition phase. Subsequently, the odor was presented alone and symptoms were measured. The conditioning effect was tested between subjects using different control conditions.[5]

EXPERIMENT I

Methods

Fifty psychology freshmen were given 10 breathing trials of 2 minutes each. All participants started with a room air trial. Next, 8 trials were administered in a semi-randomized order. This acquisition phase was different in each between-subject condition—(1) experimental/paired: 4 compound trials (odor + CO_2) and 4 room air trials; (2) explicitly unpaired: 4 odor trials and 4 CO_2 trials; (3) random: 2 odor trials, 2 CO_2 trials, 2 compound trials, and 2 room air trials; (4) CS-only: 4 odor trials and 4 room air trials; and (5) US-only: 4 CO_2 trials and 4 room air trials. The 10th (test) trial always contained the odor only. The CO_2 mixture consisted of 7.5% CO_2, 21% O_2, and 71.5% N_2. The odor used in this experiment was a diluted solution of ammonia (0.4%). After each trial, subjects completed a complaint list of 16 items.

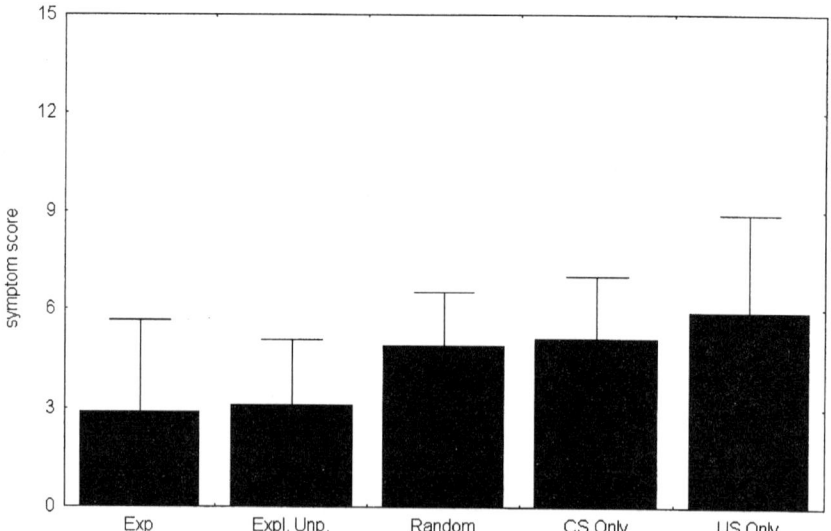

FIGURE 1. Means (± SD) of symptom score in test phase for experimental (exp.), explicitly unpaired (expl. unp.), random, CS-only, and US-only conditions.

The items all had a five-point answer scale ranging from 0 (not at all/no sensation or complaint) to 4 (very much).

For more details on materials, apparatuses, and procedures, see the published studies.[2-4]

Results

A one-factor independent group ANOVA was carried out on the total complaint scores (the between-subjects factor containing five levels). Complaints during air trials did not differ. Symptom scores were significantly elevated during CO_2 trials in acquisition. No differences were observed between the five conditions during the test trial, meaning that no conditioning effects were established: $F(4, 45) = 0.81$, n.s. (see FIG. 1).

EXPERIMENT II

Methods

Forty participants aged between 18 and 30 participated. The administered CO_2 level was raised to 10% (10% CO_2, 21% O_2, and 69% N_2). In half of the subjects, ammonia was used (0.8%); in the other half, niaouli was used and 11 trials of 80 s were run, using only the experimental and the explicitly unpaired conditions. An extra room air trial was inserted (trial 10) before the test trial (trial 11).

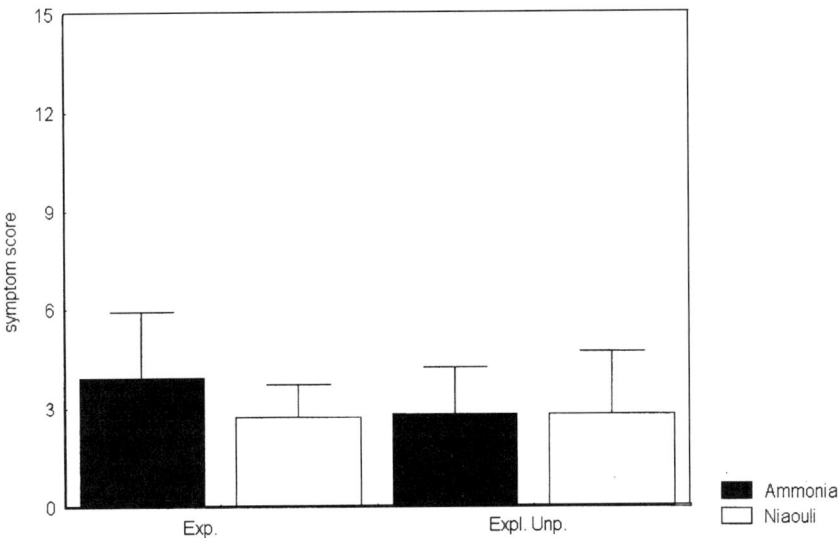

FIGURE 2. Means (± SD) of symptom score in test phase for experimental (exp.) and explicitly unpaired (expl. unp.) conditions in the ammonia group and niaouli group.

Results

Two (odor type: ammonia/niaouli) by two (condition: experimental/explicitly unpaired) analyses of variance were run on the total complaints score. No differences were found during air trials. Trials containing CO_2 significantly induced an elevated symptom score during acquisition. No differences were observed between the two conditions during the test trial: $F(1, 37) = 0.23$, n.s. for condition; and $F(1, 37) = 0.34$, n.s. for odor type (see FIG. 2).

DISCUSSION

Despite significant US effects (more complaints on CO_2 trials than on trials without CO_2), in none of the two experiments did we find elevated symptoms in response to odors in the test phase. This absence of conditioning effects in a single odor design replicates an earlier finding with a similar setup (designed to investigate generalization effects; unreported), suggesting a reliable pattern of no symptom learning in this kind of paradigm, whereas reliable conditioning effects were found in a differential paradigm. Although at present we have no clear explanation, some speculation can be advanced. A differential paradigm implies a form of discrimination learning between two odors, of which only one co-occurs with the experience of symptoms. This may cue the subjects more sharply into the critical aspects of the odor as a predictive feature; however, this may be absent in a paradigm where only one odor occurs. Once the odor functions as a critical feature, it may interact with other aspects such as affective valence. Indeed, in the differential paradigm, conditioning was only reliable when the odor was foul-smelling (ammonia). This interpretation suggests that any manipulation increasing the salience of the odor as a predictive cue may enhance the probability of odor conditioning, also in a single odor paradigm.

REFERENCES

1. VAN DEN BERGH, O., S. DEVRIESE, W. WINTERS et al. 2001. Acquiring symptoms in response to odors: a learning perspective on multiple chemical sensitivity. This volume.
2. VAN DEN BERGH, O., P.J. KEMPYNCK, K.P. VAN DE WOESTIJNE et al. 1995. Respiratory learning and somatic complaints: a conditioning approach using CO_2-enriched air inhalation. Behav. Res. Ther. **33:** 517–527.
3. VAN DEN BERGH, O., K. STEGEN & K.P. VAN DE WOESTIJNE. 1997. Learning to have psychosomatic complaints: conditioning of respiratory behavior and somatic complaints in psychosomatic patients. Psychosom. Med. **59:** 13–23.
4. VAN DEN BERGH, O., K. STEGEN, I. VAN DIEST et al. 1999. Acquisition and extinction of somatic symptoms in response to odors: a Pavlovian paradigm relevant to multiple chemical sensitivity. Occup. Environ. Med. **56:** 295–301.
5. RESCORLA, R.A. 1970. Pavlovian conditioning and its proper control conditions. Learn. Motiv. **1:** 372–381.

Deep Subcortical (Including Limbic) Hypermetabolism in Patients with Chemical Intolerance: Human PET Studies

G. HEUSER[a] AND J. C. WU

Brain Imaging Center, University of California, Irvine, California, USA

INTRODUCTION

Neurotoxic injury is known to affect memory and cognitive functions, coordination and balance, and also behavior. In addition, patients may develop sensitivity to chemicals. Their reactions to chemicals may range from increased irritability to emotional instability with "irrational" behavior, including panic attacks. Bell, Sorg, and others[1] have suggested and discussed limbic system involvement with kindling as a possible mechanism for the above reactions.

We studied PET brain scans in 7 adult patients who had developed the above clinical syndromes. All had been exposed to solvents, pesticides, or other known neurotoxic compounds and exhibited significant chronic symptoms (including chemical intolerance) and signs that continued for months, if not years, after exposure.

We started with the question of whether chemical injury and resultant chemical intolerance provide a signature or marker when these patients are studied with PET brain scans.

MATERIALS AND METHODS

All patients selected for this study were properly informed of the procedure and signed appropriate release forms. Their histories are displayed in TABLE 1.

Multiple chemical sensitivity was defined according to the criteria of Cullen.

The radioactive compound F-18 deoxyglucose (FDG) was used and was intravenously injected.

During the FDG uptake, subjects were asked to perform the Continuous Performance Test (CPT).[2] Our normal control population had also performed this same task.

The PET scans on our patients were compared to age and sex regressed normal controls derived from 56 adults with no known diseases or health problems, no history of intake of prescription or recreational drugs, and no history of alcohol intake.

---

[a]Address for correspondence: NeuroMed and NeuroTox Associates, 28240 West Agoura Road, Suite 203, Agoura Hills, CA 91301. Voice: 818-865-1858; fax: 818-865-8814.
gheuser@ucla.edu

TABLE 1. Histories of patients used in this study

Sex	Age	PET	Exposure duration	Exposure type	Disability	Irritability	MCS
M	26	10/98	1/97–1/98	New carpets Pesticides	on & off	+	+
F	39	8/98	10/95–1996	Paints Solvents	11/95–4/96	+	+
F	40	12/98	8/98–11/98	SBS	11/20/98	on & off	+
F	45	7/98	1953–1956	Nuclear plant emissions	–	+	+
			1991	Pesticides			
F	47	2/99	5/88–10/88	SBS	10/88	on & off	+
F	49	11/98	1987–1992	SBS (incl. formaldehyde)	1992	+	+
F	52	11/98	1991–3/97	SBS	3/97	on & off	+

NOTE: All patients listed above suffered from neurotoxic exposure. Some patients became ill from exposure at work and developed sick-building syndrome (SBS). All patients claimed sensitivity to a variety of chemicals (MCS). Note that many patients had become disabled as a result of exposure. The above patients had PET scans that are the subject of this poster.

RESULTS AND CONCLUSIONS

FIGURE 1 shows a typical patient whose individual PET scan was superimposed upon and compared with the average PET scan of 56 normal adult controls. White areas (yellow and red on the original coronal sections) represent significantly increased uptake of FDG ($p < 0.05$). Abnormalities shown here were similar in all 7 patients studied.

PET scans in the above patients were compared with the control group and showed significant *hypometabolism* in many cortical areas. This corresponds to areas of cortical hypoperfusion found in SPECT brain scans of chemically injured patients.[3] By contrast, significant *hypermetabolism* was found in portions of the limbic system (including the extended amygdala region) and adjacent structures. Hypermetabolism is seen to extend into the cerebellum and visual cortex, and downward all the way into the brain stem. Some of these connections are discussed by various contributors to this conference.

Since hypermetabolism can represent seizure activity and limbic system (especially amygdaloid) seizures can represent as panic attacks, and also since the amygdala is one of the most easily kindled structures of the brain, our preliminary data support the concept of limbic system involvement and kindling in patients with neurotoxic injury and resulting chemical intolerance. Thus, neuroanatomical correlation with involvement of other deep subcortical structures will have to be carefully studied.

Our tentative conclusion is that the clinical picture of chemical intolerance with its behavioral and cognitive correlates can be explained on the basis of hypometabolism in many cortical structures and hypermetabolism in deep subcortical (including limbic) structures.

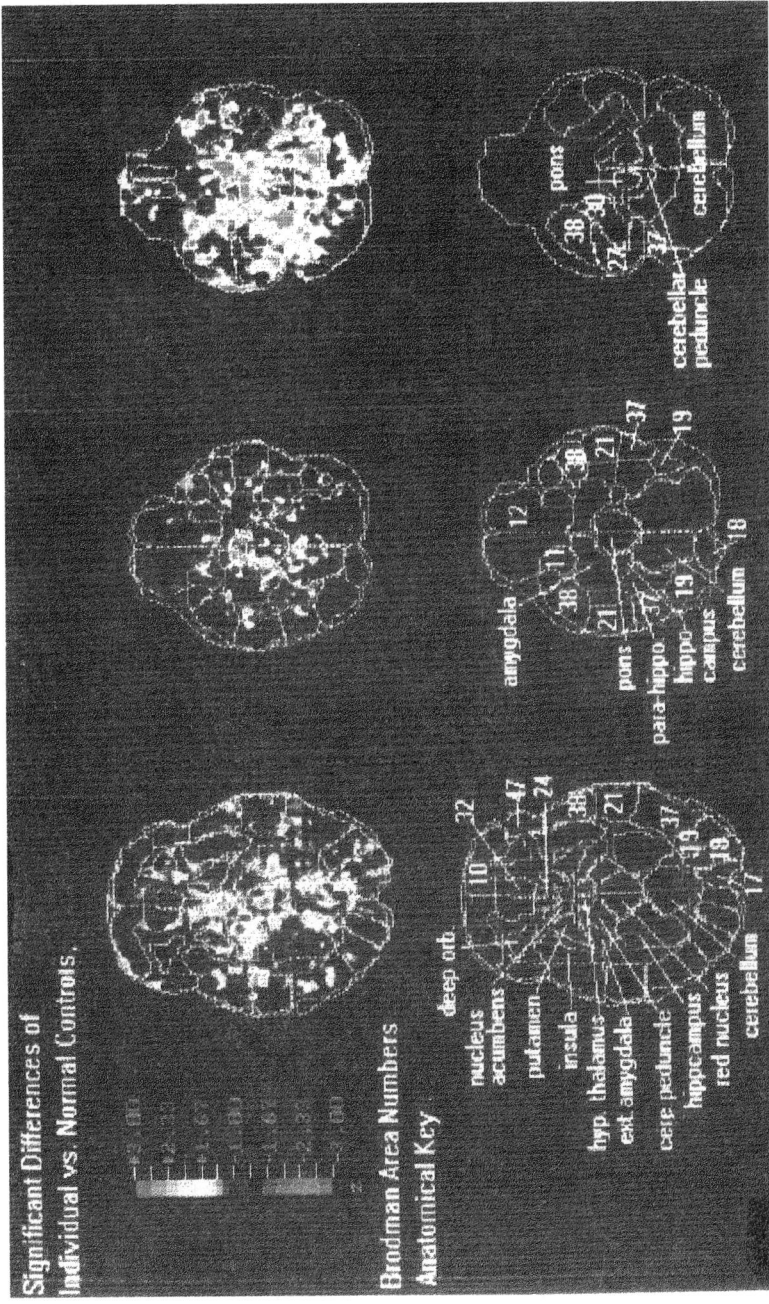

FIGURE 1. Sections and corresponding anatomical keys in areas that show significant hypermetabolism in one representative patient (F 45) with chemical intolerance. These areas are displayed in white. Upon request, a colored set of the PET scans will be sent to interested individuals.

Our PET findings were first presented in 1999 (unpublished).[4]

Other features of chemical intolerance can be explained with our finding that chemical exposure can activate mast cells and, in the extreme, lead to mastocytosis.[5]

REFERENCES

1. VARIOUS AUTHORS. 2001. This volume.
2. BUCHSBAUM, M.S. & A.J. SOSTEK. 1980. An adaptive-rate continuous performance test. Percept. Mot. Skills **51:** 707–713.
3. HEUSER, G. & I. MENA. 1998. NeuroSPECT in neurotoxic chemical exposure: demonstration of long-term functional abnormalities. Toxicol. Ind. Health **14**(no. 16): 813–827.
4. HEUSER, G. & J.C. WU. 1999. Subcortical hypermetabolism and cortical hypometabolism after neurotoxic exposure: human PET studies. Presented at the Seventh International Symposium on Neurobehavioral Methods and Effects in Occupational and Environmental Health, Stockholm, Sweden, June 20–23, 1999.
5. HEUSER, G. 2000. Letter to the editor regarding "mast cell disorder to be ruled out in MCS". Arch. Environ. Health **55:** 284–285.

Elevated Nitric Oxide/Peroxynitrite Mechanism for the Common Etiology of Multiple Chemical Sensitivity, Chronic Fatigue Syndrome, and Posttraumatic Stress Disorder

MARTIN L. PALL[a,b] AND JAMES D. SATTERLEE[c]

[b]School of Molecular Biosciences, Washington State University,
Pullman, Washington 99164, USA

[c]Department of Chemistry, Washington State University,
Pullman, Washington 99164, USA

INTRODUCTION

Chronic fatigue syndrome (CFS), multiple chemical sensitivity (MCS), posttraumatic stress disorder (PTSD), and fibromyalgia (FM) show three distinct types of overlap: each is typically induced by a short-term stress leading to a chronic pathology; all four show a set of substantial overlapping symptoms; and many patients have been diagnosed as having several of these disorders. These and other similarities have led to the suggestion that all four of these may be essentially identical, sharing a common, yet previously undefined etiology. For example, Buchwald and Garrity[1] concluded a study of CFS, MCS, and FM patients by suggesting that, "Despite their different diagnostic labels, existing data, though limited, suggest that these illnesses may be similar if not identical conditions...." Miller suggested that CFS, MCS, PTSD, FM, and several other disorders may share a common, if undefined etiology,[2] asking whether these constitute "an emerging theory of disease". One of us (M. L. Pall) has proposed a novel theory for the cause of CFS, based on elevated levels of peroxynitrite and its precursors, nitric oxide and superoxide.[3] Central to this theory are six positive feedback loops, which act such that elevated peroxynitrite increases the levels of both nitric oxide and superoxide, reacting to form more peroxynitrite.[3] By this vicious cycle mechanism (FIG. 1A), once the cycle is established, elevated levels of peroxynitrite and other components of this mechanism, notably nitric oxide, superoxide, and inflammatory cytokines, may produce the symptoms of CFS. Because the biochemical mechanisms involved here are not highly tissue-specific, some variation in tissue distribution of elevated peroxynitrite may produce the differences in symptoms often seen between, for example, classic cases of CFS and MCS.

In this paper, we focus on MCS, asking whether the proposed elevated nitric oxide/peroxynitrite mechanism may be central to the etiology of MCS. The evidence

---

[a]Address for correspondence: Martin L. Pall, School of Molecular Biosciences, Washington State University, Pullman, WA 99164-4660. Voice: 509-335-1246; fax: 509-335-9688.
martin_pall@wsu.edu

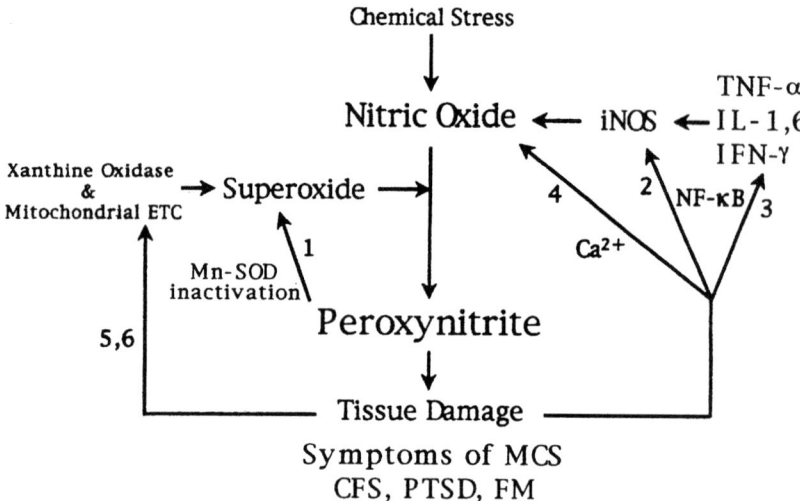

FIGURE 1A. The vicious cycle mechanism of six positive feedback loops (1–6). This figure is modified specifically for MCS/CI resulting from chemical stress and is adapted from the original proposal regarding CFS.[3] Mitochondrial ETC refers to the electron transport chain.

examined here includes each of the following: evidence that incitants of MCS act to induce increased levels of nitric oxide; evidence for induction of the inducible nitric oxide synthase in MCS; evidence for elevated levels of oxidative stress, as might be produced by peroxynitrite; evidence that incitants can induce inflammatory cytokines; and multiple types of evidence from animal models of MCS showing that increased nitric oxide has an essential role in producing the responses in these models. We also suggest that peroxynitrite may play an additional role in MCS by inducing breakdown of the blood-brain barrier.

INCITANTS MAY ACT BY INCREASING NITRIC OXIDE LEVELS

MCS incitants include a variety of volatile organics such as hydrocarbons, chlorinated hydrocarbons, other organics, and pesticides. One or more members of each of these groups are reported to produce increases in nitric oxide levels. These include benzene,[4–6] carbon tetrachloride,[7–9] formaldehyde,[10–13] and chlorinated hydrocarbon pesticides.[14] Organophosphate pesticides, which are often thought to be incitants of MCS, may act as illustrated in FIGURE 1B. These compounds are known to act as inhibitors of acetylcholinesterase, thereby leading to increased levels of acetylcholine that may act in turn to stimulate cholinergic muscarinic receptors. Such muscarinic receptor stimulation is known to produce increases in nitric oxide levels.[15–18]

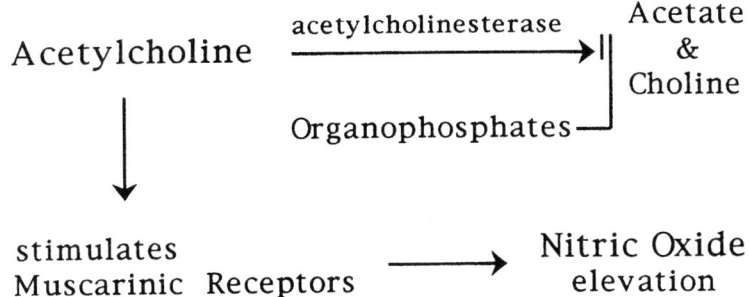

FIGURE 1B. Proposed mechanism by which organophosphate pesticides will generate elevated levels of nitric oxide.

EVIDENCE FROM MCS PATIENTS AND TISSUE STUDIES

Chemicals that induce MCS are reported to induce increases in inflammatory cytokines,[7,19,20] which are known to induce the inducible nitric oxide synthase (iNOS).[3] Further evidence for a role of elevated nitric oxide comes from the studies of Bell et al.[21] in which sera of MCS patients were reported to have elevated neopterin levels. Neopterin is a biochemical marker for induction of the iNOS because GTP cyclohydrolase I is coordinately induced with iNOS, as indicated in FIGURE 1C.[3]

The potent oxidant peroxynitrite will induce substantial amounts of oxidative damage in any disease in which it is elevated. Such oxidative damage is thought to be involved in MCS.[22,23] In one study, several antioxidants were used to treat patients with MCS, with some apparent success,[23] suggesting that oxidative damage may have a role in MCS. The blood of MCS patients was reported, in a recent study, to have elevated levels of oxidants and the serum to have lower levels of antioxidants, as compared with controls,[24] providing substantial evidence for elevated oxidative damage.

EVIDENCE FROM ANIMAL MODELS

Several animal models for MCS are based on the phenomena of neural sensitization, partial kindling, and kindling, where either repeated chemical or electrical stimulation of the limbic system produces increased sensitivity to stimulation, or leading in some procedures to spontaneous seizures (kindling).[25–29] In several studies of these MCS animal models, it has been shown that inhibitors of nitric oxide synthase activity blocked the characteristic sensitization response.[30–36] Furthermore, arginine, the amino acid substrate of nitric oxide synthases (FIG. 1C), stimulated the response.[32] Stimulation of the NMDA receptors that are known to produce an increase in nitric oxide synthesis is essential to the response.[30,32,34] Additionally, a mouse knockout mutant of the nNOS isozyme of nitric oxide synthase is resistant to sensitization.[37] Suzuki et al.[38] reported that kindling was associated with mono-

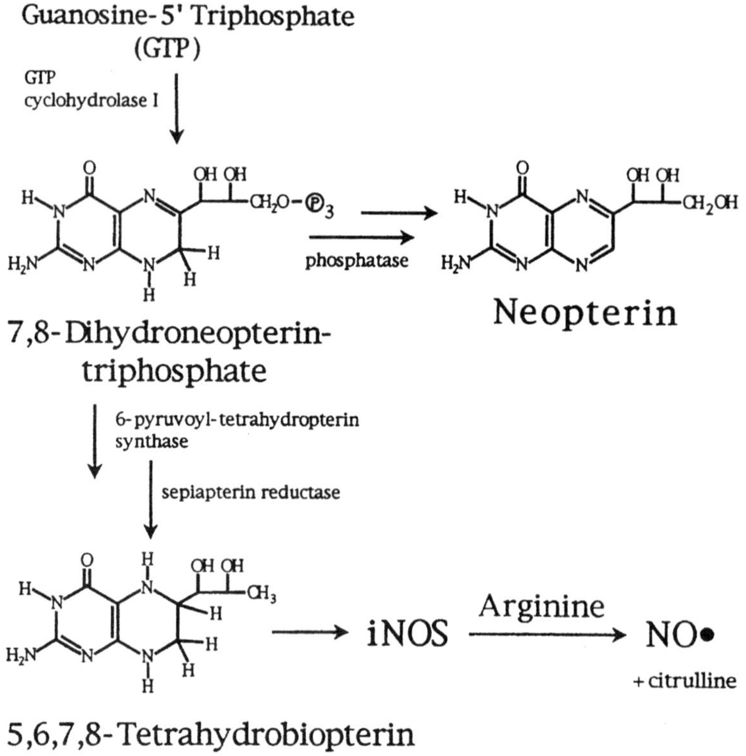

FIGURE 1C. An abbreviated scheme showing the relationship between pteridine biosynthesis and the inducible nitric oxide synthase (iNOS). As shown, neopterin is a potential biochemical marker for iNOS upregulation.

ADP-ribosylation of a protein and that this process was also increased by a nitric oxide–generating compound and decreased by several antikindling/antiepileptic drugs. These animal model studies provide compelling evidence that nitric oxide has an essential role in producing neural sensitization and kindling, suggesting that it may perform a similar role in MCS.

BREAKDOWN OF THE BLOOD-BRAIN BARRIER: A POSSIBLE ACCESSORY MECHANISM?

The proposal that MCS may share a similar mechanism to that found in CFS and PTSD suggests that dysfunction found in one of these disease states may be shared by others. It has been reported that the blood-brain barrier (BBB) breaks down in PTSD[39–41] and it is also reported that elevated peroxynitrite causes such breakdown in several diseases.[42–45] Thus, both the PTSD observations and our proposed mechanism for MCS involving elevated peroxynitrite suggest that such breakdown may also occur in MCS. Such BBB breakdown may be expected to produce a widened exposure of the CNS to chemicals and therefore a widened sensitivity to such chemicals. While it is not our contention that BBB breakdown is central to the hypersensitivity seen in MCS, this mechanism may be expected to produce hypersensitivity to a larger array of chemicals. Specifically, it may help produce the distinction between incitants and triggers, where a larger number of chemicals may act as triggers rather than as incitants, possibly due to a preceding BBB breakdown.

SUMMARY

Various types of evidence implicate nitric oxide and an oxidant, possibly peroxynitrite, in MCS and chemical intolerance (CI). The positive feedback loops proposed earlier for CFS[3] may explain the chronic nature of MCS (CI) as well as several of its other reported properties. These observations raise the possibility that this proposed elevated nitric oxide/peroxynitrite mechanism may be the mechanism of a new disease paradigm, answering the question raised by Miller[2] earlier: "Are we on the threshold of a new theory of disease?"

REFERENCES

1. BUCHWALD, D. & D. GARRITY. 1994. Comparison of patients with chronic fatigue syndrome, fibromyalgia, and multiple chemical sensitivities. Arch. Intern. Med. **154:** 2049–2053.
2. MILLER, C.S. 1999. Are we on the threshold of a new theory of disease? Toxicant-induced loss of tolerance and its relationship to addiction and abdiction. Toxicol. Ind. Health **15:** 284–294.
3. PALL, M.L. 2000. Elevated, sustained peroxynitrite levels as the cause of chronic fatigue syndrome. Med. Hypotheses **54:** 115–125.
4. LASKIN, D.L. et al. 1996. Role of nitric oxide in hematosuppression and benzene-induced toxicity. Environ. Health Perspect. **104:** 1283–1287.
5. RAO, N.R. & R. SNYDER. 1995. Oxidative modifications produced in HL-60 cells on exposure to benzene metabolites. J. Appl. Toxicol. **15:** 403–409.
6. PUNJABI, C.J. et al. 1994. Enhanced production of nitric oxide by bone marrow cells and increased sensitivity to macrophage colony-stimulating factor (CSF) and granulocyte-macrophage CSF after benzene treatment of mice. Blood **83:** 3255–3263.
7. CHAMULIRAT, W. et al. 1995. Tumor necrosis factor alpha and nitric oxide production in endotoxin-primed rats administered carbon tetrachloride. Life Sci. **57:** 2273–2280.
8. ROCKEY, D.C. & J.J. CHUNG. 1997. Regulation of inducible nitric oxide synthase and nitric oxide during hepatic injury and fibrogenesis. Am. J. Physiol. **273:** G124–G130.
9. NIEDERBERGER, M. et al. 1995. Increased aortic cyclic guanosine monophosphate concentration in experimental cirrhosis in rats: evidence for a role of nitric oxide in the pathogenesis of arterial vasodilation in cirrhosis. Hepatology **21:** 1625–1631.
10. LAM, H.H. et al. 1996. Induction of spinal cord neuronal nitric oxide synthase (NOS) after formalin injection in the rat hind paw. Neurosci. Lett. **210:** 201–204.
11. WIERTELAK, E.P. et al. 1994. Subcutaneous formalin produces centrifugal hyperalgesia at a non-injected site via the NMDA–nitric oxide cascade. Brain Res. **649:** 19–26.
12. WANG, H. et al. 1999. Peripheral nitric oxide contributes to both formalin and NMDA-induced activation of nociceptors: an immunocytochemical study in rats. J. Neurosci. Res. **57:** 824–829.
13. HERDEGEN, T. et al. 1994. Expression of nitric oxide synthase and colocalization with Jun, Fos, and Krox transcription factors in spinal cord neurons following noxious stimulation of the rat hind paw. Brain Res. Mol. Brain Res. **22:** 245–258.

14. DHOUIB, M. & A. LUGNIER. 1996. Induction of nitric oxide synthase by chlorinated pesticides (p,p'-DDT, chlordane, endosulfan) in rat liver. Cent. Eur. J. Public Health **4:** 48.
15. BACHMANN, S. & P. MUNDEL. 1994. Nitric oxide in the kidney: synthesis, localization, and function. Am. J. Kidney Dis. **24:** 112–129.
16. KONTOS, H.A. 1993. Nitric oxide and nitrosothiols in cerebrovascular and neuronal regulation. Stroke **24:** 1155–1158.
17. HARE, J.M. & W.S. COLUCCI. 1995. Role of nitric oxide in the regulation of myocardial function. Prog. Cardiovasc. Dis. **38:** 155–166.
18. VAN ZWEITEN, P.A. & H.N. DOODS. 1995. Muscarinic receptors and drugs in cardiovascular medicine. Cardiovasc. Drugs Ther. **9:** 159–167.
19. USHIO, H., K. NOHARA & H. FUJIMAKI. 1999. Effect of environmental pollutants on the production of pro-inflammatory cytokines by normal human dermal keratinocytes. Toxicol. Lett. **105:** 17–24.
20. WATKINS, L.R. *et al.* 1997. Evidence for the involvement of spinal cord glia in subcutaneous formalin induced hyperalgesia in the rat. Pain **71:** 225–235.
21. BELL, I.R. *et al.* 1998. Serum neopterin and somatization in women with chemical intolerance, depressives, and normals. Neuropsychobiology **38:** 13–18.
22. LEVINE, S. & J. REINHARDT. 1983. Biochemical pathology initiated by free radicals, oxidant chemicals, and therapeutic drugs in the etiology of chemical hypersensitivity disease. Orthomol. Psychiatry **12:** 166–183.
23. GALLAND, L. 1987. Biochemical abnormalities in patients with multiple chemical sensitivities. *In* Workers with Multiple Chemical Sensitivities—Occupational Medicine: State of the Art Reviews, pp. 755–777. Hanley & Belfus. Philadelphia.
24. IONESCU, G., M. MERK & R. BRADFORD. 1999. Simple chemiluminescence assays for free radicals in venous blood and serum samples: results in atopic dermatitis, psoriasis, MCS, and cancer patients. Forsch. Komplementarmed. **6:** 294–300.
25. MILLER, C.S. & H.C. MITZEL. 1995. Chemical sensitivity attributed to pesticide exposure versus remodeling. Arch. Environ. Health **50:** 119–129.
26. SORG, B.A. 1999. Multiple chemical sensitivity: potential role for neural sensitization. Crit. Rev. Neurobiol. **13:** 283–316.
27. BELL, I.R., C.S. MILLER & G.E. SCHWARTZ. 1992. An olfactory-limbic model of multiple chemical sensitivity syndrome: possible relationships to kindling and affective spectrum disorders. Biol. Psychiatry **32:** 218–242.
28. ANTELMAN, S.M. *et al.* 1980. Interchangeability of stress and amphetamine in sensitization. Science **207:** 329–333.
29. GODDARD, G.V., D.C. MCINTYRE & C.K. LEECH. 1969. A permanent change in brain function resulting from daily electrical stimulation. Exp. Neurol. **25:** 295–330.
30. MCNAUGHTON, B.L. *et al.* 1994. Persistent increase of hippocampal presynaptic axon excitability after repetitive electrical stimulation: dependence on N-methyl-D-aspartate receptor activity, nitric oxide synthase, and temperature. Proc. Natl. Acad. Sci. U.S.A. **91:** 4830–4834.
31. ITZHAK, Y. 1994. Blockade of sensitization to the toxic effects of cocaine in mice by nitric oxide synthase inhibitors. Pharmacol. Toxicol. **74:** 162–166.
32. ITZHAK, Y. 1995. Cocaine kindling in mice: responses to N-methyl-D,L-aspartate (NMDLA) and L-arginine. Mol. Neurobiol. **11:** 217–222.
33. HARACZ, J.L., J.S. MACDONALL & R. SIRCAR. 1997. Effects of nitric oxide synthase inhibitors on cocaine sensitization. Brain Res. **746:** 183–189.
34. PUDIAK, C.M. & M.A. BOZARTH. 1997. Nitric oxide synthesis inhibition attenuates haloperidol-induced supersensitivity. J. Psychiatry Neurosci. **22:** 61–64.
35. MCMAHON, S.B., G.R. LEWIN & P.D. WALL. 1993. Central hyperexcitability triggered by noxious inputs. Curr. Opin. Neurobiol. **3:** 602–610.
36. BECKER, A., G. GRECKSCH & H. SCHRODER. 1995. N-ω-Nitro-L-arginine methyl ester interferes with pentylenetetrazol-induced kindling and has no effect on changes in glutamate binding. Brain Res. **688:** 230–232.
37. ITZHAK, Y. *et al.* 1998. Resistance of neuronal nitric oxide synthase–deficient mice to cocaine-induced locomotor sensitization. Psychopharmacology **140:** 378–386.
38. SUZUKI, K. *et al.* 1997. The contribution of endogenous mono-ADP-ribosylation to kindling-induced epileptogenesis. Brain Res. **745:** 109–113.

39. HANIN, I. 1996. The Gulf War, stress, and a leaky blood-brain barrier. Nat. Med. **2:** 1307–1308.
40. FRIEDMAN, A. et al. 1996. Pyridostigmine brain penetration under stress enhances neuronal excitability and induces early immediate transcriptional response. Nat. Med. **2:** 1382–1385.
41. SHARMA, H.S., J. CERVOS-NAVARRO & P.K. DEY. 1991. Increased blood-brain barrier permeability following acute short-term swimming exercise in conscious normotensive rats. Neurosci. Res. **10:** 211–221.
42. IMAIZUMI, S. et al. 1996. The influence of oxygen free radicals on the permeability of the monolayer of cultured brain endothelial cells. Neurochem. Int. **29:** 205–211.
43. KASTENBAUER, S., U. KOEDEL & H.W. PFISTER. 1999. Role of peroxynitrite as a mediator of pathophysiological alterations in experimental meningitis. J. Infect. Dis. **180:** 1164–1170.
44. CALINGASAN, N.Y. et al. 1998. Induction of nitric oxide synthase and microglial responses precede selective cell death induced by chronic impairment of oxidative metabolism. Am. J. Pathol. **153:** 599–610.
45. IKEDA, K. et al. 1997. The role of calcium ion in anoxia/reoxygenation damage of cultured brain capillary endothelial cells. Acta Neurochir. Suppl. **70:** 4–7.

Index of Contributors

Baldwin, C.M., 38–47
Beck, K.D., 310–314
Beldowicz, D., 310–314
Bell, I.R., ix–xi, 38–47
Black, D.W., 48–56
Brennan, F.X., 310–314
Bushnell, M.C., 130–141

Chen, L., 57–67
Clauw, D.J., 235–253
Coderre, T.J., 157–174

Dantzer, R., 222–234
Devriese, S., 278–290, 315–318
Djuric, V., 92–102
Duncan, G.H., 130–141

Eelen, P., 278–290, 315–318
Eriksen, H.R., 119–129

Fang, J., 57–67, 211–221
Fiedler, N., 24–37

Giardino, N.D., 291–309
Gilbert, M.E., 68–91
Goldstein, B.D., 112–118

Heuser, G., 319–322
Hinze-Selch, D., 201–210

Katz, J., 157–174
Kipen, H.M., 24–37
Krueger, J.M., 211–221
Kubota, T., 211–221

MacPhail, R.C., 103–111
Mao, J., 175–184
Mayer, D.J., 175–184
McEwen, B.S., 265–277
Melzack, R., 157–174
Miller, C.S., 1–23

Moldow, R.L., 310–314
Mullington, J.M., 201–210

Nemery, B., 278–290, 315–318

Obál, F., Jr., 211–221
Okiishi, C., 48–56
Ottenweller, J.E., 310–314
Otto, T., 291–309
Overstreet, D.H., 92–102

Pall, M.L., 323–329
Patarca, R., 185–200
Pollmächer, T., 201–210

Rainville, P., 130–141
Rivier, C., 254–264

Satterlee, J.D., 323–329
Schlosser, S., 48–56
Schwartz, G.E.R., 38–47
Servatius, R.J., 310–314
Sorg, B.A., ix–xi, 57–67
Swindell, S., 57–67

Taishi, P., 211–221
Tschirgi, M.L., 57–67

Ursin, H., 119–129

Vaccarino, A.L., 157–174
Van de Woestijne, K.P., 278–290
Van den Bergh, O., 278–290, 315–318
Veulemans, H., 278–290, 315–318

Willis, W.D., Jr., 142–156
Winters, W., 278–290, 315–318
Wu, J.C., 319–322

Zhu, G., 310–314

OHIO UNIVERS
to return

have